THE
EARLY SESSIONS
Book 4 of The Seth Material
SESSIONS 149-198
4/26/65–10/13/65

THE EARLY SESSIONS

The Early Sessions consist of the first 510 sessions dictated by Seth through Jane Roberts, and are expected to be published in a total of 8-10 volumes. For information on expected publication dates and how to order, write to New Awareness Network at the following address and request the latest catalogue.

New Awareness Network Inc.
P.O. BOX 192
Manhasset, NY 11030

Internet Address: http://www.sethcenter.com

THE SETH AUDIO COLLECTION

Rare recordings of Seth speaking through Jane Roberts are now available on audiocassette. For a complete description of The Seth Audio Collection, write to New Awareness Network Inc. at the above address.
(Further information is supplied at the back of this book)

THE
EARLY SESSIONS
Book 4 of The Seth Material
SESSIONS 149-198
4/26/65–10/13/65

© 1998 by Robert Butts

Published by New Awareness Network Inc.

New Awareness Network Inc.
P.O. Box 192
Manhasset, New York 11030

Opinions and statements on health and medical matters expressed in this book are those of the author and are not necessarily those of or endorsed by the publisher. Those opinions and statements should not be taken as a substitute for consultation with a duly licensed physician.

Cover Design: Michael Goode
Photography: Cover photos by Rich Conz and Robert F. Butts, Sr.
Editorial: Rick Stack
Typography: Juan Schoch, Joan Thomas, Michael Goode

All rights reserved. This book may not be reproduced in whole or in part, without written permission from the publisher, except by a reviewer who may quote brief passages in a review; nor may any part of this book be reproduced, stored in a retrieval system, or transmitted in any form or by any means electronic, mechanical, photocopying, recording, or other, without written permission from the publisher.

Library of Congress Cataloging-in-Publication Data

Seth (Spirit)
      The early sessions: volume 4 of the seth material / [channeled] by Jane Roberts ; notes by Robert F. Butts.
      p. cm.–(A Seth book)
      ISBN 0-9652855-3-7
      1. Spirit writings. 2. Self–Miscellanea
      I. Roberts, Jane 1929–1984. II. Butts, Robert F.   III. Title
      IV. Series: Seth (Spirit), 1929–1984 Seth book.
      Library of Congress Catalog Number: 96-69349

ISBN 0-9652855-3-7
Printed in U.S.A. on acid-free paper

I dedicate The Early Sessions
to my wife, Jane Roberts,
who lived her 55 years
with the greatest creativity
and the most valiant courage.
-Rob

SESSION 149
APRIL 26, 1965 9 PM MONDAY AS SCHEDULED

(In the 135th session, Seth gave me a little puzzle involving a Saturday evening and the number 5. Since then I have noted two occasions where the two conditions might apply. I have been mentioning the incidents to Jane just before session time, in case Seth cared to comment on them, but to date he hasn't dealt with them. I do not know whether either of the incidents is the one he referred to, or whether the correct one still lies in the future.

(Last Saturday, April 24, Jane received another letter from F. Fell, publisher, and mailed her answer today. This is mentioned briefly in tonight's session.

(Jane's manner this evening was quite intent throughout the session. She spoke at a good rate for the most part, even with pauses, and toward the end of the session her voice became loud. As usual she spoke while sitting down and with her eyes closed. Her voice was normal in tone and volume to begin with.)

Good evening.

("Good evening, Seth.")

A short personal note to Ruburt.

After his birthday, immediately after, the day following, is an excellent day to give up his smoking habit. It is the most favorable day to begin such a venture, for him.

Immediately following the birthday his energies are more certain of themselves. The subconscious remembers the struggles of physical birth, and immediately following his birthday is a time of expansion. This is the end of the personal message to Ruburt.

(Jane's birthday is May 8. She was born in 1929.)

As for you, Joseph, within two weeks you will have completely recovered from the effects of your recent illness.

Now, regarding again the nature of action, I would like to discuss action in relation to the dream reality, for you are intimately familiar with action in dreams, and your practical experience will enable you to understand the true nature of action more clearly.

We mentioned that there are always actions within actions, and made it clear that all action does not necessarily involve motion that is apparent *as* motion to you. Actions may be thresholds or openings for other actions. To one extent or another all actions involve unfoldings. The action of dreaming itself is partially a physical phenomena. There is then, comparatively speaking, the outside action that makes dreaming possible, the action that *is* dreaming.

There are then truly endless varieties of actions within the dream, which is itself a continuing act. There is, most simply, within a dream the creation of images. These images then also act. They move, speak, walk, run. There is at times a dream within a dream, where the dreamer dreams that he dreams. Here of course the dimensions are even more diverse.

Many of these actions performed by dream images are muscular ones, physical manipulations. But many of these actions are also mental manipulations, or esthetic realizations and even esthetic performances. These dream images are not one-dimensional, cardboard figures by any means. Their mobility in terms of perspectives and within space is far greater than your own.

You perceive, however, but a very small portion of these images which you have yourselves created. You simply cannot bring them back into the limited perspectives of your own present field, and are left with but glimpses and flimsy glimmerings of images which are actually as actual, vivid, and more mobile than those in the physical field.

I have mentioned that what I call the dream universe is indeed composed of molecular structure, and that it is a continuing reality, even though your own awareness of it is most usually limited, for quite necessary reasons, to the hours of your own sleep. There is a give and take here, for if you give the dream universe much of its continuing energy, much of your own energy is derived from it. There is, between the physical field and the dream universe, an interdependence that is not at all unusual, for all fields are indeed dependent one upon the other.

(*Seth began talking about dreams as far back as the 15th session, about dream locations in the 44th session, about the subconscious and dreams in the 92nd and 93rd sessions, etc., among others.*)

Nor is the dream universe a shadow image of your own. It carries on according to the possibilities inherent within it, as you carry on according to the possibilities that exist within the physical field. The possibilities for action <u>vary</u>, however, within these two fields as they vary within all other fields. You may say that in sleeping you focus your energies to form a different reality than the reality of waking physical matter.

You focus your awareness in altered form into another universe, that is in every way as valid and <u>permanent</u> as your own. It is also as <u>changing</u> as the physical universe. A small amount of energy only is focused upon the physical field during sleep, enough simply to maintain the physical body within its physical environment.

I have much more to say here, but you may take your break.

(*Break at 9:26. Jane was more dissociated than usual for a first delivery. She knew, she said, that she was moving along at a good pace. She could have kept going, but stopped so I could rest my writing hand.*

(She resumed at a slightly slower rate at 9:37.)
The dream universe and the events within it are, therefore, as meaningful as those events that occur within the physical universe.

In many respects actions within the dream universe are indeed more direct than in your own. It is because you remember but vague glimmerings and disconnected episodes that dreams appear, sometimes, chaotic or meaningless, particularly to the ego, which censors rigidly much of the information that the subconscious does retain.

For most people this censoring process is valuable, since it prevents the personality from being snowed under by data it is not equipped to handle. The ability to retain experience gained within other fields is the trend of further development. You are at least however to some extent familiar with this field of dream action, and every man intuitively knows his involvement here.

The feeling of unreality is not felt when the dream experience is being participated in by the dreamer. At that time the experience is felt to be real, and some dreams indeed are more vivid than waking experience. It is only when the personality passes out of the dream experience, or the dream universe, that the dream experience in retrospect may appear unreal. For now, again, the focus of attention and energy is in the physical universe. Reality then is a result of the focus of energy and attention.

I used the term "pass out of" the dream universe purposely, for here we see a mobility of action easily and often accomplished, a passing in and out that involves an action without movement in space. The dreamer is acquainted intimately, and has at his fingertips so to speak, a memory of his previous dream experiences, and carries within him the many inner individualistic purposes which are behind his dream actions.

On leaving the dream state, he becomes more and more aware of the ego, and creates then activities which have meaning to it. In the deep dream state the inner purposes are more involved. As I have mentioned however, all dream symbols have meanings to all portions of the personality.

(See the 92nd session in particular, in Volume 3.)
The dream universe has molecular construction, but this molecular construction takes up no space as you know it. The dream universe, while composed of molecules, is not composed of matter as you know it. The dream universe consists of depths and dimensions, expansions and contractions, that are more clearly allied, perhaps, to ideals that have no need for the particular kind of structure with which you are familiar.

Obviously, time in terms of continuity, is not an element of importance in the dream universe, and this is one of the reasons for the lack of physical structure. The intuitions and certain inner abilities here have so much more freedom that it is unnecessary for molecules to be used in any _imprisoning_ form or structure. Action is more spontaneous within the dream universe, more fluid. The images appear and disappear much more quickly because value fulfillment is allowed greater reign.

The slower physical manifestation of growth that occurs within the physical field involves long-term patterns filled by atoms and molecules which are, to some extent, then imprisoned within structure.

(*See the 71st session [in Volume 2] among others.*)

In the dream universe however the slower physical growth process is replaced by psychic and mental value fulfillment, which does not necessitate any long-range imprisonment of molecules within a pattern.

This involves, simply, a quickening of experience and action relatively unhampered by the sort of time necessities inherent within the physical universe. Action itself therefore is allowed greater freedom. This is not to say that structure does not exist within the dream universe, for _structures_ of a mental or psychic nature _do_ exist. But structure is not dependent upon matter as in the physical universe, and the motion of molecules is more spontaneous, and an almost unbelievable depth of experience is possible within what would seem to _you_ a fraction of a moment.

I will have more to say concerning the connection between the two fields and their manifestation in action, for one of the closest glimpses you can get of pure action is action as it is involved within the dream universe, and in this mobility as the personality passes into and out of the dream field. Within your own universe you deal with the transformation of action into physical manipulations, but this involves but a small portion of the nature of action, and it is my purpose to familiarize you with action as it exists more or less in its pure form.

In this way you may be able to perceive the manners in which it is transformed into other fields that do not involve matter as you know it.

I suggest your break.

(*Break at 10:18. Jane was more dissociated, as usual. As before, her manner had been very intent. When she resumed she retained this intentness, coupling it with a good rate of delivery and a voice that was her loudest in some time. Her voice did not boom out, however. Resume at 10:30.*)

Your own universe expands as an idea expands, in ways that have nothing to do with space.

The whole reality of the dream world, or of the dream universe, lies along these lines. Within it fulfillment and development are not dependent upon permanence of _physical_ matter, however, and are not at all dependent upon any concept like that of your physical time. There [are] therefore possible bursts of developments, that have matured within perspectives that are not bound up in time, and that would appear spontaneous to the waking self.

But these developments, nevertheless, are the results of actions that occur in many perspectives <u>at once</u>, and not developments that occur as within the physical system, through actions that happen in a series <u>seemingly</u> strung out moment after moment.

Now basically even the physical universe itself is so constructed, but for all practical purposes, as far as general perception and experience is concerned, time and the physical growth development apply, so that we find the ego portion, particularly of the human personality, is to a large extent dependent for its maturity and development upon the amount of time that the physical image has spent within the system.

A certain portion of physical growth, in terms of a series of physical moments, is therefore necessary for value fulfillment to show itself within a physical organism. Within the dream field and within many other systems, this series of moments is unknown. Development comes not from a series of actions strung out along a single line, one before the other in lengthwise fashion. Instead development is largely a matter of value fulfillment, which is achieved through the perspectives of action, through traveling within any given action, and following it and changing with it. To make this clearer, I have said that action exists within limitless perspectives, and that you are mainly familiar with it as it is materialized along a single line of continuity within the physical system. You experience action then as if you were moving along a single line, each dot on the line representing a moment of your time. But at the imaginary point on your line that represents any given moment, action moves out in all directions. From the standpoint of that moment point, you could imagine action forming an imaginary circle with that point as an apex. But this happens at the point of every moment.

There is no particular boundary to the circle. It widens outward indefinitely. Now. In the dream universe, in all systems of such nature, development is achieved not by traveling your single line, but by delving into that point that you call a moment. The physical laws simply do not apply here, within such a value fulfillment system. Basically your own physical universe is at the apex of such a system itself, and it is only because of the purpose and nature of the particular apex that experience <u>appears</u>, from my viewpoint, to be so slowed down. The particular point, in one manner, is being pursued by you in such a slow fashion that it <u>appears</u> to be a series of happenings strung out in a thread of continuity. You experience action as one happening after another, <u>not</u> because of the nature of action itself but because of the nature of your own structure and perception.

This is in itself, you see, a form of value fulfillment, since you are perceiving one simultaneous action as if it were a series of separate actions. You are delving into one action, and within it continually creating action within action. This is however, or this can be, while fulfilling, also limiting.

I have intended to get into this subject thoroughly for some time. You may now as you prefer take a break or end the session.

("Well, I guess we'd better end it then.")

I have then another small note for Ruburt. He may if he prefers do his psychological time in the afternoons, when you are here, Joseph. Indeed now regularity is good, particularly since I have limited his time.

The letter to the publisher is a perfectly acceptable one.

This has been an excellent session. My most fond regards to you both. Joseph—

("Yes?")

Your health will indeed improve. You will live to be a very hearty old gentleman.

("How old was I in Denmark?")

When you died?

("Yes.")

Eighty-three. I will continue the session or close it as you wish.

("We'll close it then. Good night, Seth.")

(*End at 11:02. Jane sat quietly for a few moments before opening her eyes. She was well dissociated. She also reported that during this last delivery she had experienced another concept from Seth. For other recent experiences see the 141st-143rd, and the 148th sessions.*

(*Jane made a quick drawing of the concept she received tonight. I helped her as much as I could from her description of it. It should be stressed that often Jane finds these experiences difficult to put into words, let alone onto paper. What she "saw," she said, was an approximation of a mental diagram involving a circular string. Closely paralleling Seth's description on page 5, there would be a series of dots on the circle. Each dot would be intersected by another circle, with dots upon this, and each of these dots in turn would be intersected, etc., so that there could be an infinity of expansions. If time permits I will try to make a more finished drawing of this idea.*

(*Jane's voice remained strong until the end of the session.*

(*For some material on travel through concepts and impulses and time, see sessions 131 and 135. [A note: All underlined words are called for by Seth.]*)

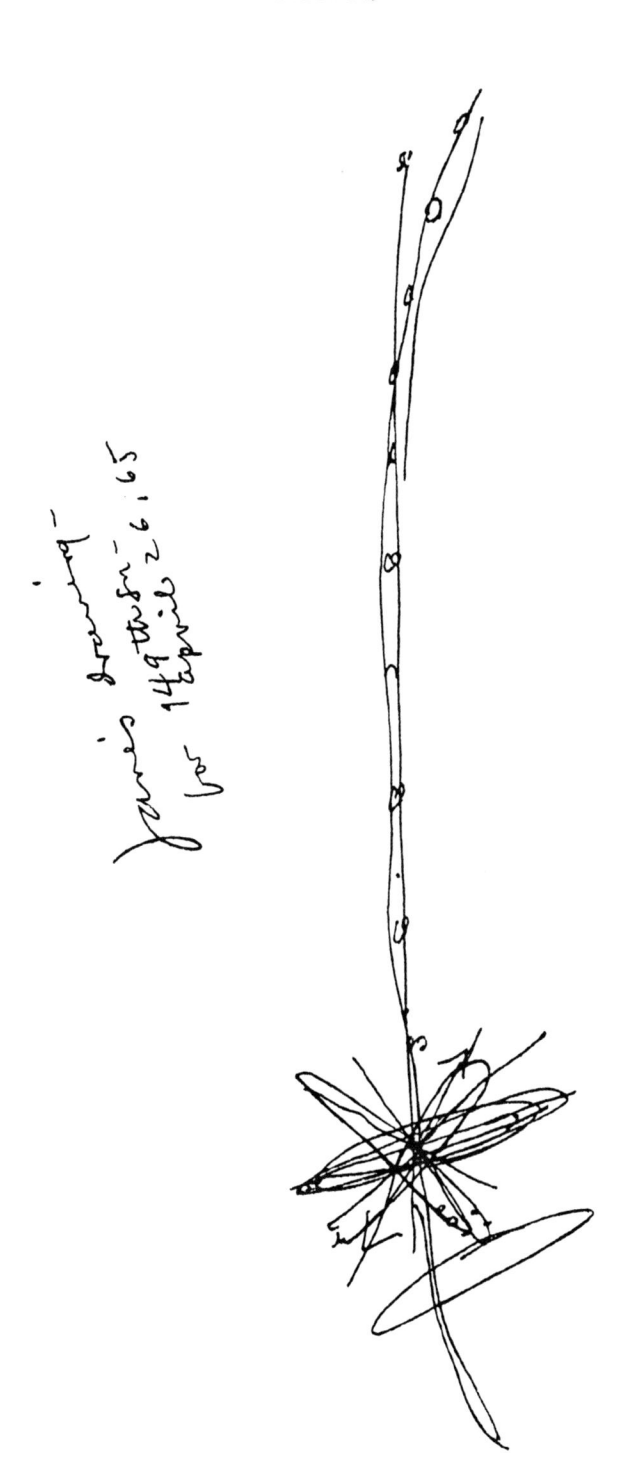

SESSION 150
APRIL 28, 1965 9 PM WEDNESDAY AS SCHEDULED

(This afternoon, frightened by a grim tale of lung cancer involving an acquaintance of ours, Jane made an abrupt effort to stop smoking. The acquaintance was a heavy smoker. Jane went so far as to throw away a half-used pack of cigarettes.

(It might be noted here that the 87th session dealt rather extensively with Jane's death from cancer in a previous life in Boston, and stated that she would not die of the disease again. Jane was a woman medium in Boston a century or so ago, according to Seth, and possessed clairvoyant knowledge of her own death, at 82 or 83, from cancer.

(Following Seth's recent okay, Jane has begun trying psychological time on a fifteen-minute basis, either in the afternoons or evenings. She has not as yet achieved many results. Nor is she yet back on a regular daily basis.

(Jane spoke this evening in a very quiet voice that often bore quite humorous, if gentle, overtones. She took many pauses, some of them very long. It soon became apparent that the session would not be a long one. She waited well over a minute to begin speaking after she sat down and closed her eyes.)

Good evening.

("Good evening, Seth.")

I am having some few difficulties here, with our balky Ruburt, but I presume we can handle it.

To think that all these years his good disposition has been dependent upon the cigarette between his lips, and not upon any native good spirits. Alas.

He will do all right, even if I do rib him now and then.

(Jane now took another long pause.)

Now. We will endeavor to continue speaking of some matters discussed in our previous session. A moment point basically consists not of any particular given time division, but is within your system a convenient term that expresses or represents the range of reality that can be conveniently embraced without undue strain.

Within what you call one moment, many such perceptions flash through to affect any given individual. However there is within your system a lapse before the organism can effectively organize these perceptions. My idea of a moment point is only an approximation of your physical moment. I am trying to make it plain here that the range of action is what is important. A moment point _is_ a range of action.

(Jane's pause was again very long. Her delivery had been broken by many other short pauses.)

He, Ruburt, feels so deprived. I had originally suggested the day after his birthday to end his smoking habit, simply because it would be relatively easy for him at that time. However, the benefits are well worth whatever passing discomfort he fancies he feels. The personality hangs on to his small indulgences, but good sense will rule the day.

I suggest your first break, and we will see what we can do.

(Break at 9:18. Jane was dissociated about as usual, she said, for a first delivery. She resumed in the same slow manner at 9:26.)

All realities are the result of psychic organizations. All time structures within them represent the range of action which can be conveniently perceived.

Ruburt's subconscious has been thrown into a panic, and indeed feels cheated, since it had been preparing itself for the May 9 date, particularly since that date was mentioned here. But Ruburt may as well now continue with this heroic endeavor, although I fear that it will cost us this session. It would perhaps have been more convenient if the effort had been started on other than a session night, but in any case I expect to see the endeavor succeed, and certainly do not mind missing a session for this purpose.

He is stubborn, as we have discovered, you and I, and this stubbornness will also work for him. There is no reason why he should not succeed, and he will succeed in letting go the smoking habit. Do not fret because of this brief session, Joseph. It is well worth the while. This evening however Ruburt's subconscious is in a rather chaotic state, and I shall not attempt now to carry on a regular session.

It is true that Ruburt's health will show definite improvements. The sinus condition has always been to some extent aggravated by the smoking habit, and there are also other conditions which will largely vanish. Perhaps we can make up this session, or perhaps we can make it up in an entirely different fashion. In any case, you may possibly hear more of me in one way or another before our next regular session. Ruburt, incidentally, will be in good shape by then. My fondest regards to you both. Good night, Ruburt, you soldier, you.

("Good night, Seth."
(End at 9:40. Jane was dissociated as usual.)

SESSION 151
MAY 3, 1965 9 PM MONDAY AS SCHEDULED

(Jane has resumed smoking again, and we wondered whether Seth would comment on this during the session. The session was held in our living room rather

than in our back room, because of a lawn party being held in back of the house.

(Our windows are now usually open, with the advent of better weather. This admits traffic noise also, and as we prepared for the session we were quite conscious of the difference compared to the quiet back room.

(As usual Jane spoke while sitting down and with her eyes closed. She also spoke more rapidly than she has for many a session; my notes indicate she delivered the first monologue entirely without pauses. It soon became apparent that the unaccustomed traffic noise was having its effect, also. Jane began speaking in a rather normal voice, but before long it began to deepen and strengthen. The volume increased a little, but the lower key and a peculiar heavy monotone her voice acquired cut across the noise. I heard her without difficulty. She maintained this heavy voice for most of the session.)

Good evening.

("Good evening, Seth.")

There is much to be explained along many lines which we have only begun to touch upon, for all things are correlated; and there is indeed a correlation between our moment points of which we have spoken, the spacious present, and that portion of the whole self which you call the subconscious.

We are dealing here principally, and in the main, with the essence of action, and essentially all apparent divisions are arbitrary for the sake of explanation. The moment point is in itself arbitrary, an artificial division. As we have said, the moment point for you is actually composed of the amount of action which you are capable of assimilating within your present framework, for the moment point is indeed a portion of the spacious present.

(For a more graphic interpretation of what a moment point might be, see Jane's description of the concept she received from Seth in the 149th session.)

The subconscious, and in fact all portions of the self with the exception of the ego, are capable of assimilating a wider area, so to speak, of action. Therefore to these other portions of the self, time has a much different essence than it has for the ego. The ego is indeed many things. It can be defined in relationship to many other aspects of reality. In relationship to action, and moment points, the ego is indeed that portion of the self which stands at the apex of the moment point, and is limited by the moment point. The ego is in this context the portion of the self which is utterly focused upon, and imprisoned by, the moment point.

The ego is that portion of the self which experiences time as continuity, and to whom experience is a series of stimuli and responses carried on one after another. And yet this is in itself a division, so to speak, or a kind of value fulfillment, for the simultaneous nature of a given action is here experienced in slow motion, as a child must learn to walk before the child can run.

The subconscious however is not so limited. If you consider the ego at the apex of the moment point, and imprisoned therefore within the realm of its own before-and-after, cause-and-effect experience, then you can imagine the subconscious reaching further outward and seizing upon many other moment points. It should be easy to see then why the focus of the ego is so sharp and brilliant. Within its limited scope there is intensity of stimuli and response. Indeed, the ego is that portion of the personality which is plunged into a specific and intense preoccupation with a given field of action or dimension.

The subconscious, reaching outward, reaches also inward. For while there is no real past or present or future within the spacious present, there is indeed an infinity of inward and outward; and again, of actions within actions, and there is no end to these actions for they are self-generating. The other portions of the inner self reach then even further in all directions, and they therefore envelop many moment points. To many portions of the inner self then, what you would call a moment would correspond to an almost limitless number of moments, for even physical time has no meaning without experience without action.

Your whole concept of time is built about your own capacity for perceiving action; as this capacity for perceiving action grows, so indeed do the dimensions of time grow. Conceivably therefore one moment of your time would indeed be experienced by the whole self as centuries.

This should lead you to understand why physical time is basically meaningless to the subconscious, and why the inner self has at its command a knowledge of past lives and past endeavors; for the inner self, dear friends, these lives are not in the past, nor is the life of the ego necessarily present to the whole self.

For to the whole self all personalities that compose it exist simultaneously, and personalities that would appear to you as future personalities are experienced by the whole self in the same dimension as it experiences personalities that you would call past personalities. For all your ideas of time are illusion, not merely philosophical illusions, but delusions as far as any basic reality is concerned.

It is only the ego that steps from moment to moment, as a man who walks from puddle to puddle. It is only the ego who drowns in time. Therefore, since only the ego is momentarily imprisoned within the focus of your plane, it is only the ego who probes so slowly into simultaneous action, perceiving it bit by bit and sip by sip. So now you will see what I meant when I spoke about the limitless self, for the whole self is not so bound. The whole self could and does perceive a limitless number of such moment points simultaneously. And now hear this:

(Jane reached over to rap on my writing table for emphasis, a practice she used to indulge in when she still paced endlessly about the room while delivering the material.)

The whole self not only perceives these limitless moment points, but being a part of action, each whole self projects fragments and personalities from itself to all these points, creating therefore other egos, other intense focus points which are independent, which work out their own destinies and experiences, which in turn perceive any given moment point in slow motion.

I now suggest your break.

(Break at 9:31. Jane was fully dissociated—way out, as she put it, probably as far out as she has ever been. She was aware of her voice phenomena, she said, and her subjective reaction to it was very similar to the way she felt during the Father Trainor episode: she felt carried away by the voice as though she was inside it, in a very light weightless state. In Volume 3, see the 131st session for information on the Father Trainor experience.

(The heavier overtones of Jane's voice had subsided to some degree by break time, but it still had good substance. Jane maintained this reduced characteristic as she began dictating again, at a good rate, at 9:42.)

It must be stressed that there are no sharp boundaries, however, between the various portions of the whole self.

There are shadings and variations and that is all. The inner ego is that part of the inner self which is closely allied with the outer ego, in that it is to some degree a director of function and activity. But it is not sharply focused. It looks inward. Here we run into some language difficulty.

The inner ego looks inward, yet in looking inward it looks outward toward those vast portions of the self. Because there is always action within action, and because of the three dilemmas of which we have spoken earlier, the new personalities projected outward into other fields of perception, or other moment points, these other personalities in turn create new ones, and the cycle is again repeated.

Time, physical matter, these are but portions of action as perceived in one particular fashion. The basic stuff, or the basic action of the universe, is one. It is perceived differently, and therefore reality constantly wears a different face. It is speeded up or slowed down according to the scope of perception.

(It might be interesting to note here that Seth began talking about action in the 13th session, January 6, 1964: "Love and hate, for example, are action," and "In your plane, action is the main word of importance," etc. See Volume 1, page 71.

(See the 138th and 141st sessions for material on the three creative dilemmas.)

It is almost impossible to explain clearly, through the use of words, this massive complexity, for all fields of activity are self-generating. Even the dream field is self-generating. No consciousness can bring itself to destruction. It can only cease experiencing a certain portion of action. This is a rather important point.

The multiplicity of human experience would be impossible were it not for the inner self, and for the heritage that speaks through the cells of every human being. The perspectives and psychic relationships that make up the human personality simply could not have resulted through action within your field alone. It cannot be stressed too strongly that experience <u>within</u> the self can lead to at least some understanding of the nature of action in its pure form, for within your physical universe action is to some extent frozen, insofar as your perceptions of it are concerned.

Yet within your own psychological experience you can perceive its fluid nature. The material that I have given you concerning the three dilemmas will be most helpful here.

There is much that you simply cannot perceive at this point. There is much that mankind as such will never learn, simply because such knowledge is beyond the reach of the ego. But there is much that you do not know that you can learn.

A note here: Ruburt may try the psychological time experiments twenty minutes daily; and indeed yes, the time of the day should be uniform. I would suggest now that he seriously begin to schedule this with his daily activities. It is best that you be in the house with him, Joseph. And indeed, for your own edification your life in general will be much more comfortable within what I would call a short time; though to <u>you</u> this may be two years, before a noticeable change is apparent.

("In what way?")

I am speaking in financial terms. The changes themselves will begin earlier, but you will probably not be sure of them yourself until the time that I have given. I will not go into any other personal matters this evening, however, as it was not my intention.

I suggest a <u>short</u> break, and I will continue with our other matters.

(Break at 10:05. Jane was dissociated as usual for this delivery, and although her voice had maintained its rather deep monotone she had no particular feelings about it now.

(Jane has been trying psy-time lately, though not yet on a regular basis. She seems to think fifteen minutes is not quite enough for her to achieve results as a matter of routine, although she enters a trance state readily enough.

(Of course Jane and I have for some time been aware of the possible differences

in meaning between Seth and ourselves, over interpretation of the word "soon". Sometimes the situation has been rather humorous, other times not. A good case in point would be the 104th session of November 4, 1964. In it Seth stated that Jane had already made a sale, yet she did not receive confirmation of the sale of her ESP book until April 19, 1965. See the 147th session.

(Jane resumed in a voice not quite as strong at 10:13.)

Art often appears timeless to the ego because it often merges within it a greater number of moment points than the ego can ordinarily perceive.

In such cases the artist captures the dominant essence, and through the energy which he has given the art, it then makes such an effect upon the ego, which could not ordinarily perceive so much.

Despite the fact that I had not intended to deliver any personal material this evening, a small note to you, Joseph: you should now once again concern yourself with your painting. It is very necessary to your own concept of yourself in many ways. Not only do you impart energy into a painting, but you also derive energy from a painting even while you are working on it. I had indeed meant to mention this earlier.

Now. Each moment point is a field or dimension. You perceive certain very limited aspects of a given number of such moment points. The same moment points may simultaneously be experienced in an entirely different fashion, and to a different set of perceptions. These moment points would appear quite different than they appear to you.

There is a delicate connection here with the dream universe that is somewhat difficult to explain. The dream universe, however, pervades many other fields. It does not exist outside or apart from your own universe, but simultaneously with it. It appears, and is a reality, to all aspects or portions of the self, and often it is only within the dream universe that the personality can change focus easily or efficiently enough so that he can perceive the variety of roles that he himself has played.

I mentioned the chemical relationship between your universe and the dream universe. There are like relationships of one kind or another that tie together all fields and systems, from the largest to the most minute. The freedom of the inner self, then, is never determined by time as you know it. It is determined <u>by time as you do not know it</u>.

There are such manipulations within various systems that change other systems. Your own behavior and action within the dream universe definitely affects the physical universe. From one field of activity then you have changed another, and without ever knowing, in many cases, that you have done so. In the same manner do the activities of the physical universe alter the dream system.

SESSION 151

It is virtually impossible for me to explain all these inner workings. We will have to wait until you can experience concepts for much of that.

These moment points _may_, for simplicity's sake, also be thought of as reference points from one system to another. Do you see now a connection here with camouflage, as explained in early sessions?

(_"Yes."_)

The moment point will be seen as camouflage, which simply means that it will be perceived differently according to the perceptors. Definitions have little meaning unless they are related to other issues. For that reason I will try whenever possible to relate terms with which _you_ are familiar in ways so that their relationships will be clearly seen.

There will be much more here also concerning moment points and value fulfillment. For this, value fulfillment, is the reason behind the existence of all systems, and of all experience within your field. I mentioned that value fulfillment seems, and is to some small degree, dependent upon time as you know it, but this merely reflects upon the manner in which _you_ perceive time, and in no way alters the simultaneous nature of value fulfillment, which grows in dimension but is not dependent upon time as you know it.

Once more I suggest a brief break, and I will continue—with of course your permission.

(_Break at 10:38. Jane was dissociated as usual. Her voice was not as strong, now, as it had been, yet was still above her usual volume. She resumed in the same manner, with few pauses, at 10:46._)

I will shortly close the session.

I believe I should once again suggest, Joseph, a daily short walk for you. Such suggestions may appear trivial, yet they are not, and will prove most beneficial. There is indeed a value fulfillment within the enjoyment of nature that can release you from many restraints.

Inner action, in terms of psychological reality, is every bit as important as physical action; more important. It would be most unfortunate if either or both of you let physical action on the part of others stand in the way of beneficial action on your own parts.

(_I assume this statement refers to my getting upset this evening by the actions of our neighbors. I realized their actions were trivial, yet also felt they were thoughtless. From talking to Jane, I gathered she felt we should watch our reactions to others, so I let it pass. Still I admitted that I was upset._)

There must, or should be, particularly in this season, an acquiescence toward growth and release in general, and this can be triggered, though such triggering should not, ideally, be necessary to the enjoyment of nature. For nature is fluid. It is <u>fluent</u>. It is ever responsive, and it does not set up barriers.

The experiments that you have done in projection were most beneficial to you in the past. Throw your consciousness outward into nature, and your inwardness will be replenished. The power and necessity to feel is a strong necessity within all planes. I have never suggested to you that you close off from this.

When <u>all</u> your sensitivity is directed into sensations of misgiving, then however the balance is wrong. Spontaneity of feeling will almost automatically allow you greater freedom, increased mental and physical health; and balance will then be very well maintained.

I tell you that you are indeed headed for more comfortable times, but this does not mean that there is not very much within your own daily life now to be thankful for. Spontaneity will open many doors. I am speaking of emotional spontaneity.

There is much more that I could say to you now concerning this, but I will not. Do not refuse those joys that are available to you. You have nothing to make up for now, in this respect.

I will close because you are, I believe, somewhat tired. But because I am your friend, pay heed to what I say. My fondest regards to you both. You must be open, even to maintain the strength of the ego itself. But when you are not open, not only are you imprisoned by the moment, but you are not able to enjoy even that fully.

If I speak sternly, it is merely as a precaution. You know that I am fond of you both.

("Good night, Seth."

(End at 11:02. This time Jane was fully dissociated again.)

SESSION 152
MAY 5, 1965 9 PM WEDNESDAY AS SCHEDULED

(This morning Jane had an experience that pleased her greatly. Putting herself into a light trance state, she used appropriate suggestions before she went to the dentist to have her teeth cleaned. Such cleaning has always been very painful for her because of heavy tartar deposits, but today she withstood an hour's heavy scraping with practically no discomfort.

(Her dentist was so puzzled by her exceptionally good reactions that in the middle of the session Jane had to explain her apparent insensitivity to pain; usually it takes two trips for her to achieve the same results, with the use of Novocain. Today she had no anesthetic of any kind, and in addition her dentist reported he was able

to do a much more thorough job.

(Jane said she thinks her practice with psychological time experiments had much to do with the ease with which she put herself into a good state, since she achieved it in about five minutes. Nor were her gums sore at all afterwards.

(Jane also had another success involving her cooperating subconscious. Last Saturday afternoon she lost a package downtown while shopping. It was late in the day before she discovered this, and she just had time to make the rounds of the stores, all of whom reported nothing found and turned in. At home that evening she questioned her subconscious with the old pendulum technique, and learned she had left the package in the dressing room of a certain store—one which had already said no package had been found.

(Jane called the store Monday, and was told the package had been found. I drove her down to the store for it Monday evening. She plans to use these two experiences in her ESP book. Jane tells me that she now has little talks with her subconscious, requesting its help. I have been experimenting also with subconscious communication, at times with excellent results, and also using the permissive "I can" approach, rather than the commanding "I will" approach.

(Lying down for a nap late this afternoon, Jane heard a loud noise within, then felt what seemed to be a blow within her head—that is, a rather strong jolting without any external cause. The experience was so vivid she found her head rocking back and forth on the pillow, like a "flower on a stem." She has felt this jolting before, for instance on April 28, 1964, and on April 30, 1964, just before her "Saratoga experience", but not recently. See Volume 2, pages 64-65.

(I have begun a schedule of daily walking and sketching trips to the nearby river, and find it most refreshing.

(The session was held in our small back room, and again Jane spoke while sitting down and with her eyes closed. She displayed no particular voice effects. Her pace was a good one, though not as fast as last session's.)

Good evening.

("Good evening, Seth.")

We find here a situation this morning in which Ruburt achieved excellent communication with his own personal subconscious, spoke with it, giving it credit for being as important to the whole personality as the ego.

He spoke to his subconscious therefore as a partner and an equal, which indeed it is. It was because of this approach, among other things, that the results achieved were so successful. Nor after stating his case did he then badger the subconscious.

The personal subconscious and the ego are indeed equal partners in the formation of any given present personality. Ruburt's results are evidence that his training is bearing fruit. Once such a relationship is set up between the ego and the subconscious, then communication in general between the two will always improve. The subconscious, even the personal subconscious, is much freer from the moment point than is the ego, and it can inform the ego of important developments which can be of great help.

This sort of communication also comes close to action in a fairly pure state. There is also another result of such relative ease of communication between the ego and the subconscious, in that the subconscious, which is listened to and taken into consideration by the ego, will have relatively little need to make its wishes known in other, perhaps less pleasant ways. Illnesses and various minor and major physical symptoms are often caused as the subconscious tries to speak out, in an effort to make itself heard by the unheeding conscious mind. If the conscious mind consults with the subconscious, such nagging or sometimes explosive efforts will not be needed.

The pendulum is an excellent manner for reaching the personal layers of the subconscious. Unless a trance state is adopted, it is much less effective as a manner of reaching those layers that lie, so to speak, beneath the personal subconscious. For practical purposes it is excellent policy to check often with the personal subconscious through use of the pendulum.

As a humorous sideline here, I might add, only halfway in jest, the following suggestion.

When you purchased attire, testing it out first with the pendulum would actually be very effective. The pendulum ideally would be held above the garment in question. The point would be to discover the reaction of the subconscious. Believe it or not, the personal subconscious is extremely sensitive to color, and to certain vibrations given off by color and by fabrics. It responds to the clothing you wear, to the clothing worn by others with whom you come in contact.

This applies particularly to color; and also it responds strongly in a positive or negative manner to natural fabrics, such as wools and cottons.

("Can you tell us good colors for Jane and me?")

I was going to suggest, for practice, that you yourselves find out from the pendulum. I would like you to become familiar with the experience of conversing with this portion of your own personality. I would like you to become intimately aware of this not-so-silent partner.

This experience will be most beneficial. It will enable your present personalities to operate in a much more enjoyable esthetic, psychic and practically efficient manner. As you realize, I have little to do with the personal layer of Ruburt's subconscious. It is merely something through which I pass.

I have explained through which layer of the subconscious I come, but my <u>origin</u> has nothing to do with any portion of Ruburt's subconscious, not even those vast areas beneath the personal subconscious.

I am going to say more here concerning those characteristics of Ruburt's whole self, which allow me to communicate with your field. Here, however, I merely wished to make the point that this communication between your own egos and your own subconscious must depend upon yourselves, and the easier the communication between the ego and the personal subconscious the greater the strength, abilities, potentialities and value fulfillment of the present personality as a whole.

There are many small beneficial ways to use the pendulum, if you work with it seriously. It may be held over certain foods to see if you may be allergic to them. These are indeed questions that I could answer for you, but again, I prefer that you establish this intimate working relationship with your own personal subconscious. The experience itself will be of great value.

Later you will not need the pendulum. The habit of communication will then operate without it. All the information, for example, that I gave you earlier, very much earlier, concerning say your refrigerator, and the unsuitability of its location at that time, such details could have been received through the pendulum.

(Jane now took a long pause, by a good length the longest of the session. For the most part her rate of delivery was excellent. For the session dealing with the refrigerator see the 30th, in Volume 1. It was unscheduled.)

There are also for example, times of the month when you are both more actively inclined toward various activities, and less inclined toward others. Such periods can be discovered through the pendulum.

I suggest your first break.

(Break at 9:32. Jane was dissociated as usual for a first delivery. She resumed at a good rate and in an average voice at 9:42.)

Contrary to current opinion, the subconscious is far from rigid.

It is indeed more fluid and resilient than the ego. It is the failure of the ego to listen to the inner voice of the subconscious that causes many difficulties. The ego would wish the subconscious out of existence. It does not want a partner. It wants to master the entire personality.

For a portion of the self that is relatively so powerless, this is quite presumptive. It is obviously no coincidence that almost the entire survival of the organism is held under the responsibility of the subconscious. To be somewhat prosaic here, it is nevertheless true that the whole efficiency of the personality can be improved if the inclinations of the subconscious are taken into consideration, in the manner of clothes and accessories and living surroundings in general. The personality is simply not pulling against itself so much.

<u>The ego thwarts the subconscious often out of mere perversity, to prove its superiority</u>. You might also ask the pendulum, or the subconscious through the pendulum, about the times of the month, if any, when you may be more open to psychic phenomena. But here, check with me concerning the answers that you receive.

Such easy communication with the subconscious will also allow the subconscious to be more flexible, in allowing various information through to the ego from the deeper layers of the whole self. As a further benefit there will be increased joy, and a feeling of oneness with the self, and with reality in general.

Ruburt is only learning now not to scold and badger his subconscious. Again, all of this involves action within action. Now. It is the intuitive, spontaneous and psychically exuberant nature of Ruburt's whole entity, for one thing, that makes it possible for me to communicate with you both.

The whole self of which Ruburt is a part is an extremely elastic one. The various portions of this whole self reach outward and inward with much more resilience than most. Therefore this whole self surrounds many more moment points simultaneously, using one moment point in particular as a reference or entry point.

I can then, therefore, enter the limits of your psychic comprehension. This is a very simplified version, but I must, so to speak, therefore journey through the various areas of Ruburt's whole self, or inner self, until I reach a point where entry into your consciousness is possible. This happens to be the third undifferentiated layer of Ruburt's subconscious.

(*Seth devoted the 88th session to the layers of the subconscious, especially Jane's third undifferentiated layer. He discussed his source and structure to at least some degree in many sessions, among them the 128th, the 24th, etc.*)

I am usually able to escape the personal subconscious area in general. However, as you know I speak only for convenience, for there are no real barriers to separate these layers. They are simultaneous areas, that merge one into the other. For an analogy you may say that upon some occasions, though few, Ruburt's personal subconscious layer expands so that I must travel through portions of it, and at other times it contracts and bothers me not at all.

Again, it goes without saying that I am not physically traveling through like a man on horseback through foreign territory. The traveling involves merely a change of focus, both on my part and <u>some</u>what on Ruburt's part, for he is far from inactive, far from being a passive receiver.

Translations, and faithful ones, of my communications are constantly made by a certain portion of his inner self. Nor is your capacity here a passive one. Your psychic energies help him make these translations. At times you join together to enlarge your psychic environment, allowing me to come within its limits.

This will all be explained in particular, rather than general terms at a later date. Suffice it to say here that such communications, again, represent the characteristics of motion in a more or less pure form. I will have something to say also, perhaps at our next session, concerning Ruburt's experience this afternoon.

These moment points, incidentally, serve as reference points often from one field of activity to another, as openings or entryways. Such a moment point has a peculiar molecular structure, that is a result of intensification of action, and basically has nothing to do with the moment point <u>happening</u> to coincide with what you call a physical moment.

I will go into this directly. First however I suggest a brief break.

(Break at 10:09. Jane was dissociated as usual. Her pace had been good, with few pauses. See page 16 for a description of her psychic experience of this afternoon, referred to above.

(Jane resumed in a voice a bit deeper than usual, and at a good pace, at 10:20.)

There is of course another point to be here considered, since I mentioned very much earlier that the <u>three</u> of us are offshoots of the same entity originally.

(See the 54th session, in Volume 2.)

Therefore, to some extent we are part of one vast sphere of action; and it is relatively more easy, therefore, for us to communicate. You in particular, Joseph, can benefit through the development of an easy access of communication with your own personal subconscious. Our Ruburt is indeed at times heavy-handed. At times he badgers <u>you</u>, but his remarks concerning the importance and indeed the strength of joy, should be well taken.

Joy and the spontaneous expression of it will always bring increased strength and resiliency to the personality. It also brings deep and abiding satisfaction to the subconscious, which is much more joyful than it is given credit for. The subconscious, for example, the personal subconscious, takes great pleasure in its manipulation of the physical fibers in locomotion. The expression of joy also makes the ego more resilient, less fearful, less resentful of diverse conditions when they occur. The emotion itself is an automatic signal that unites the conscious and subconscious in shared experience.

(Jane now took a very long pause. It was one of her few pauses during the session.)

It is, as a rule, lack of knowledge on the part of the ego as to the nature of reality, and its part in it, and the resulting fear, that often prevents a personality from accepting spontaneous expression of emotions in general. The capacity to feel is important. When one fears to experience seemingly unpleasant emotions, the personality also tends to set up an emotional pattern of rejection that seriously cuts down, also, not only on the expression but the very perception of joy.

This does not mean that the personality must be completely swept away by an emotion, though this is what such an ego fears. Emotion replenishes even the ego. Emotions demand resiliency, and resiliency is both the result of spontaneity, inner assurance, and discipline. <u>All</u> this is action, for the personality itself is composed of action, and is constantly changing. This is action, therefore, delighting in the expression and form of itself.

I think that you will find this particular session most beneficial. The desire to set yourself apart from emotion, and coolly appraise it, is merely an indication of the ego's characteristic nature. It tries to separate itself from action, to view it objectively, and to see itself as something apart from action.

Since it is itself action, such an attempt is basically doomed to failure. Yet the very attempt <u>causes</u> the formation of the ego. Once this apparent separate ego is formed, and once a fair amount of stability is maintained, and a new identity arrived at, the initial desire and energy will maintain the ego in its position during its existence in any field. Since this existence of separate identity <u>is</u> assured, attempts should then be made so that the ego can better participate in its realization of action, and the emotional life is very important in this respect.

In any fairly normal personality the intellect will indeed stand guard. There is no need to fear identity's complete immersion into emotional sensation. Such emotional experience actually strengthens not only the ego, but it opens communications between the ego and the subconscious, and allows for a much greater flow of energy from the primary source of action.

This energy, incidentally, can be most effectively used for creative work. I could have given you much of this material earlier, but I wanted you to understand the basic reasoning behind the material, and for this a knowledge of the nature of action was necessary.

You may as you prefer, take a short break, and I will continue the session, or you may close it.

("We'll close it then.")

Then my fondest regards to you both.

Again, I recommend that you continue your walks, and that Ruburt put his psychological time experiments once more on a regular basis.

("Good night, Seth.")

(End at 10:44. Jane was fully dissociated.)

SESSION 153
MAY 10, 1965 9 PM MONDAY AS SCHEDULED

(Jane's psychic experiences continue. While lying in a drowsy state early Sunday morning, she heard the words "twelve-o-five." They were spoken very slowly, in a husky whisper of a male voice, and seemed to originate just outside her ear. She heard nothing else. Checking with the pendulum, she got the answer that she had received random telepathy.

(This morning before the alarm rang, Jane found herself having an experience in which she was standing amid gray-white smoke. She knew she was not dreaming, and was possibly in a drowsy state again. She smelled the smoke. She appeared to be the observer here, yet felt a quick sense of panic, and when this appeared the experience ended. She saw nothing else and heard nothing.

(Jane is trying to get back on a regular basis of psy-time experiments. Both of us are making an effort to work regularly with the pendulum, as suggested by Seth.

(Jane's pace tonight was much slower than the previous two sessions. Again she used pauses, a few of them very long. She spoke while sitting down and with her eyes closed. Her voice was average.)

Good evening.

("Good evening, Seth.")

We find, on Ruburt's part, a much less violent reaction to springtime than the reaction which in the past was more or less characteristic with him.

The previous overviolent response was caused by a difficulty, among other things, in handling chemical changes, both in the atmosphere and in the physical body. The difficulty, however, was caused by a psychological tension, and an inability to utilize added energies.

You are both acquiring a facility in communication between the ego and the subconscious, which is enabling you to increase the efficiency of your overall behavior.

I have been wanting to speak further concerning the inner ego, for we have not discussed this issue in any depth. The inner ego is formed about characteristics and abilities that have been dominant in previous personalities, characteristics which the entity has developed through its experience in various lives.

The inner ego is focused inward, with as much intensity as the outer ego is focused outward. This inner ego is in many respects a composite, as indeed to a lesser degree the outer ego is a composite.

The inner ego, however, while conscious of itself, has returned to a subjective position within action, and views itself as a part of action. The outer ego, if you recall, views itself as apart from, or separate from, action. The inner ego contains the various purposes toward which the entity, as seen in its various personalities, has been working to achieve.

The inner ego has experienced, then, objectivity, and has returned to a subjective state. It is a relative storehouse of energy, and it is capable of aiding the outer ego when certain conditions arise. The inner ego may be termed the unfamiliar "I". In many cases it is the I who dreams, bringing valuable information to the personal subconscious, information that may be then used for the benefit of the outer ego itself.

I have often said that all these divisions and separations are arbitrary. All exist one <u>within</u> another. Apparent boundaries are not boundaries, but only differences in the focus of attention. Even this inner ego is not the same from one given moment to another, for it is not a static thing, but is a part of continuing action. It is much more familiar with the subconscious and with the dream universe, and with the inner self, than it is with the outside ego, however.

To some extent it also acts like a director of experience and action. It is not actually composed of the past egos, but of those dominant aspects of the various personalities. The inner ego, as action, thrusts in an inward direction; that is, back toward the originating impulse. The outside ego thrusts outward. They are two faces, therefore, and form one of many spheres of action, one pulling inward and one outward.

As the outer ego is constantly creative, so is the inner ego. The focus in which the creativity occurs is merely different. The subconscious could be thought of as a nucleus, surrounded by the inner and outer egos. Certain tensions are maintained here, and all communications, incidentally, are the results of tensions.

Tension is action's inherent impulse to know itself through further action. All actions are the result of tension. Without tension there would be no existence. Tension therefore is a creative state. A lack of understanding concerning tension will always lead an organism to fight against itself.

The ego, the inner ego, the subconscious, the whole self, and even the entity, these are all states of tension.

I suggest your first break.

(Break at 9:29. Jane was dissociated as usual for a first delivery. She resumed in the same normal voice, but at a faster pace, at 9:38.)

The inner ego, however, through the subconscious, may at times encourage the development of abilities that will better allow the whole self to achieve balance and fulfillment.

The outer ego is very seldom aware of the inner ego, and the subconscious is indeed a vast area dividing them. We are discussing now the outer ego in relation to the inner ego, and describing a situation in terms of relationships. Other relationships would show both the outer and inner egos in a different light. Relationships are also the result of tensions, and each action sets up a new tension.

No action can be considered by itself. There is no solitary action. Such a possibility is basically meaningless. Nor does a tension exist in isolation. In all of these matters there is also constant pulsations of action within the outer ego, the inner ego, and all the other aspects of the whole self.

We have not touched in any degree concerning further possibilities here, but as there is no real or actual boundary between any of these areas of the whole self, so there are no <u>actual</u>, definite boundaries between any given whole self and another, nor between any given entity and another.

The boundaries are functional units rather, and functions may blend one into the other. For practical purposes there are apparent divisions. In basic actuality there are no such divisions. This will be dealt with very thoroughly at a later date, but it is an important point to keep in mind.

It is therefore obvious why one action affects all others, so intimately that it is basically impossible to speak of one action in isolation. Tension is a condition of action, and an inherent quality of action. The possibilities of action are limitless. Regardless of the origin of any given action, it will never be entirely dissipated. It may pass beyond or through the system in which it originated, but its existence will not cease.

Tension is infinite. Your time system is indeed the result of tension as it is distorted within your own system, yet the distortion itself, as you see, creates a new reality. And that reality then continues to operate, forming like realities of the sort that can exist within the given conditions already set up by the original distortion.

Distortion, in this respect, has a different meaning than the sort of distortion arising from a misreading of information. Yet in some respects it is similar. An original action can never repeat itself in an identical fashion. Its attempts to do so, never successful, result in a kind of distortion, and this distortion then becomes the basis for a new reality.

The reality then tries to recreate itself in identical fashion, fails, and is again distorted into a further facet of basic reality. This holds true under all circumstances and under all conditions. Recall here the material concerning identities in general.

(*Among others, see the following sessions: 136 to 139 in Volume 3.*)

A very simple analogy will arise as an artist attempts faithfully to reproduce a landscape. The attempt is obviously doomed to failure, since the necessary actual perspectives in which the landscape exists are denied to him as working materials. He cannot create an actual reproduction of a living landscape.

Such a landscape would have to take up as much physical space as the original. But more, it would have to take up an <u>identical amount</u> of physical time, in terms of past physical existence, which is clearly impossible.

Such a landscape would have to be composed of the actual elements that compose the original landscape. The artist would have to assemble mountains of rocks, an infinity, that is infinity of molecules, all equally impossible. The best he can do is create a distortion of the original landscape—a creation of an approximation that can comfortably exist within the limited perspectives with which he can work, and using the materials that are at his own command.

The painting that results is a new reality, but it is also a distortion of the original landscape. The artist may hint at time within his painting, but he cannot capture the physical eons that might be contained in the mountains themselves, which he wishes to reproduce.

However his painting contains new realities, and distinctive ones, that would be alien to the original landscape. The actual trees, had he <u>really</u> been able to reproduce them, would then undergo their seasonal changes. The trees in his painting, being artificial reproductions, do not undergo the same physical changes, even while the atoms and molecules that compose the canvas itself, and all the pigments, constantly themselves change.

The painting, therefore, is both a distortion of reality, and the creation of a new reality. Likewise all realities are formed.

I suggest your break.

(Break at 10:07. Jane was well dissociated. She had spoken at a faster rate. She also said that as she spoke she had received the feeling of a concept from Seth. It was difficult for her to put into words. It had something to do with her perception of two identical masses of landscape, one being meant to duplicate the other. At the same time, she said, the duplicating mass would have to displace <u>another</u> equal mass to make room for the duplication.

(Jane remarked that whenever she receives a concept she always will remember at least the gist of the material she has been delivering, even when she has been deeply dissociated.

(Jane resumed in a normal voice and at a slower rate at 10:20.)

Mankind is to some intimate degree acquainted with this attempt of action to recreate itself, for human reproduction is here a case in point, each individual attempting to create a replica, the attempt doomed to failure, but the attempt itself resulting in a distortion of the original action; that is, a distortion of the original individuals, and in the creation of a new reality, this process then being repeated indefinitely.

The distortions are then creative. The nature of action itself is such that tension is one of its positive characteristics, and the tension is the element that causes action to seek expansion in terms of an attempt to duplicate itself.

We come therefore to the fact of creative tension. The individual in his psychological state is familiar with creative tension, often in its pure state. So quickly however is the tension transformed into a distortive creation that the sensation of creation is mistakenly accepted as the tension itself, rather than seen for what it is. Creation is the result of tension, though instantly new tension is set up, since tension is a characteristic of action. And each creation, being action, will instantly set up new tension.

It is possible, with some discipline, to become familiar with this state of tension from which new creation will so quickly arise. Familiarity with this brief state of tension will allow an individual to use it more efficiently. He can ride it like the crest of a wave.

The act of creation occurs, itself, not at the peak of the wave of tension, but as the wave dissolves into the fulfillment of itself. The exhilarating sensation is the tension. The sensation is usually mistakenly applied as if it accompanied the creation itself, but the creation is the final act, so to speak, of a given tension.

The creation is, therefore, the relaxed fulfillment of a tension. This can have practical results, for you will be able to recognize and use the tension itself toward purposeful goals. It can be dissolved or set at rest in <u>any</u> action. Recognizing the tension itself will allow you to choose the action that will result, to some degree.

Creative distortion, in its relationship with action, affects therefore the creation of thoughts. The principle of creative distortions is mainly responsible for the fact that no identical thought is ever transmitted from one individual to another. Here the material that I have given you on telepathy should be considered.

(See the 136th and 137th sessions, among others in Volume 3.)

The thought received in telepathic communications will not, therefore, be the exact thought that was transmitted, but a close approximation, a creative distortion, actually created by the receiver. There are, as I mentioned, no duplication of identities.

Now. Compare a thought, an original thought, with our original landscape. The problem would be then the same problem with which our artist was concerned.

Say for example that our individual "A" wanted to transmit this thought to "B". The thought is as much a reality as the landscape. It is as much a part of individual "A" as the landscape is part of the physical earth. Our imaginary artist could not <u>rip</u> the landscape out of the earth, or bring it to his studio. He could not create an identical landscape because he did not have at his command the perspectives or materials necessary.

Likewise, our individual "A" cannot rip the thought out of the context of his own inner electrical system. He cannot send it to individual "B". He can send an approximation of it, for the attempt to transmit the thought automatically changes the thought itself. He sends an approximation of the original thought, and this approximation is further changed by "B's" action as he attempts to receive it. Have we this clear now?

("Yes."

(Seth asked the question because I fell behind in my notes on the above paragraph, and had to ask for its repetition.)

In a like manner for example, the act of dreaming itself changes both the dreamer and the dream. The act of doing anything <u>at all</u> automatically changes the doer. The reality of any action automatically determines that the action will change.

The creative dilemma, the creative distortion, is of course itself an action that is resolved in further acts. These are basic principles concerning the nature of action, principles that are carried through within any system. They are valid therefore within your own system, within the electrical system, within the dream system, and among all others.

The action involved in these sessions, for example, changes us all, yet truly none of us perceive the nature of the entire action of which we are a part. I, for example, cannot perceive the <u>entire</u> future consequences of any one action. I may perceive the entire consequences of any given action within your system or my own, but it is impossible for me to perceive a given action's consequences as it is felt within all systems, for each action occurs within all systems simultaneously.

I may use the word future, but I use it only to express that which is beyond my present perceptive limits. It is almost impossible to speak of a single, simple action, though I may do so for convenience's sake.

You may if you prefer end the session; or I will continue, after a short break, into some further material along these same lines.

("We'll end it then.")

Our next session then will be concerned further with the nature of action, and I will speak concerning the complexity of what may appear to be a single action.

My fondest regards to you both. I expect you will both get quite springy with the spring. I am in fine fettle.

("Good night, Seth.")

(End at approximately 10:50. Jane was well dissociated. She said Seth felt very good, and could have carried on indefinitely.)

SESSION 154
MAY 12, 1965 9 PM WEDNESDAY AS SCHEDULED

(Jane has begun her psychological time experiments, though she is still not on a regular day-to-day basis. Her experiment mentioned by Seth at the opening of the session was not a spectacular one by any means. It involved what Jane calls merely her "good state". In more exceptional cases this escalates into her version of ecstasy.

(This state is one of thrilling or tingling, or of a singing sensation, that can either suffuse the whole body, or perhaps locate itself in one side of the body or in one limb. Both of us have experienced it in varying degrees during psychological time, sometimes intensely. I have also experienced it outside of psy-time. It can indeed be a thrilling experience, making one feel about to be swept up and away. We have been aware of its relation to sound, since we soon learned while in the state that any sound, be it of running water somewhere in the house, or a robin's call, would momentarily impart an upsurge to the sensation within the body. Thus sound, even though detected by ear, would act also as a stimulus to the body's detection of the same sound via feeling.

(For some material on this sensation on Jane's part, see the 39th and 50th sessions in Volumes 1 and 2, and the attached notes. For the same thing on my part, see sessions 24 and 35 in Volume 1. There are many other accounts of it scattered through our psy-time notes preceding various sessions.

(Yesterday, deliberately, I mentioned to Jane that Seth had not given us any more material on the inner senses for many sessions. What I meant of course was that he had not catalogued the later material under the various inner senses, as he had originally designated them. I felt that he would eventually do so. Checking the various categories of material against the original list of the inner senses, it was usually easy to see where the two fit together.

(Jane spoke while sitting down and with her eyes closed. Her pace was average, with pauses, her voice quiet.)

Good evening.

("Good evening, Seth.")

If you recall, many sessions ago, [the 24th] we discussed feeling sound.

Ruburt experienced this in his psychological time experiment this afternoon, and it reminded me that more material definitely was needed here.

Basically, the physical body has the potentiality for perceiving stimuli on a generalized basis. I mean by this that although the eyes are for seeing, the ears for hearing and so forth, the <u>potentials</u> of the physical body include the capacity to hear, for example, through any given portion of the bodily expanse.

The same applies to seeing, and obviously to feeling or touching. It goes without saying that this potentiality is very seldom realized, but it is part of the human heritage. It is the learning process that conditions you to translate a given stimuli into data that will be picked up by a given physical sense; that is, translations always occur in any case.

You may see an automobile for example with your eyes, and hear its sound through your ears, but it is also within the human capacity, ideally speaking, to hear the <u>sight</u> of the car, and to see the <u>sound</u> of the car. Practically speaking these capacities have been overlooked in human development simply because the ego hit upon the present method of perception, and clung to it.

In other species within your field, however, some of these various methods have been chosen and utilized. Many animals for example literally <u>see</u> through the sense of smell. They quite literally perceive what you would call the sight of another animal, through the use of the sense of smell.

They build up multitudinous variations of odors to build the likeness of a structure complete in its translations as to size, weight and so forth. Sound, then, can be felt as well as heard, although you might say in such cases that the sound is <u>heard</u> in the depths of the tissues. This however being an analogy.

Now for a moment we will return to our material on action, and you may perhaps see why this fits in so well here. No action is identical to any other action. An action is never entirely dissipated, though it may pass beyond its particular field of origin. This transference, incidentally, from one system to another, necessarily changes the action itself; but for simplicity's sake we may say that an action has its reality within many systems simultaneously.

The sight of our imaginary automobile, therefore, is perceived by you as a visual stimulus, because you are conditioned to perceiving it in such a fashion. But it is also possible to perceive our automobile in entirely different fashions within different realities, and from various perspectives.

It is even possible for the physical individual to train himself to change the nature of his <u>own</u> perception of such objects. It is not a question of the car having certain properties, being real to one perceptive view and therefore necessarily <u>unreal</u> to another. To a very large degree, the portion of <u>any</u> reality that you can perceive is determined largely not by the given, so-called real object itself, but from the perspective, and because of, the senses with which you perceive it.

The scent image built up by the animal is every bit as real as the visual image. Action cannot be caught and held, and the nature of <u>perceiving</u> an action changes the very nature of the action itself. It is indeed, here again, that tension causes such a change.

Ruburt, in feeling sound, merely experienced the sound from a different perspective. You have had this experience more frequently perhaps than Ruburt, Joseph.

While we are somewhat on the subject, I have not forgotten that we have left behind our discussions on the inner senses, and really with good reason. When we return to the inner senses again, we will be able to discuss them in further depth because of the material that we have covered in the meantime.

I suggest your first break.

(Break at 9:26. Jane was dissociated as usual for a first delivery. She resumed in the same quiet manner at 9:37.)

Since perceiving an action is itself an action, the perceiving must because of its nature to some extent distort the object of perception.

Again, in this distortion we see the creation, however minute, of a new reality. The universe is cohesive, but it is also more various than you know even now. The nature of our object, our automobile for example, is indeed largely determined by those who perceive it, for it is different things in reality, and not one thing. Electrically it has an identity, and would be perceived as an entirely different phenomena from within an electrical system, where there would be no perceptors of physical data.

Within your field the automobile is perceived mainly as a physical object. Within some systems the same automobile would appear to be no more than a shadow. Within some systems the automobile would not be perceived at all, unless it were in motion. In other systems it would not be perceived at all, unless it were <u>not</u> in motion.

These various conceptions of the automobile would also apply of course to the perception of any physical beings within the car; that is, their reality would also be perceived differently, according to the perspective systems which viewed them.

You must indeed for practical reasons pretend as if the automobile had no reality except the reality with which you are familiar, but this is not the case. I mentioned feeling sound because this is a capability that lies latent within your own physical system, but this same sort of a juggling of perspective data is what happens, generally speaking, when inhabitants of a different system perceive realities that also have an existence within your own system.

It is really a building up of idea into a whole pattern that can be perceived by the camouflage senses. Any reality therefore will be variously perceived, and the nature of the reality will necessarily be distorted in the very attempt to perceive it. Here again we have our creative tension, whereby a new reality is formed as a result of the distortion itself. Within your system colors may be perceived as sound. Their connections with human moods is only too apparent.

They may also be <u>tasted</u>, as well as <u>sniffed</u>, and these experiences are actually to some fair degree carried on continually beneath awareness, all adding up to the individual's perception of a given color. Colors may even be perceived through an inner sense of balance. Their stability or instability is, therefore, subconsciously appreciated.

Emotions may even cause a color reaction. <u>Any</u> reality, regardless of which system it originates within, will appear to some degree within all systems. Even within your own system, though perhaps on a subconscious level, all emotions have a reality in color. They have, as you know, a chemical reaction which is sniffed by other animals.

From your odor, an animal instantly builds up an image of the state of your psychological condition.

I am not going to hold a very long session this evening. Rather than give you fairly frequent short vacations, I may at times close a session early. We still come out ahead in terms of time. We are heading here indeed, slowly but surely, toward a thorough discussion of the inner senses, which could not be given until you had a good background in the nature of action itself. For you should be able to see now that the inner senses allow a more faithful perception of basic reality than the outer senses could ever give.

Reality is indeed not necessarily that which is constant within the various <u>appearances</u> of reality through all systems, as it is the perception of the whole picture of reality, or the sum of all reality as seen within the various systems. This involves quite a complicated point, and implies a complicated position; for true reality would not be completely either the reality of an automobile, say, as it appears within the physical system, or as it appears within the electrical system. It would not be that which appears identical to the two systems, but it would be indeed the sum of the realities of all systems, as applied to our weary automobile.

The inner senses, by being free of camouflage information, are more or less (in quotes) "pure" perceptors, perceiving with but little prejudice of many realities while being imprisoned by none.

I suggest here a short break.

(Break at 10:05. Jane was well dissociated. She resumed at a somewhat faster rate at 10:15.)

Concerning Joseph's point about sound; sound alone, entering the body, instantaneously changes it.

Any <u>perception</u> instantly changes the perceiver. It also changes the thing perceived, and this we will discuss at a later session, for it involves the other side of the coin, so to speak.

Any action, any reality, irregardless, constantly and instantaneously changes. There are no exceptions to this rule. Any appearance of permanence is illusion.

I will indeed now close our session, the reason mainly being that Ruburt has been oriented in a quickened fashion toward our work since he began his book again, and he has used additional energy in doing so. I am always conscientiously aware of his condition at any time. It is only the transition here that has caused the additional use of energy, and he is readily adapting himself so that he will not be under strain. Our sessions have been highly compact as of late also, and intensified in energy content.

As always, my heartiest good wishes to you both, and one small note for Ruburt's edification: a beef bouillon in mid afternoon would serve him well. Incidentally, his system automatically as a rule seeks those foods that tend to build up the particular sort of energy that he uses in the main. As a rule therefore, proteins are indeed a most beneficial food to him, and it is for this reason that he automatically seeks them out.

Other personalities do not benefit in the same way from proteins, and should not use them as a <u>main</u> portion of their diet. This however does not apply to you, Joseph.

I will now close, my spring pigeons.

("Good night, Seth.")

(End at 10:25. Jane was dissociated as usual.)

SESSION 155
MAY 17, 1965 9 PM MONDAY AS SCHEDULED

(Jane has received her contract for her ESP book from Frederick Fell. For several days she has been debating over the terms it contains, liking some and not too fond of others. We have discussed it together also.

(This evening Jane checked with her pendulum technique, and learned that it would be best for her to sign the contract as it stands. Mr. Fell has already made some

changes in the contract, as requested by Jane. The pendulum also advised her against a trip to New York City at this time. I asked myself the same questions with my own pendulum, and received the same answers. The upshot of all this was that by session time we had about decided to sign the contract.

(Again Jane spoke while sitting down and with her eyes closed, in a normal voice with some pauses.)

Good evening.

("Good evening. Seth.")

The relationship with Frederick Fell will be a good one, although the present contract reflects the publisher's caution, as well as the money already received reflects an impulsive belief in Ruburt on the publisher's part.

The caution can later work to Ruburt's advantage, in that Fell is usually cautious in business relationships. The impulsiveness caused him to forward the money already received, however. Undoubtedly Ruburt could receive better clauses if he pressed for them. At this point however, it will be to his advantage to leave matters as they are.

A later trip to New York, perhaps when the manuscript is completed, may however prove most beneficial. Also a lively concern shown by Ruburt in his letters as to publicity matters and promotion, with mention later of other books in the field that he plans.

He could indeed press for better clauses now, but in one way he would lose a certain advantage. He is an unknown quantity to the publisher to a large degree. His letter, however, did make an impression upon Mr. Fell. Ruburt is the underdog at this point. He has however gained several advantages, as you know, in altering the terms originally offered.

The book will be successful in terms of beginning to establish Ruburt in reputation, and also successfully in financial terms. Because this contract is less than Ruburt could press for, the next contract will be a much better one, since the publisher will then feel rather embarrassed concerning this contract.

Ruburt of course should make his own decision, with your help. I am stating simply what I see.

(Jane now took a very long pause, sitting quite still for well over a minute.)

A trip now would not be nearly as advantageous as a trip later. Ruburt's concern should be with his manuscript. After this book he will be in a much better bargaining position. The added worries involved are not <u>now</u> worth the mental and psychic strains that they would cause.

This could reflect in the book itself. In one way he will not be making as much money as he could if he insisted upon changes in the contract. On the other hand the important thing here is that the book be completed with full psychic and creative powers, without distraction. The book will be an important one, and in the overall the money difference will not be great enough to tip the scales. The experience in the business will be invaluable in any case.

The most important clause, the option clause, has been settled in Ruburt's favor. He has done very well, actually, in maintaining fairly decent equilibrium.

I here suggest your first break.

(Break at 9:18. Jane was dissociated as usual for a first delivery, remembering some of the material in a general way. She resumed in the same quiet voice at 9:34.)

This endeavor, the book, should be carried on now unceasingly, with periods of complete relaxation or change weekends. But the work should be intensive during the week.

There should be no vacation unless Ruburt takes the manuscript with him and works upon it. This would work out very well both for him and the book. His natural energies will carry him along here, and these energies will be reflected and caught in the book itself.

It is to his advantage that the earlier publisher did not take the book. It is the subject matter of the book that intrigued both publishers, plus Ruburt's belief in the book. But it was <u>also</u> the subject matter, to some degree, that made Mr. Fell cautious, and that finally caused the earlier publisher to turn it down.

(Jane now began to cough. She had been sipping some fruit juice at break. The coughing was not violent but it became persistent. She sat with her eyes closed for a minute or two while she tried to control it.)

I suggest a break.

(Break at 9:39. Jane had been dissociated, but toward the last realized she was coughing. Seth, she said, took a break so that she could rest. She drank some water, remarking that as far as she could remember this was the first time she had ever so interrupted a session. Without checking each session, I agree.

(Once again Jane resumed in the same quiet voice, at 10:44.)

A paperback edition will indeed appear.

I wanted this evening to discuss these matters, since you have **both been** concerned with them. I am aware of the work done on the book so far, **and find** that it is indeed quite remarkable.

The Seth book will be finished at the correct time.

Ruburt may trust the pendulum, although care should be taken as far as predictions are concerned, though with training the pendulum will give valid answers to predictions.

Our Wednesday evening session may well be somewhat longer than usual, since for this one I was mainly concerned with discussing the practical problem at hand, since it is important that the air be cleared in this respect.

Do you, Joseph, have any questions of your own concerning the book?
("No, I think we've covered everything I had in mind.")
The main points, I believe, have been taken care of.

I will here again suggest that Ruburt return to a definite scheduled psychological time habit. The walk to the river is an excellent idea for you both. And your suggestion, Joseph, concerning suppers there, is a very good one. You will both find it effective and refreshing.

Ruburt's predictions and his dream records will again improve. To some degree he was tied up in knots, although his condition is far superior to what it would have been under the same circumstances at any time in the past. For short periods, sunbathing will be restful for him.

("How about the way we use the pendulum to check our predictions, after the event? Is that a valid use of it?")

The pendulum can be used to check predictions, although such a study will involve long-term experimentation. Any material proof of this sort is extremely difficult, since oftentimes you pick up a generalized picture of coming events, so to speak, and the words that you use are so literal that they cannot convey the whole picture sufficiently enough so that validity can be proven, in your terms. By all means continue.

Ruburt now is in a very relaxed state. I will leave him in it, and close this short but most fruitful session. Wednesday's session however will be a long and compact one. Longer perhaps in time than usual, and even more compact in terms of material delivered.

Our spring and summer sessions should be particularly enjoyable to us all. If you have any questions, however, I will answer them.

("How come the pendulum will sometimes say Jane or I made valid predictions, when we don't see any connection consciously?"

(For many months now both Jane and I have followed a practice of making perhaps half a dozen predictions for the following day. Usually each one consists of three or four words at the most. On the day the predictions were made for, we check them against what we can consciously remember of the day's events. It is great fun to make them, and was Jane's idea originally.

(Lately we have begun using the pendulum to "verify" the validity of our predictions, and our interpretation of them. To our surprise, we have discovered that the pendulum does not always agree with our conscious interpretations. At times it will agree with our predictions and our interpretations. At times it will not agree with our interpretation of what it calls a valid prediction. And at times it will state that a prediction is valid, when we can see nothing during the following day's events to tie to the prediction.)

The range is very large, oftentimes too large, for the conscious mind to perceive a particular segment of it. Clairvoyant material comes constantly. Some of it is used and acted upon. Other portions are discarded simply because the particular information is not pertinent.

Tell Ruburt that he can now rest assured concerning the book.

My best and fondest regards to you both. Ruburt has used much energy in worrying about the contract in general. For this reason I wanted to discuss it this evening, and because his energies were momentarily depleted I am holding a rather short session.

We will return to our regular sessions, and to a continuation of our discussions. You will both be better off however for this evening's session, and I think you will notice an assured, calm, yet sure increase in Ruburt's energies. You are doing very well, incidentally. I bid you now both a fond good evening. And if Ruburt does not watch out, then I will charge him 10 percent as his agent.

("Good night, Seth.")

(End at 10:06. Jane was very well dissociated.)

SESSION 156
MAY 19, 1965 9 PM WEDNESDAY AS SCHEDULED

(Jane had no idea of the material for the session. She spoke while sitting down and with her eyes closed, in a quiet voice, and with pauses. Her voice was very amused as she began the session; she smiled as she spoke.)

Good evening—

("Good evening, Seth.")

—my springtime robins, though you are not as plump as springtime robins, nor is your chirrup quite as melodious. Nor, for that matter, is my own.

I have watched with some amusement the proceedings of the last few days, as Ruburt involved himself with his contract, hemmed and hawed, worried it and clucked.

I am not one to say I told you so necessarily. However, I did tell you so, not only concerning the book sale, but also concerning the fact that it would be advantageous for Ruburt to leave his gallery position. His ability to focus direction of energy in his writing has vastly improved, due to the last months' labors, and will show in his book.

(Seth suggested Jane leave the gallery job in the 82nd session, August 27, 1964, and she soon did so. In the 92nd session, September 28, 1964, Seth predicted the sale of Jane's book on ESP by name. Today Jane signed her contract for the book, and will

mail it to F. Fell tomorrow.)

Now, we will speak again concerning action.

Our material on the fifth dimension seemed almost infinite to you at the time. That is, the fifth dimension appeared infinite in its complexity, but you see that it is but one dimension within an infinite number of dimensions. For there are infinite possibilities in the patterns which action can of itself form.

(See the 12th session for Seth's first discussion of the fifth dimension.)

I do not intend to number indefinitely, or list, an endless number of dimensions of actuality, though we will go into this later to some small degree. I am much more concerned for now that you understand the dimensions of action as they exist within the dream world, within psychological realities, and within other scopes with which you are yourselves somewhat familiar.

Your experiments with the pendulum are quite helpful to you, in that the subconscious is allowed, through its own action, to make itself more readily available. Your own conscious awareness is increased because you are then aware of inner actions with which the conscious mind had not been familiar. Here we have a coming together of actions, a joining and an immersion of one action within another: the action of the subconscious in answering questions put to it by the conscious mind, (use brain rather than mind), and the <u>acceptance</u>, which is itself action on the part of consciousness, of the answers received.

Here the self, by becoming part of greater action, increases its own ability to deal with action. The principle that action acts upon itself is extremely important when we are dealing with psychological action. The principle that action is self-generating, and that it cannot be withdrawn, is also vital in connection with psychological action.

Energy cannot be <u>retained</u>. It must be discharged. The very attempt to deny an action automatically changes the nature of the action, and also changes the nature of the individual who attempts to deny it. All energy seeks to materialize itself, which is another way of saying that action must act.

In the psychological realm it goes without saying that a repressed emotion is never really repressed, since action cannot be retained. It must change. The cause of such difficulties lies not in the repression of an emotion, for this is impossible. The emotion in one way or another, will out, but the difficulty lies in the <u>attempt</u> to repress the emotion. This attempt is itself an action.

There is a term used occasionally to the effect that an emotional block is like a wall. The analogy is an excellent one. I have told you earlier that there are other kinds of structures beside physical structures. Emotions and thoughts have their own structures, that may be manipulated in the same manner that physical objects are manipulated, generally speaking.

An action has reality, as you know, within every possible field of activity. An emotion has an electrical and chemical structure. This is extremely important. It is not a structure that takes up space as you know it, obviously, but it is a structure nevertheless, and could be compared to the appearance of dream locations.

(In Volume 2, see the 44th session for material on dream locations.)

Emotions are a quite natural portion of action, and left to themselves are fluid. They have electrical validity, and shape. When an attempt is made to reject an emotion, this does not affect the emotion half as much as it affects the individual involved. The act of rejection in itself is detrimental and doomed to failure.

I suggest your first break.

(Break at 9:30. Jane was dissociated as usual for a first delivery. She resumed in the same quiet manner at 9:39.)

You may perhaps come closer to understanding how these psychological structures are manipulated if you consider the same sort of structures as they exist as dream objects in sleep.

If you toss a ball in a dream, neither the self that tosses the ball, nor the ball, exist in any space structure as you know it. In somewhat the same manner are emotion structures handled. A refusal or a denial, an attempt *not* to handle a particular emotional structure involves action. The refusal itself is an action.

(Jane now took a very long pause.)

What you have here is an attempt to objectify, or stand apart from action in such a refusal. This is not the fault of the subconscious, but a fault of the ego, which refuses to assimilate or accept a given action. As you know, it is the ego who exists as a result of such objectivity. All the qualities that make up the ego are objectified to that degree, but they are collected about the ego with the ego as center. When the ego however refuses to accept an emotion as a part of itself, it tries one of two actions.

Either it attempts to return the emotion to a subjective state, or it attempts to objectify it further away from itself. In either case the ego is at fault for not assimilating or accepting the emotion. It is easy to see then that the ego is itself a series of actions, that it is a collection of more or less similar actions, selected from a larger mainstream of other actions.

You will recall that the ego, while disliking change, is nevertheless dependent for its identity upon change. The ego to a large degree, therefore, chooses during its development those characteristic actions which will form its nature. Because the ego necessarily changes however, actions or emotions which at one time it chose as acceptable, at a later date so to speak it may attempt to deny.

The habitual pattern or characteristic nature of the ego may then be led to refuse to accept an emotion, at the same time that a pattern has already been set to receive the particular type of emotion. Here the ego fights against itself. Such an emotion may of course be given release through dreams, but this is of limited value to the ego involved, since the ego does not accept the reality of dream existence.

The strength of the ego actually depends on the flexibility with which it can accept and assimilate ever more complex actions, and give them a unity of its own. An action or emotion not accepted by the ego, but nevertheless a part of it, will always drain energy from the main core of the ego, despite the ego's denial, and energy that cannot therefore be used by the ego for the purposes of its own purposeful action.

The rejected emotion, in other words, will express itself in any case, but it will do so then as a rebel, outside of the organizational directives of the ego itself. Hence for example, actions that appear senseless to the ego are often the results of such unassimilated or denied emotions. At one time or another such emotions were acceptable to the ego. There was an attraction, or the emotion would not have been permitted to enter into a realm close to ego control.

Inclinations with which the ego has very little liking, for example, are very seldom a problem for the ego, since they remain generally outside of the ego pattern, never having been chosen by it to form a characteristic part of the ego pattern. Obviously, to some degree every conceivable sort of inclination is latent to the ego, but it is apparent that each ego has its peculiar set of adopted characteristics, its set of characteristics that it <u>sometimes</u> accepts and sometimes rejects; and it is obvious that some characteristics simply seem alien to any given ego.

It is therefore with the second alternating group of characteristics that most such problems arise. An ego who can, and has at one time or another accepted as part of itself a violent and unruly desire to kill, for example, will not automatically reject the emotion of hatred. He may dislike it, but he will recognize it as a part of himself during whatever period it is assimilated. An ego which once accepted such an idea of violence, and knew it as a possibility of action, such an ego, if he then rejects the conception, can no longer afford, ever, to recognize this once acceptable emotion, for he is only too aware of the action that <u>could</u> have at one time developed.

It is in this area that such conflicts arise. The man, or ego, who has never really accepted such violence as a part of his action pattern, will usually have no conflicts in this particular line, simply because the inclination was never a strong part of the ego's inner image, and is more or less discarded automatically, along with all those other characteristics or inclinations which are not in his ego pattern.

This is obviously somewhat simplified, in that the ego constantly changes, and the above examples must be read carefully or their meaning could be misinterpreted. Actions may _appear_ to be separate, but they are all part of other actions, this being of course the basis for all organization, including that of the ego and the inner self.

Again, it must be remembered that no real boundaries exist, only diversity of function.

I suggest your break.

(Break at 10:17. Jane was dissociated as usual. She resumed in a very slow manner, taking many pauses, at 10:30.)

All boundaries, therefore, are apparent boundaries, boundaries in appearance only.

Groupings of actions of any kind merge into other groupings, both within the physical field and outside of it. All apparent units are merely formed by functions, the functions of action. In this context the ego is also a function of action. There are of course also functions within functions, which should be obvious.

The ego itself attempts as its function to be the director and center of other functions. The ego, while considering itself apart from action, is obviously not apart from it. As dreams allow the inner self great freedom, and as in dreams great perspectives of time are available, and great freedom in space, though no space as you know it is involved, so it is possible for the ego itself to achieve the experience of freedom from time and space, if it would only allow itself for a short while to relax the intensity of its objective focus.

It could still do this and retain its own nature, merely by allowing into its awareness the reality of other actions as a part of its self-image. There is for example no basic reason why the subconscious and the ego cannot communicate to a much larger extent than is now usual. Such communication would result in the acceptance of additional energy and action by the ego, and an expansion of the ego's self-image.

It was necessary for the ego, in its origins, to objectify itself as much as possible. Now however the stability of the ego, generally speaking, as a part of the human personality is established. It can now afford to be much more elastic, to include, in other words, more and more of reality within its awareness. Such an inclusion would be most beneficial. It would of course however to some extent change the ego, and any change is resisted by the ego.

Nevertheless the course of future events will move in this direction. It must. The ego must change in this rather basic manner, including other realities within its scope of awareness. There is no basic reason why it cannot add its directive energies to other aspects of the personality, and if it could so expand it would, theoretically, be possible for the ego to become aware of many experiences which have been impossible for it in the past.

The hope and the possibilities here, as well as some of the dangers, lie in the fact that the ego does indeed change, and is not one specific reality but a series or group of actions, with direction, that have the potentiality for unlimited value fulfillment. The ego will never be less than it is now. It may very well be more. Possibilities for development here are very great, but most such possibilities lie still in the future, and only, so far, as possibilities. There is nothing that will force the ego to enlarge the scope of its awareness.

Ruburt may now, if he wishes, work on his psychological time in the morning. I wanted that particular routine broken up for a while, but now if it is more convenient he may return to his old schedule; that is, that same time of day, but twenty minutes should still be the limit.

We will shortly launch into a new discussion, though there are still some matters to be cleared in our material on action. I will now close the session, or if you prefer you may take a short break and continue.

("We'll close then.")

My best regards to you both, and a most fond good evening.

("Good night, Seth.")

(End at 11:00. Jane was dissociated as usual.

(Seth referred to Jane's endeavors with psychological time because she has been having trouble establishing an effective routine for it in the afternoons. She always found it natural to try it between eleven-thirty and noon, after she had put in her morning's work writing, and before I get home from work.)

SESSION 157
MAY 24, 1965 9 PM MONDAY AS SCHEDULED

(Before the session began, Jane said she felt much more restless than usual. Once again she spoke while sitting down and with her eyes closed. Her voice was average, her rate of delivery average also, but with pauses. She actually began speaking at 9:02.)

Good evening.

("Good evening, Seth.")

The nature of action cannot be altered.

I am speaking now of the basic nature of reality, and not of any particular action, for particular actions can indeed be altered by other actions, and no given action occurs in a solitary manner.

This last is extremely important. Actions are perceived as realities according to the nature, not of a given action, but according to the nature of the perceiver. His viewpoint and his field of reference will at all times color to some extent or another the nature of the reality which he perceives.

This may sound contradictory. We have stated that a reality remains as it is, unchanged even though the perceiver, because of his sense apparatus, may perceive it in a limited or distorted fashion. While this is to some extent true, we can now delve into the matter somewhat more fully. In our later sessions for example, we have mentioned that the desire for duplication must always result in a distortion, but this distortion is also the basis therefore for a new reality.

Now, putting these two statements together, you see that an individual will perceive basic reality, in the main, only from his own reference point, and through his outer sense apparatus. His perception of basic reality in one way does not change the nature of that reality or of that action, as it exists independently of his field of reference. However, the very distortions that occur in his attempt to perceive this reality results in a new reality. What he perceives then is legitimate, for his very perception of it is the basis for its existence.

Would you like a break?

("No."

(*My head had been bothering me today and yesterday. The effect was something like an allergy or cold, although the pendulum told me it was neither. The condition was very annoying.*)

Any individual reacts to a reality as he perceives it to be, and he perceives it to be since he has himself created it from basic reality. The very distortions therefore form many of the characteristic differences which for him gives his reality its peculiar nature. Those whose actions set them apart drastically from others within your system, and who seem in one way or another mentally unbalanced, are often told that they must relate themselves more clearly with reality as it exists.

This however is not their problem, for like all other individuals they perceive a reality that they have created. Their problem therefore is a distortive one. It is not related to their attitude toward reality as a whole, but it is intimately connected with the reality which they have created. They are indeed relating to <u>that</u> reality very well. The reality, however, is much more distorted than usual, and this is one of the main problems.

It is only because their realities are so distorted that the difficulty is discovered. I mentioned many sessions back that your physical universe, so taken for granted, is actually at least as diverse and multitudinous as the dream system. Within the physical universe you merely focus upon similarities and ignore the vast differences that exist. Each reality is completely unique for every individual, and through his own actions he attempts therefore to communicate the nature of this reality of his to his fellows.

We have discussed the ways in which telepathy operates in this respect, and we have to some extent discussed the ways in which the appearance of cohesiveness is maintained. In many cases the individual who is called mentally unbalanced is simply one whose individual reality is so composed that it is impossible for others to find in his expression of it any similarity with their own. The error is one of inadequate idea construction.

I suggest your first break.

(Break at 9:29. Jane was more dissociated than usual for a first delivery. At times during the delivery her voice had risen a bit in volume. She resumed in a good voice, still with pauses, at 9:35.)

I will now direct my remarks to you, Joseph.

It is not advantageous for you to work with the pendulum over a half-hour per day. A daily routine involving a half-hour's work with the pendulum will do you good.

Further work with it at this time turns to an introversion with the personal subconscious, and an overinvolvement with it as far as overall focus is concerned. The half-hour is sufficient and beneficial. A deeper involvement however at this time serves to focus your energies in a bunch, so to speak, in the personal subconscious, blocking creative energies that come from deeper layers of the inner self. The half-hour however will allow you, in a smooth manner, to communicate with this important area of the self in a way that will not block other energies, and that will be beneficial.

I would also suggest for the present that you deal with other matters than your health; then you may return to the subject, and I will be glad to further elaborate upon what information you receive. My further suggestions are that you return to painting or sketching, and you will find that your energies will now be allowed much more freedom.

What you have been in danger of doing is using too much energy oriented toward the past, and this will also show itself in your physical reactions. Your trouble of yesterday and today does indeed <u>originate</u> because you have not been painting, but one of the reasons that you have not been painting is that energy has been used as a searchlight into the past, searching for certain origins.

The quest is a good one. You have simply concentrated upon it too deeply. You have learned much, both in relating yourself to inner reality and to outer relationships, and the error is understandable. The outer relationships are serving you well, for you are already storing up many ideas for your work, for your painting, that have at least partially come as a result of your perception of others.

It is in your nature to use much of your energy in artistic creation. You must then turn it outward in this manner. From the wealth of inner data your nature demands that you form new gestalts, and in painting them you automatically relate them outward. You need the inner data and the journeys inward, but these must always be of a disciplined nature, and not overdone.

More energy indeed can be held in the personal subconscious in such a manner than can be used in studying other areas of the inner self, for it is in the personal subconscious that energy blockage most frequently occurs. This does not mean that you should cease in that direction. A smooth and disciplined schedule will serve you well here. I would indeed suggest however that this half-hour schedule not include your weekends.

And now I suggest your break. I am with you however quite strongly this evening.

(*Break at 9:55. Jane was well dissociated. The restlessness was still apparent to her, also. She said she felt at times like getting up and pacing about as she talked, even with her eyes closed.*

(*Actually, I have been painting for the last two weeks, following my final recovery from my illness of late March and early April. This apparently had not been sufficient to satisfy the literal-minded personal subconscious, hence my coldlike symptoms. I have also been investigating with the pendulum to some extent, and can say that usually the periods did not last more than half an hour a day.*

(*Jane resumed in the same manner at 10:06.*)

You should find the above material most helpful.

You have indeed been trying too hard with the pendulum, which sets up its own kind of resistance. At your present stage of development with the pendulum you get a reaction that could be compared to a closed circuit, where the energy is directed into the past, into the personal subconscious too abruptly, and too intensified, and is not yet allowed the release of discovering full causes, which would then release not only that energy, but the energy that has in the past gone into the formation of various physical ills.

At a later time, you see, the difficulty will automatically be passed, there will be a freer flow of energy, and a quicker release of it. Even in your desire to discover such original causes of physical ills, a part of you sets up resistances, new ones, which take additional energy.

The half-hour schedule will allow for a disciplined, smooth and automatic self-discovery which will not drain your energies. You have indeed additional energy at your command, but the focus in the personal subconscious prevents you from using it. You will find that your condition is now improving and will continue to do so. And all of this also involves a practical lesson in the nature of action.

Enough cannot be said along these lines regarding the nature of your expectations, for according to the manner in which you expect your reality to behave, in that manner shall it be.

Out of the goodness of my heart, Joseph, I will bring the session to a close.

("Well, I'm okay."

(I did feel much better, and in any case did not want a short session if we could avoid it.)

Then if you are certain we will continue.

("Alright.")

These incidents in the past, that appear as the original initiation of an illness, they represent points, or kinks, where energy is not smoothly used, but tends to bunch up because of a resistance. Now obviously the particular energy does not bunch up, but a pattern remains in the personality where energy is spent in resistance, and not in efficient action, and not in effective idea constructions.

The ego, for reasons of its own, does not want to accept an action which has already occurred, and does not want to admit it within the framework of its own reality. The point of resistance becomes woven into the personality framework, the problem being not of the subconscious, but again of the ego's denial or attempt to deny a portion of its own reality.

The event is not assimilated. It becomes to all intents and purposes a dead end, isolated from the acceptance of the whole ego, and the most advantageous solution here is, of course, that the ego in one manner or another is made to accept this particular portion of its own past.

We have this evening been somewhat led astray, indeed, ourselves, from the main nature of the subjects at hand. We will however closely examine the nature of action for a brief time further. You have for now a sufficient basis in its characteristics so that we can begin with other discussions, and shortly we will do so.

I will now end the session, or you may take a break as you prefer.

("We'll take a short break then."

(Break at 10:25. Jane was dissociated as usual. She said the restlessness had subsided somewhat, yet still lingered. She resumed in a somewhat louder voice. As she sat back down and closed her eyes, she remained quite motionless and quiet for perhaps two minutes before she began speaking. Resume at 10:39.)

Ruburt should also now find that he begins to recall his dreams once more, and his predictions will also begin to show their validity.

In his case, extra reserves of energy have been used in practical concerns over his book, although to deal with them he has drawn upon additional energies. There is still here a certain holding back, with which we must <u>all</u> contend. Unfortunately the knowledge that his book <u>will</u> be published, while bringing him much satisfaction, has also served to remind him of the manner in which he fears many might look upon both our sessions and his past endeavors in this field.

We are largely over this hump now, and the actual writing of the book in its entirety will actually serve to strengthen his confidence in this respect, since the validity of our sessions will be stressed as he reads material for his book. At its completion he will be much more committed than he is now, and indeed our sessions will attain added depth through his acquiescence.

There will never be on my part any attempt at <u>any</u> sort of invasion. We may indeed take time out shortly, not only to go into our own relationship more thoroughly, but also to discuss other such relationships in general. You should both find such a discussion rewarding. Other aspects of Ruburt's abilities will also let themselves be known within the near future, when he himself lets this come about. His own book will allow him to reassess the nature of our sessions. It will do neither of you harm, and might do you both good, to discuss our sessions personally with some other persons whom you have mentioned.

I will give Ruburt some reinforcements shortly. I will now close our session. We may indeed try a few very simple experiments shortly, simply for a change. My fondest regards to you both. I am emotionally close to you both this evening.

("Good night, Seth.")

(End at 10:55. Jane was well dissociated. She wasn't sure she wanted me to put this down, but she felt that one of Seth's experiments might involve her opening her eyes while she was sitting down in a deep trance—so that <u>Seth</u> might look out of them.)

SESSION 158
MAY 30, 1965 11:06 PM SUNDAY UNSCHEDULED

(Our regularly scheduled session for last Wednesday, May 26, was not held because Jane had developed a heavy cold. The pendulum told her this came about because of her concern over the contract and money matters involving her ESP book. Since then Jane has received her signed contract from the publisher, with money due,

and now feels better.

(Peg and Bill Gallagher visited us sometime before 9 PM this evening. Peg is a reporter for the Elmira Star-Gazette, and will do the news story about the sale of Jane's ESP book. After the conversation had turned to matters psychic, Jane played the tape recording of the Father Trainor episode of last February 11. In Volume 3 see the 131st and 132nd sessions, and the notes on pages 261-63.

(Jane said later that listening to the tape did not "bother" her very much, although she felt some emotional and psychic reaction. On the tape she manifested many voice changes, while reading G. K. Chesterton's narrative poem Lepanto, *that were quite reminiscent of the way the deceased Father Trainor had read it. Afterward Jane endeavored to answer a question of Bill's by reading a few lines from the poem aloud. Because of her cold and her still impaired voice, she thought she could get through a few lines at best.*

(This was her last conscious thought. Immediately the same voice effect again manifested itself in no uncertain terms, and Jane then swept through the long poem without pause. Her voice did not bother her; indeed it became very loud and powerful and dramatic, very vibrant. She remained seated. She held the book in her right hand, and used many gestures with her left hand that were unlike her usual mannerisms. Almost at once it became apparent that the psychic phenomenon taking place, whether or not it involved a medium's contact with Father Trainor, was much superior to the version already on tape.

(Since we had been taken by surprise by this development, we had made no plans to record the reading. I hesitated to interrupt, remembering Seth's comments about the value of spontaneity. Jane's eyes were open, but much darker and more luminous than usual. At times the almost deafening power of her voice, and its emotional content, were indeed thrilling. At the end of the reading Jane closed her eyes; when she opened them again she was out of the trance. She said she was subjectively aware of the gestures she executed with her left hand, yet she felt the hand was not really hers at the time. She felt that it was a fatter hand, belonging to a much heavier arm. Father Trainor, in the photograph we have of him, was a very heavyset man. Bill Gallagher felt that while she was reading Jane spoke with a brogue. Father Trainor was Irish.

(After this our conversation turned to what Seth might say about the origins of Bill Gallagher's ulcer. The ulcer had bothered him all day while Peg and he attended a family gathering. Jane announced that she felt the rapport in our group was favorable, that Seth could hold a session now if we requested it. Not long after this she asked me to get my notebook. The session then began with Jane sitting in the same chair, facing us.

(Her eyes remained closed this time, but she was very active in her delivery,

using many voice effects and gestures—the most active, I think, since she began to deliver material while sitting down and with her eyes closed. Jane said later that the presence of Bill and Peg seemed to give her extra psychic energy somehow; that she felt a greet freedom while giving the session that was most enjoyable. Seth has remarked in the past about the special value and character of unscheduled sessions.

(Jane's voice was rather loud, and it was to become much louder. Seth expressed much amusement at the beginning of the session.)

I give you all here this evening my most sincere regards, and I give greetings like a most enthusiastic host to our visitors.

We will not indeed at this time go into all the circumstances involved in the illness about which we have been questioned at this time. Nevertheless, we do here find a personality who has been, in this life, from an early age, involved in a most complicated network of emotional involvement, concerning both mother and father—and do I speak too quickly for you, Joseph?

("Yes, just a bit.")

(Actually I was writing as fast as I could. Jane smiled broadly and momentarily leaned back in her chair.)

I await as always your pleasure.

("All right.")

Nevertheless these relationships have a cause, basically, in past relationships having to do with other lives in the seventeenth, eighteenth, and fourteenth centuries, when this family was unfortunately involved in other relationships which are even now only working themselves out.

There is much that the personality can do to help his own situation, as indeed we shall see; we also find an involvement here between both families of the man and the woman in past existences, and for this reason a very close psychic framework has been built up here.

The physical condition, having its basis in past relationships, nevertheless can indeed be settled to the personality's satisfaction.

May I here add for our friend Ruburt's satisfaction that the performance of which he was so skeptical, was indeed, despite all his protests, quite legitimate. Now he can stew over that.

(This we take to be a reference to the Father Trainor episode of earlier this evening.)

Without carrying us into a long and lengthy session, it would be impossible for me to go into the complicated relationships involved in the psychic history of the personality whom I will here call Manuk, which is the male as he now sits before me. The solution of the problem is in his hands, and recognition on the part of the ego, which has not assimilated past knowledge, will do much to settle his condition.

I will say this much. There was, I believe, an afternoon in 1940 or 1942, either in a barracks or in a solitary room, which in <u>this</u> life, had something to do with stirring up the present condition. That is, in making it possible for the condition to later show itself.

I will here suggest a brief break, always being considerate of our Ruburt's condition, and if you prefer I will continue for a short time.

("All right.")

(Seth/Jane was most amused.)

I must here express my gratitude indeed that Ruburt deign to allow this unscheduled session, particularly since we missed our own last scheduled one. But I shall not badger him, as I believe indeed he badgers himself enough. I will now take my leave and give you a short break.

<u>I should</u> warn you that I am indeed feeling rather humorous myself this evening, and we have been so besieged with weighty matters that I have not had the opportunity to express myself in the more sociable fashion that I would like. So I take this opportunity to give my greetings to you both, and I will now as promised let you take your break.

(Break at 11:27. Jane was fully dissociated, having no memory of what she had said. Her voice had been strong and varied throughout the delivery; she had smiled much and used many gestures, half of the time sitting on the edge of her chair. At times her voice had boomed out.

(Jane resumed in the same active manner at 11:31.)

There was indeed, also, an incident that occurred when the woman was six years old, having to do with the resulting fear of a feline family.

<u>It</u> had to do with a circumstance. A school was involved, and I believe classmates. The woman's ego will not recall the event at this time, though later it may. Classmates were involved, and a spitting cat that belonged in a house nearby the school.

I want here, Joseph, to make one note for our own benefit, that should be included with our material on the nature of action, if indeed our two visitors will for a moment forgive me. Are you ready?

("Yes.")

Now, involving the performance on Ruburt's part this evening, we have here once more another example of the nature in which action is changed by itself. For indeed, as it was possible for Ruburt to some slight degree to allow her friend to speak, nevertheless the action involved in the whole situation nevertheless changed not only Ruburt, but also necessarily changed her Father Trainor, in that <u>any</u> action of its own nature can never remain the same.

His personality, that is the Father Trainor personality, was of necessity changed by this communication in the same manner that any experience will always change any personality.

An aside here: the incident involving the woman had mainly to do—I suggest here, my esteemed Joseph, that perhaps you watch Ruburt's features. And I would also like to mention the fact that indeed the woman in our gathering, Aniac, does indeed have abilities that are not being used, and possibilities for energy focus which she would do well to explore.

Were it not for the relationships between these two, then indeed the condition of the male would be more critical; and here we come to an interesting point.

Do I speak too fast, Joseph?

("No.")

(*Jane, smiling, leaned forward in her chair, eyes still closed, to question me solicitously. Actually, I was just about managing to keep up with her speed of dictation, but disliked interrupting to ask her to slow down since Seth was obviously in a rare mood—as witness his hopping, almost excitedly, from one topic to another. This manner was far different than our usual quiet, almost sedate sessions. Certainly Seth, or Jane, felt a keen enjoyment.*)

(*Seth had also referred to Peggy Gallagher's undeveloped psychic abilities in the 63rd session. This however is the first session Peg and Bill have witnessed.*)

In a past existence the male in this room, during in fact two existences, was an extremely intelligent female of high standing. The woman was in the last existence a male. The husband in the immediately last existence was also a male, but in two lives previous to that he was a female. A wealthy one in one life.

(*Jane now took one of the few brief pauses of the session.*)

It is true, generally speaking, <u>generally</u> speaking, that those personalities who fear their dependent leanings may develop ulcers. Dependent feelings are quite universal, however, and it is obvious that all human beings do not have ulcers. As far as the particular case is concerned, you will feel well for the rest of the evening.

(*Here, her eyes still closed, Jane pointed at Bill Gallagher. At last break I had poured a glass of milk for him.*)

I will now, because I am such a good host, not bore you with an extended monologue where you find yourselves in the position of not daring to utter a word, so I will give you a break, or I will if you prefer continue.

("We'll take the break.")

(*Jane smiled broadly.*)

For your benefit, my dear Joseph, I am seeing to it that Ruburt is in good condition. Far be it from me to add to his considerable burdens.

(*Break at 11:48. Jane was again well dissociated—"far-out", as she puts it. She had no memory of the material. Bill said his ulcer was, now, not bothering him.*

(*During break the conversation turned to Jane's feelings toward Seth, her ESP book, and related matters. Once again she expressed concern about the public's reception of the material. I thought her attitude at times somewhat ambiguous. Jane made some statements about her reputation resting upon the validity of the material, etc.*

(*When she resumed dictating, she expressed another change of mood. This time she was very grim. Her voice boomed out; the loudness, the determined tone of displeasure persisted. She was again very energetic, gesturing often.*

(*I had been trying to keep an eye on Jane's features, but her speed of dictation kept me too busy for more than an occasional glance. I had noticed nothing striking, certainly, or out of the ordinary, since Seth requested that I watch her. Resume at 12:00.*)

We have had <u>well</u> over a hundred sessions to date, and I have here been once more subjected to the multitudinous and weighty doubts of our stubbornheaded Ruburt.

While indeed <u>I</u> try to understand his ways, nevertheless I find it most difficult to understand on his part these mountains of self-doubt. I am hardly a portion of his personality. <u>Were</u> I a secondary personality of his, I would exhibit those characteristics that are inhibited in his personality, though I must admit I find it difficult to discover where he is inhibited. A less inhibited personality is difficult to find.

You both know, for I have told you time and time again, I am no misty—

(*Now, as if by way of punctuation, Seth/Jane's voice really shouted out:*)

—potbellied Buddha image, nor indeed any manifestation of your conception of a ghostly spirit that drifts in out of the night. It is only your own ignorance, and if you will excuse me, the superstition of the multitudes, that would give you the idea that I am some ghost of a nether world.

If you do not know when you hear them facts that are facts, then it is certainly not because I have not told you.

Are you ready for me?

("Yes.")

(*Once again Seth had been racing along, and I had asked him to wait.*)

I have gone along, you must admit, with extreme good will, and suffered indeed all of Ruburt's most painful and conscientious objections. The fact merely remains that I am who I am, and I am not Ruburt.

Not only that, it is simply a fact that your scientists will indeed discover, and no misty, magical superstition, that consciousness, of itself and because of its nature, forms physical matter. Because I once inhabited physical matter, as you all do now, does not mean that I am now some esoteric, occult creature of dim spiritualistic rather doubtful origins, who manages to invade gullible and neurotic consciousness.

Are you ready?

("Yes.")

I have better use for my time, and Ruburt certainly has better use for his own. From the beginning I was indeed grateful that Ruburt was not—

(Now Seth's voice really boomed out, even louder than before.)

—of a gullible, pseudomystical type of temperament. Nevertheless I cannot help but grow annoyed when I am literally besieged with the protests meant to insist upon his sanity, the point being that if <u>he</u> is sane, then I must be some nefarious seven-eyed monster. He does indeed give acquiescence for these sessions, and I am indeed fond of you both. I have been aware that you do not care, particularly, for the opinion of your fellow men. But our <u>Ruburt</u>, who has <u>never cared</u> for the opinion of his fellow men, now rises up in great worry. What is he afraid of?

Indeed the answer is only too obvious: the great writer fears to be found out; and why? Because the words he speaks are not his own. He knows only too well the importance of these sessions, and I am not afraid of his ego, for even his ego knows.

(Seth/Jane's voice was loud and scathing.)

I will now suggest your break, and I will discuss to some greater degree data concerning your guests. And if I took time out for this discussion, it is indeed because for once I have grown impatient. For much of this on Ruburt's part is indeed pretense—not conscious pretense, but pretense. He knows full well not only the importance of the sessions, personally, but he knows the far-reaching consequences of these sessions, and he is indeed quite <u>able</u> to deal with the consequences.

Tonight's session, Joseph, is a rather important one, and the woman who is attending our session is also quite important, in that her abilities are helping me to come through with, I might say, crystal clarity.

Nor do I here mean to depreciate Ruburt either, for I also am only too aware of those psychological tests which shall be put to us; and it should be obvious to you that in this respect your precious privacy is indeed invaded, and <u>will be</u>. None of you shall regret this night.

I am quite capable of continuing on without a break, but out of the goodness of my heart, Joseph, I will give your fingers a rest. You may take a break. If you and your guests are agreeable I will continue. Or if you are fatigued, you of course may be excused.

(Break at 12:21. Jane was indeed fully dissociated. She was not aware that she had been taking herself to task so vehemently. Her manner had quieted somewhat just before break.

(Bill Gallagher's ulcer was not bothering him. He said he felt fine, and that it was a most welcome situation. I had not observed any change in Jane's features, the few times I had managed to take a look. Bill however remarked that he thought he had detected a change; he thought Jane's lower jaw line had become more rounded, losing a little of its angularity. As it happened Bill could see Jane full-face from his position on the couch. I sat beside him and saw more of the left side of Jane's face, and Peggy from her position was looking at the right side of Jane's face. Peggy also thought she noticed some change.

(In Volume 1, see the 68th session for some material on facial changes in Jane.

(I was quite pleased that in spite of the fast and furious pace of most of the session, my writing hand was holding up remarkably well. I didn't know whether Seth was helping me out or not; he didn't mention it in those terms, and unfortunately I neglected to ask.

(Jane resumed in an active manner again, but with a somewhat quieter voice, at 12:30.)

It is obvious that the ulcers are at this time serving a purpose for the personality. The purpose must be uncovered. It will be beneficial if we give, if you will forgive the term, and if Ruburt will forgive the term, a life reading.

Such a life reading would involve incidents from both past and present lives, including circumstances which, taken all in all, tended to bring about the illness. Such a malfunction is very seldom the result of circumstances that relate to one existence only, but you see they do involve—are you ready?

("Yes."

(Once again I had to ask Seth to slow down.)

—a characteristic method, and an unwholesome one, of satisfying needs, a characteristic method which has been built up through personality patterns that have been adopted through many existences. For example, in one past life you attacked quite forcibly the female physical organs: an ovary with which you had great difficulty.

(Jane had pointed to Bill. Her eyes remained closed.)

We find here a swing between aggressiveness and dependency. In the female existence of which I am speaking, it was the aggressiveness which the personality found distasteful; and in this existence we find the dependency, which you see does not fit in with the personality self-image.

If indeed it is understood that this personality, as with many personalities, has been materialized in feminine form, then these perfectly natural dependent feelings are found to be merely residues from previous personality patterns. And a word here should be said, indeed, concerning the distortive ideas that arise concerning dependency and passivity.

Am I going too fast?

("Just a bit?")

—for we find in all cases that creativity rises first in what you would term passive terms. The aggressive reaction is actually but the termination of a passive creativity. It is your confusion of terms, and the distortive nature of human understanding concerning sexual give-and-take, that makes you think that dependency is weakness. For in many cases dependency is a passivity that leads to creation.

What appears to you as aggression in these terms is merely the tail end, or the <u>apparent</u> manifestation of creation. The male personality then finds himself unable to accept so-called passive subconscious manifestations with ease, this being in part the result of feminine existences.

However, the personality does not seem at this time able to realize that this inhibited passivity is indeed the basis for <u>all</u> resultant aggressive behavior.

I can hardly in one evening undo the distortive errors of a lifetime to date. It would be most advantageous if other sessions were held for the particular purpose of delving into the problem, but this session alone has already prepared the self to know the self, and here the personality will take strides forward. The condition will improve. Of this I am certain.

I myself am in fine fettle. However I realize that I am somewhat freer than you, and I will indeed, my Joseph, end the session at your request.

("All right.")

I am most pleased to meet with you both, and I have no doubt that we shall indeed have other communications in these sessions. There is, Joseph, an importance here that you have not seen, but perhaps at our next session I will make it clear.

My best and heartiest regards to you all. I found this evening's session most enjoyable. My fondest good evenings.

("Good night, Seth."

(End at 12:47 AM. Jane was again fully dissociated. It now took her a few seconds to open her eyes and keep them opened; they flickered several times first. Seth had been by far the most active yet since Jane had begun to speak while sitting down and with her eyes closed.

(We have always thought of the 33rd session as furnishing the most dramatic display of voice changes on Jane's part, both in volume and a lower register. I would

say that tonight's session saw Jane surpass those voice effects as far as sheer power and staying ability went by some little margin; but I do not think her voice dropped as low. Nevertheless it was very vibrant and strong, and Jane now told us she felt no aftereffects, her cold notwithstanding. She said that before the Father Trainor demonstration she had been concerned about her voice being able to give a session tomorrow night, Monday, let alone tonight.

(Bill's ulcer was still not bothering him, and he was still free of symptoms at 1:20 AM when Peggy and he left for home. Bill again mentioned that he thought he saw a change in Jane's features while she was speaking, especially in the jawline and the shape of the face in general. I had noticed nothing. My writing hand felt only a mild fatigue.

(Jane and I talked for a few moments after Peggy and Bill said good night, and I then walked back to the studio to put these notes away. I heard Jane call me out to the living room. When I reached her she was again sitting in the Kennedy rocker; she asked me to get my notebook once again.

(This time I sat at our living room table in my old accustomed place. Jane began to speak from the rocker but had uttered only a few words when she got up and took a chair at the table with me. I saw that her eyes were now open, and very dark and luminous. She was staring right at me. It will be remembered that in the 157th session Jane had mentioned that she felt Seth might try to have her speak with her eyes open soon, and while in a deep trance. In that session also, Jane had felt very restless, perhaps presaging such a change.

(Jane's glasses were off as she looked at me, and she was also smoking. Her voice was very dry and quiet; at the time I thought this was because her cold was finally interfering with her voice, but events will show how wrong I was about this.

(I felt an immediate intimate involvement now that was quite new to me in the sessions. I would say this subjective feeling was enhanced because Jane was not actively pacing about as she used to with her eyes open, but sitting comfortably at table with me. I also knew that she was in a deeper trance. The direct stare of her eyes, very large, very dark, was at times disconcerting. This effect of course was heightened, now, because I began to feel that I noticed a change in her features.

(In trying to be objective, I can say that perhaps the change I became aware of was partly observed, partly subjective. Jane's features were quite animated. Whereas I had not observed any changes in the first half of the session, I now thought her features lost some of their feminine characteristics and became more angular and drawn, as though a masculine presence was making itself seen deliberately. I believe her facial planes appeared to be somewhat older to me. I felt that possibly I was being observed by a masculine personality through the eyes, deliberately. The sense of involvement with a personality other than Jane's usual one, which I know so well, was quite strong. I was, actually, more concerned with trying to decipher <u>what</u> change I was observing, than wondering if there was a change to be seen.

(*Resume at 1:25 AM, once again at a rather fast rate.*)

My dear friend, we have been in the immediate past involved in a low point, involving Ruburt's psychic activity.

It is partially due to characteristic seasonal variations on his part, and it is because this evening happens to represent the upward thrust of his abilities that I am taking advantage of the opportunity involved.

There is much concerning the laws of energy which I have not yet explained to you, and so it is inevitable that our sessions are dependent upon his abilities to utilize energy. He has indeed done very well. But for a while yet we are still dependent upon his utilization of energy.

Indeed I do occasionally, as you saw this evening, badger him, but for his own good; and we are closer this evening than we have been for some time. Closer, in fact, than we have ever been, and I am permitted here with Ruburt's eyes quite open, to sit with you and chat.

There were changes in his features this evening, and I tried to tell you to watch for them, but your notetaking apparently left you little time.

I never want to take too much of his energy, and you are indeed a watchdog in this respect, as is right. Nevertheless, I felt that it was legitimate to take this extra time to speak with you, since there are few occasions when Ruburt's psychic abilities and energies are sufficiently attuned so that we can work together in this manner.

He has realized for a while that it would be possible for me now to speak while we—that is, he and I so cooperated that his eyes were open, and yet his trance was deep, much deeper than in our early sessions, where the exterior circumstances might appear the same.

(*Jane had been staring steadily at me while she spoke, and this in turn impelled me to look at her as often as I could while I wrote. Her posture in the chair was an easy one except when she leaned forward to make a point, yet the feeling I had of another personality being entwined with hers persisted. I was discovering that it took some getting used to.*

(*As she continued speaking, Jane now got up to pick up a pack of cigarettes from the coffee table, then returned to her chair as she lit it.*)

The physical changes in his features were fairly obvious, and I am indeed sorry that you did not perceive their nature. I do not know if you can perceive the difference in the emotional proximity this evening between us now. And if I do badger Ruburt as I did this evening, it is because I too have an emotional reaction in all of this.

There is what amounts at times to a wall that separates us, as far as emotion is concerned, and this is our Ruburt's doing, though of course he does not do it deliberately. Again, the strength and indeed the stubbornness of his ego, made the sessions possible, for without it in the beginning there would have been difficulty in maintaining necessary stability.

When I badger him it is for shock value, for in that way I can get through to him. If I take so much of your time this evening, it is only because I know the effort on your part will result in beneficial aftermaths that will more than repay you for this weighty schedule.

I will take advantage when I can, that is when Ruburt allows me to make contact so well.

You may take a break. If you are not too tired I will continue.

(*Break at 1:39 AM. Jane was well dissociated and did not remember any of the material. Her voice was practically a whisper now. When she stopped dictating her eyes closed, then blinked several times. When she looked at me again she was out of her trance.*

In spite of her whispering voice Jane said she felt all right. My writing hand was beginning to feel tired. The feeling of change in her features and personality had persisted through her delivery. It once again manifested itself when she resumed, still in a quiet voice and with her eyes open again, at 1:49 AM.)

I do not as a rule advocate stretching our schedule in any degree. However this evening, <u>when</u> we find Ruburt's abilities at a high level, it behooves us to take advantage of them.

You need not feel that you must rush, Joseph, for Ruburt, in taking our notes. There is an intimacy in tonight's communications that has been rather unfortunately lacking. This in time will be remedied.

I regret that you must be so involved in your notetaking. This evening's session, all in all, will be most beneficial to Ruburt, and I hope it will be beneficial to you. I must work along the lines of his development. This involves us in many circumstances that are necessary. I cannot get around him as far as his abilities are concerned. I <u>will not</u> push him. We would lose in the long run. The spontaneity of the whole night's adventure, including the Father Trainor episode, was advantageous. He, Ruburt, is basically with me all the way, but he has Jane to contend with.

(*Jane made a humorous gesture toward herself. She was smoking, and now took a sip of wine.*)

I have been with you this evening in a manner which has not been possible lately. We have been involved in variations of the trance state, while at the same time anxious to continue our material, so that the two ventures have been tied into one. It has taken me a while indeed before we could reach this point of more intimate communication.

And your ideas this evening have been most legitimate. We need still now and then a touch of spontaneity in our sessions, now that the routine is assured, and I hope that we will achieve it.

Since we are involving you in such additional work, I will leave it to you to tell me when you are tired. Do you want to take a break?

("No, that's all right."

(Actually I was getting tired. It was one of those situations in which it was easier to keep going, however, than to stop and then start again. My writing hand felt a kind of numb fatigue, and my eyes burned from cigarette smoke; but Seth/Jane, staring at me and smiling from so close by, seemed set and able to go on forever.)

I quail before your quite human limitations, and if I smile it is not indeed within ridicule—

("All right.")

—but in gratitude for your fortitude. However, taking into consideration your willingness, I do suggest a break.

("Okay."

(Break at 2:00 AM. Jane was fully dissociated. She ended the delivery with a broad smile. She said that emotionally she "doesn't know who she is," this evening.

(Through this delivery, as before, I was still markedly aware of a change in her features that I thought probably part physical, part subjective. It was as though the Jane I knew so well had taken a step away from me and allowed another personality to come forward, bringing with it some slight physical change and a much greater psychological change. I was still intrigued that Jane could be in such a deep trance, yet so active and responsive in talking to me. She had no memory of the material.

(During this break, since Jane's voice had again been very low and dry, almost a whisper, I made the unfortunate remark that her heavy smoking this evening was responsible. This brought on her most spectacular voice display of any of the sessions to date, bar none. She began speaking in a voice that was at least as loud as that used in the Father Trainor experiment earlier this evening, and that was loud indeed. Resume at 2:05.)

The hoarseness on Ruburt's part is not because of the endless cigarettes which he has smoked, for I could indeed continue along these lines, and with this voice, as long as I desired.

("All right."

(I was already wincing, thinking of our neighbors on the floor above us, and below too. Earlier in the evening we hadn't minded voice displays, but now I immediately became conscious of the power of Jane's voice. I began to feel embarrassed.)

It was out of due consideration for your sleeping neighbors—

("That's a good idea.")

—that the whisper was involved. Tonight his abilities allow my communications to come through so well! But I could indeed <u>blow apart the rooftops, in theory, if I so chose.</u>

(To my genuine amazement, Jane's voice became even more powerful. This was an escalation in volume that was based on strength, sheer power. There was no hint of strain involved as she produced this blast. I would not have been at all surprised to feel the ceiling vibrate over my head as she spoke the last sentence above.

(Jane laughed as she finished the sentence. She stared intently at me as though daring me to ask her to be quieter. Her voice now surpassed by a good deal the Father Trainor experiment. It was not a deeper voice particularly.)

This has nothing to do with Ruburt's distasteful habit of smoking cigarettes—

("Don't you wish he'd quit smoking?")

—but if you are looking for voice changes—

("Oh, no.")

—I could indeed give them to you so that there would be no doubt as to the origin of the voice involved. I could indeed, if I <u>were</u> so inclined, give you voice changes that would have the neighbors down upon your shoulders—

("You're doing pretty well right now."

(The strange thing here was that by now even I realized that Seth could do just what he said he could, that he still had not hit the top of his, or Jane's, ability to produce a really stunning effect. I have no real way of measuring the magnitude of what I was hearing, beyond stating that it enveloped me completely. I not only felt that everyone in the apartment house could hear the voice, but that it was audible on the street. I am still surprised that no one banged on our door and asked for quiet.

(Now, also, the voice had dropped somewhat in register. Jane grinned and leaned toward me.)

Do you require a trifle more? I am quite prepared to deliver. It is because Ruburt's own voice is so unmelodious with his cold that any effects of that nature—

(Now Jane gave a great shout.)

—which you will receive this evening will be revealing!

I would suggest because of the lateness of the hour, however, that you do not this evening request such signs.

("Oh."

(And, magically, Jane's voice dropped to its previous near whisper. By contrast this in itself was almost deafening.)

May I then return to our more conventional whisper?

("Yes."

(Since Seth was obviously having such a good time needling me, I very nearly yielded to temptation and told him to pull out all the stops as far as voice effects went. I was curious to see what he could really do, through Jane. But I didn't have the nerve, considering the hour and other people.)

There is an emotional action, Joseph, in this session that is important; for our sessions deal with many layers, and I regret that this one layer is at most times neglected. I am endeavoring to give this evening's session an emotional gestalt that will be an experience in itself, and in itself a lesson.

You may if you prefer cut tomorrow's session for this one, but I would suggest that you continue with the session as long as you can, for the benefits will more than make up for your discomfort.

Ruburt presently feels no discomfort. He may be slightly tired tomorrow, but that is all. The emotional rapport built up between us will reinforce our sessions in general, and you know how important this can be. I must still work within the realm of his energies, and I do not even now believe that you realize how much more effectively he is using those energies, nor what strains our sessions have put upon his ego, which he has managed to triumph over.

You may take a break. I feel on the one hand that I am overstaying my welcome. On the other hand I know too well that this session will be more than worth your while. I suggest however that you take a break.

(Break at 2:18. Jane was again well dissociated, although she realized her voice had been sounding out. Her eyes closed briefly at the end of the delivery, and when they opened she was out of her trance. In being so preoccupied with noting the great voice effects, I had been, I realized, less observant of the facial changes I had been aware of earlier; but there had been no doubt of the emotional interchange.

(Although I was tiring I was ready to go along with Seth's request to keep going. I thought Jane looked good. She appeared to feel no fatigue particularly, and was greatly interested in questioning me about what I had seen and heard.

(My feelings of relief at the quieter voice were almost premature. Seth couldn't resist a few more blasts when Jane resumed, and these are indicated. These bits were loud, but didn't quite hit the previous peak. They always were accompanied by a smile and an implied dare that I egg him on. I didn't. Resume at 2:25.)

We will now close, or begin to close our session.

You do well, Joseph, to watch out for Ruburt as you do. He does however allow himself freedoms, as this evening, and on other occasions which are most beneficial.

There will be other evenings like *(louder, to soon quiet down)* this evening, and there will be other demonstrations that will be of quite legitimate purpose. For on all occasions we find a desire for proofs and for signs, and <u>although</u> I find such desires on the one hand childish, on the other hand I find myself realizing that there is to some extent a legitimate claim, particularly on Ruburt's part, considering the limitations of the human egotistical nature.

I can indeed feel you quail at the volume of my voice *(louder again)*, considering the ungodly hour *(louder yet, really loud, blasting out with a smile, to soon quiet again)*, and so I will lower it. But I would like it understood that now, if I so chose, there would be no doubt *(louder, very loud)* as to my identity *(and now also deeper)* or my abilities.

(And I thought that if Seth really showed what he could do, cars would probably stop in the street outside; seriously.)

With Ruburt's consent however, and I have it, I could make such a blast of masculine voice that you would indeed be embarrassed when the neighbors complained *(louder)*. It is to show my humorous consideration for your feelings that I do not so indulge *(louder)*.

Therefore, though I sincerely regret, and with deep sympathy for your desires, I will here close our session—but only because I so sympathize with the lamentable weakness of your fingers. I have not been able to come through personally so well in quite a while; and if our situations were reversed I would not shut you off.

("Oh yeah?")

I will therefore leave it to you as to when our session will conclude. I have Ruburt, for once, cooperating to a laudable degree; and there is much, seriously, that I can say along these lines. In any case I will not be responsible for five fingers lying weakly on the table, broken and disjointed because I have so misused them. If I were you—

("Yes?")

—I would be thankful to have them available.

("I am.")

It is this impossibility of speaking in normal tones, in normal conversation with you, and indeed with Ruburt, that does annoy me at times. If you knew of our histories in detail, it would not surprise you, and there would be much more that you would understand.

You may now as your prefer, and of course irregardless of my feelings, end the session or take a break.

("I'm ready to quit, I guess, sorry to say."

(I said this in spite of Seth/Jane's exaggerated display of self-commiseration. I half-expected another voice blast, but it did not materialize.)

You blackmail me with your human limitations. Why do you not utilize your recorder to a greater degree, particularly for such unscheduled sessions?

("We got out of the habit."

(Actually time plays an important role here. To type up notes from a recording means I have to spend as much time, <u>again</u>, listening to a session. This expenditure is then increased each time I have to stop and rerun a section to pick up a missed word, or because the dialogue simply runs so rapidly, etc.

(I thought of recording this evening's session earlier, as stated, but did not do so in the interests of spontaneity, a quality to which Seth attaches great value. To be ready to record an unscheduled session we would have to have the recorder set up and ready to go at a flick of a switch, constantly. To date our unscheduled sessions haven't been that frequent by far, and there are actually few unusual effects to be noted.)

You still have simply no idea, Joseph, of the benefits that <u>you</u> and Ruburt receive through such communications. And unscheduled sessions are apt to be more important at times, in certain ways, than other sessions.

My energy, unfortunately from your viewpoint, is comparatively endless.

("Yes.")

(Seth/Jane made this statement with a grin.)

Perhaps if you continue I will take care of your precious fingers. In any case, come to a halt.

(Break at 2:45. Jane was well dissociated, and remembered none of the material. Her eyes closed, then opened again as usual.

(My writing hand was tired, but since I had decided I could go on if necessary, I said nothing more about ending the session.

(Jane's voice had been quiet for some time now, and it remained so as she resumed at 2:46, again with her eyes open.)

I will indeed close, but you will find that the benefits of this session are more long-lasting than either of you can now suppose.

I would not, Joseph, take advantage, either of the hour, which is later, nor of you, nor Ruburt's willingness this evening, if I did not know that the action so involved would more than repay you. And the emotional qualities that we have achieved are also more important than you know.

("Good night, Seth.")

(End at 2:48 AM. Jane was dissociated as usual. Again she closed her eyes briefly to bring herself out of the trance. Her eyes had been very dark and luminous all evening.

(And even now, at the end of the session, I had been still strongly aware of something different about her, of a strong emotional involvement and immediacy. Her voice, her mannerisms in speaking, the steady way she stared at me, all contributed

to this feeling.

(And once again, let it be noted that Jane suffered no aftereffects of any kind from this long session. Her cold was not affected either for better or worse. She had no voice fatigue. The next day she was not tired, etc.

(It can also be noted that in the second half of the session Seth made no reference to my watching out for physical changes in Jane, as he had when Peggy and Bill Gallagher had been present. Bill and Peggy had seen changes. I observed my own set of changes later. It is my thought, at least at the moment, that Bill's observations and my own would not coincide. This may be explained later.)

SESSION 159
JUNE 2, 1965 9 PM WEDNESDAY AS SCHEDULED

(Due to the very long unscheduled session of last Sunday, May 30, our regularly scheduled session for the next day, Monday, May 31, was not held. This was more to save me work in finishing up notes than because of any tiredness on Jane's part. She had no ill effects from the session.

(Jane has been back on a regular schedule of psychological time now for a while, on the restricted twenty-minute schedule set by Seth. She experiments just before noon. She usually achieves what she calls an excellent state, and this is as far as the experiments have carried her.

(Jane's cold still lingered to a lesser degree. She was coughing, but made no mention of not wanting to hold a session. Her cold had been worse when she held last Sunday's long unscheduled session.

(Jane had no idea of the material for the session beforehand. For variety's sake she wanted to hold the session in our living room again, as we used to do regularly. I was somewhat concerned about interruptions but as it developed there were none.

(Jane spoke while seated in the Kennedy rocker, and with her eyes closed for this first delivery. Her voice was rather quiet, although easily heard above the traffic noise. She coughed briefly occasionally, and used pauses that were not very lengthy. She opened the session with a smile.)

Good evening.

("Good evening, Seth.")

I was not certain, after our last so-lengthy session, that I would be greeted with open arms this evening.

I know that indeed our last session so involved you, Joseph, in lengthy notetaking, and typing chores. I do regret the amount of such work that is necessary. In the last section of our previous session in particular, I attempted to make a more direct emotional communication, and to some extent succeeded.

We also of course experimented to some degree with Ruburt's state. He carried on for me very well, and his abilities have once more shown a good degree of advancement. I tried again to speak with you on a much less formal basis. To some extent there must always be some barriers here, but we can with practice overcome many.

There is a certain knack necessary on Ruburt's part, a difference in the way in which energy is used, a variation of <u>method</u> between sessions in which rather objective material is presented, and in those sessions where we attempt to make a more personal type of contact.

The guests of the other evening were most advantageous, their attitudes objective; not gullible people, nor on the other hand were they the type who will not admit the results of their own experience. The woman has a large store of energy which she is using with above-average efficiency, but she <u>also</u> has abilities which are not being used.

The man is using his own energies less effectively, since so much of them are being consumed in nervousness. He has not learned to conserve his energies, but to use them at <u>all</u> it seems that he must allow them almost to explode, so that there is little reserve. This is unfortunate, but can be corrected.

Both of these personalities however are basically constructive, creative, and a relationship between the four of you should work out very well, not only on a short-term, but on a long-term basis, with advantages for all.

The ulcer problem can indeed be solved by the personality himself. An attempt however should not be adopted by the personality, if possible, on an intense or desperate level. This, or any such too-intense effort will tend to make additional drains upon needed energy.

The ulcer simply can be cured, but this will involve on the part of the personality a disciplined program of self-understanding. Certainly such a program will be worthwhile. We do not want, for example, the personality to <u>plunge into</u> a solution. Instead what is advisable is a gradual but definite program that will result in a legitimate and a long-lasting cure.

I will suggest a brief break, and with your consent we will speak a while longer on this particular matter.

(*Break at 9:21. Jane was dissociated more than usual for a first delivery. She said she felt like opening her eyes a couple of times, or rather that Seth did. Her voice was rather dry and hoarse at times but was not strained, and became no worse during the session. She did not appear tired.*

(*I was a little tired, however, from the extensive typing involved from the last session, and reminded Jane that some of her comments regarding this were not good suggestions. She agreed. She had lit a cigarette during break, and now when she resumed speaking she held the cigarette in a hand. I thought this meant she might be getting ready to open her eyes while delivering material. But she resumed with her eyes closed, in the same quiet dry voice, at 9:27.)*

Now indeed we will overcome our Ruburt's poor suggestions.

There are many aspects of our sessions, some that we have developed well, others that we have only begun to develop, and others that are yet to be developed.

All of them will be important, and all of them will serve to add dimension to the reality which the sessions involve. This could indeed be thought of in terms of value fulfillment. The sessions also will be helped in general by variety, always of course within our framework.

(Jane now smiled again, then opened her eyes. They were again dark and luminous as she looked at me. This however was not the intent stare of the last session, but a more conversational and quiet one.)

I will help you and your poor fingers when it seems advisable. You yourself are learning to substitute good suggestions for bad ones, and it will help you further to keep this in mind.

I did indeed wish to experiment, though not on a spectacular basis, along the lines that we are using this evening. I now and then enjoy sitting at a comfortable table with you, with *his* eyes open, and it is good training for Ruburt.

I intend to speak more concerning your friend, we can initiate a program for him. It will perhaps seem like a conservative program, and he will do all of the work.

We may not expand this program this evening. When we do he will see that only good can come from it. It will not involve medicines or drugs. It will involve perhaps more than anything else the task of slowly changing the focus of his attention and energies, of turning energies that are being used in a self-destructive manner into constructive channels.

This is the main problem. The reason that these energies are being used against the self must and will be uncovered. I will also have, if I am asked, suggestions for the woman in their relationship, that will be most beneficial. I mentioned that the reason for the difficulty had been built up.

(Jane, now, looked at me but occasionally. Her voice remained quiet. She used pauses less often and they were short ones. She spoke while looking casually ahead for the most part, and performed such ordinary chores as putting out her cigarette, sipping from a glass of wine, sometimes rocking back and forth, etc.)

The personality in the past, in past existences that is, had a history of hitting out at the organs of the various physical bodies that were its home, as other personalities sometimes have histories that include turning destructiveness outward against others. Such tendencies again are of long standing, and adopted for various reasons having to do with characteristics of the underlying personality.

These cannot be recounted, again, in one evening; nor would such a performance serve any purpose at this time; listed, so to speak. There are considerations that connect them that must be discussed, if any good will be done. The need for the ulcer was aggravated in the fairly recent past, but the personality is basically flexible enough so that adjustments can be made.

There will also be suggestions given as to needed adjustments on the part of the personality during his business hours. In other words, there are small but important adjustments that can be made within the framework of his present working life. Also perhaps an adjustment here on the woman's part that will aid him.

I am going into this because the problem has obviously become an organic one. As a beginning I would suggest that your friend read our material concerning the formation of physical matter in general, the formation of the physical image, and the physical organs. If he can see that he is indeed responsible for the condition of his physical body in the most practical manner possible, then it will be much easier for him to picture his own cure.

I will now suggest your own break.

(Break at 9:50. Jane was well dissociated. She blinked several times without closing her eyes for any length of time, then she was out of her trance.

(It remained a quiet and easy session even when Jane's eyes remained opened. In a slightly louder voice, she resumed at 9:55.)

I am not going to hold a long session, feeling that I have indeed taken much of your time already this week.

I am going to take this instance of your friend's illness however to make a few points of my own, some that may not be too well received. A cure of any kind will never depend upon any given treatment. <u>It will in all cases depend upon the belief on the part of the sufferer that he can be cured</u>. It will depend upon his desire to be cured. It will depend upon the <u>strength</u> of the purpose that an illness serves. It will depend upon, in the last analysis, <u>the individual's own ability</u> to mobilize his own energies, <u>for only these will effect a cure</u>.

<u>Any</u> physician of any kind can only help a sufferer mobilize these energies and direct them. A sufferer has adopted an illness into his own self-image, through suggestion, which to a large degree he himself has given. He has caused the illness, whether it be organic or otherwise, <u>and only suggestion</u> will rid him of it.

It is indeed quite time for us to discuss the true nature and reality of what is so loosely called suggestion. We have indeed spoken much concerning the focus of energy, and a sufferer is truly entranced with the idea of his illness, and it is only this which basically allows the illness to continue. He focuses upon it both consciously and unconsciously.

An illness is a failure to solve a mental or psychological problem in the correct manner. As long as the illness continues the problem remains unsolved, and a vicious circle is maintained because of this unwholesome balance. The sufferer focuses upon the illness, therefore avoiding his task of functioning upon the problem.

The energy that would be used to solve the problem instead is spent maintaining the illness. It is therefore necessary that an attempt be made as soon as possible to solve the problem, which of course must first be discovered by the ego, which has avoided it.

This first attempt to discover the problem, automatically and because of its nature, immediately aids the sufferer in changing the focus of his attention away from the symptom, which he has himself formed, and already the symptom is weaker.

The trouble with many health programs for recovery is that they cause the sufferer to focus upon his illness more than ever. The unsolved problem is therefore pushed further away. Our program for your friend will almost immediately include a brief but effective suggestion that should be given before sleep, and at various times during the day.

We ourselves will be concerned for a while with the nature of suggestion in its relationship to action. It should be most beneficial material, practically speaking, and will also add to your knowledge and carry our discussions toward certain directions that I have in mind.

If I am, myself, subdued this evening in contrast with my activities in our last session, it is only because I would give you both a needed rest. I particularly enjoyed the session myself. I will now give you a break. I will end the session if you prefer, or I will continue.

("We'll take a short break then."

(Break at 10:15. Jane was again well dissociated. She said that when speaking with her eyes open she is not as sharply aware of the transition from a trance state to a nontrance state. Now, she felt as though she could quite easily slip back into a trance, although she did not feel Seth.

(Jane resumed with her eyes open, in an average voice and at a faster rate, at 10:20.)

So-called suggestion causes not only sickness but health.

The term itself is a very poor one. We will go much more deeply into this as the whole discussion continues. Needless to say, suggestion operates as strongly and as realistically and as practically within an atom, or a toad, or a leaf, as it does in man.

Our material concerning the construction of the physical universe and of physical matter in general may now, perhaps, give you an idea of how important suggestion is. Also consider our material on expectation, for indeed expectation comes closer, as a term, than does suggestion.

Our focus of energy is vital, both yours and mine. Expectation to a large extent determines the manner in which we will use this energy, and the types of constructions that will be formed. Your friend's ulcer for example <u>is</u> his problem in its entirety, constructed into the physical matter of his own organism.

This is to be taken literally.

The problem, as a mental manipulation, has not been settled. The resulting construction, therefore, is a faithful replica of this distortion.

(Jane's eyes now closed. She continued speaking without interruption, and her eyes remained closed for the balance of the session.)

In some types of illnesses such distortions are mirrored or reflected, so to speak, many times within one organism. We will have much more to say along these lines.

I will indeed now close our session. For Ruburt's benefit, may I here add that in my remarks of our last session, I was speaking of our sessions only, and did not mean to take credit for any of Ruburt's own creative work. I am saying this in gentle tones, to avoid upsetting him further.

(Jane spoke with a smile.)

Again, my heartiest and most fond wishes to you both. Ruburt incidentally would do well to be even more aware than usual, since he is at a peak now of psychic activity.

Your painting will now spur you on.

("Good night, Seth.")

(End at 10:32. Jane was dissociated as usual. She did not realize that she had closed her eyes before the end of the session. My writing hand felt little fatigue.)

SESSION 160
JUNE 7, 1965 9 PM MONDAY AS SCHEDULED

(Again we held the session in our living room, as we used to do. There were no interruptions. Jane had no idea of the material for the session before she began speaking, on time. She sat down as usual, with her eyes closed for this first delivery. There

was quite a bit of traffic noise even at this hour, and Jane's voice had a stronger edge, as though to cut through it.)

Good evening.

("Good evening, Seth.")

I would like to make a few remarks concerning such spontaneous sessions as we have had, and particularly concerning our last spontaneous and witnessed session.

In the past we have held few such spontaneous sessions. When Ruburt's condition is such that a particularly good trance can be achieved, and when the emotional climate surrounding you is advantageous, then we can do much.

It is advantageous to take our opportunity when <u>possible</u> at such times. I have been strict concerning our schedule, since conditioning must be set up, and while we always allowed for some spontaneity, it was necessary that Ruburt develop greater efficiency in his handling of the trance state.

There are obviously many occasions when his condition is unusually suited to hold a spontaneous session, but when the emotional climate is not for one reason or another correct, or when other elements, practical ones to you, may prevent a session.

As a general rule a spontaneous session will be an excellent one. It goes without saying however that discretion must be used, and I will not come through without your consent. The consent however on your parts may be conscious or unconscious. If however you consciously do not want a session, and express yourselves in this direction, then no session would be held.

When no conscious decision has been made, I would be following your subconscious wishes in such a manner.

Now, to return to an earlier discussion. What you call suggestion is indeed expectation. You should understand by now how the physical image is constructed. This construction is from the inside out. The inner self attempts to construct a physical image in line with its own self-image. Any errors of construction have their origin not in the inner self, but in either the personal subconscious or in the ego.

(The traffic noise was now even heavier. I thought it was bothering Jane, since she seemed to be sitting in a rather tense position in her rocker. Her voice grew a little louder.)

As errors and mistakes creep into the physical organic system, bringing forth mutant genes and distortions, so also these mutant genes and distortions are, on a smaller scale, the result of inner distortions within the consciousness of the individual genes.

The same sort of distortion occurs on another scale, in the duplication of any given illness or destructive organic or gross misfunctions. What you call suggestion should ideally come from within the self, and not from outside the self.

I suggest your first break.

(Break at 9:16. Jane was dissociated, but not as well as usual for a first break. She said the traffic noise bothered her, but that she would make an effort to see that it didn't continue to do so.

(Jane's eyes had remained closed for the first delivery, but they opened soon after she began speaking again. She was also smoking. As during the last session she looked at me occasionally, but for the most part looked casually ahead without staring fixedly at anything. Her eyes were dark, her voice a little heavier and louder. Resume at 9:22.)

I can indeed arrange our evening in such a manner that your traffic will bother us not a bit.

When we have gone into the nature of action still much more thoroughly, then you will be able to use such knowledge for quite practical purposes, and to your advantage. For as you know, you do not perceive <u>all</u> aspects of action by any means, and it can indeed to some extent be up to you to <u>choose</u> those aspects of action with which you will be concerned, and those which you would ignore.

This in no manner affects the nature of those actions which you ignore. However, to all intents and purposes it changes action in so far as <u>you</u> are concerned with it. This would therefore imply a choice on your part, in a manner that you do not now enjoy. For you can then choose to perceive advantageous action, as well as you can choose not to perceive action which for any reason or another you choose to ignore.

This obviously implies powers of discipline and discretion. The <u>ability</u> therefore will not come until you can handle it.

Suggestion would of course play a part in the development of these abilities. It is difficult, even though we are so far into our sessions, to give you any full understanding yet of what is involved in the basic nature of suggestion, but as we go deeper into the subject there will be experiments that you both can try.

I have often mentioned that the divisions in our subject matter are <u>often arbitrary</u>, and for practical purposes of discussion only. The word suggestion is in itself so bound in your minds with other matters that even I find it difficult not to let the subject matter become suggestive of matters that do not really belong under discussion.

(Jane leaned forward to tap on the table for emphasis. She smiled. She now acted as though immune to the traffic noise, and I realized that at times I too had

forgotten about it as I wrote along.)

You think for example in terms of good and bad suggestions, and I have on occasion used the terms myself, in order to make a point clear. However what you call suggestion, left alone, is a part of the inner impetus of action, which is translated in all areas of consciousness outward.

What <u>interrupts</u> this inner impetus could be compared to what you call poor suggestion. It is indeed distortive. It represents a blocking of impetus. It interrupts what should be a simultaneous and <u>easy</u> flow of inner impetus outward, in your case outward to physical construction. The particular negative words spoken or thought are but indications of this break of impetus. The break occurs first, and it is for this reason that what you call negative suggestions therefore are acted upon.

The negative suggestions therefore are symptoms of an inner block of energy and impetus. They represent a rift that has already occurred. It is rather important that I make this point clear. It goes without saying that these which you call negative suggestions are in themselves actions. They represent however dead eddies, the motion that means nothing in dead waters. They are impeding actions.

Many, many occasions arise when action could be so impeded, and is not.

(Now Jane's eyes opened briefly. She looked at me, then closed them. Her eyes had been closed for the last few paragraphs.)

What you call a negative suggestion is never acted upon unless the <u>inner</u> block of energies has <u>already</u> occurred. Suggestion, as I understand it, is the culmination of the inner voice that urges action into ever more diverse and creative patterns.

We will have much to say concerning impediments; and impediments, incidentally, are what you call negative suggestions. And yet remember that these impediments are themselves action.

I now suggest your break.

(Break at 9:45. Jane blinked a few times, then came out of her trance. She said she had been a good deal more dissociated for this delivery. She had not been conscious of traffic, nor had I.

(When Jane resumed dictating her eyes remained open. She was smoking. Again, her glances at me were casual. She had used pauses before this break, but now she spoke quite a bit more rapidly. Resume at 9:50.)

What you choose to call suggestion operates unceasingly within all aspects of action.

It is this that allows the body its physical manifestation. It is this that allows for all change. It can be called on one level instinct, on other levels it is much more. When it operates at its most efficient level suggestion is indeed the inner affirmation. Without the ego we do not <u>have</u> what you call negative suggestions, for when action is left to itself it flows unimpeded, seeking its fulfillment along its numberless unimpeded ways.

Your own experiments in psychological time have allowed you, to some extent, to experience within yourselves such unimpeded action. You know now that the ego, because of its nature, attempts to set itself aside from action. It obviously cannot do so. The ego, being part of action, nevertheless affects the nature of action as seen in the various manifestations of the whole self.

The personal subconscious can be thought of as a threshold between the ego and the inner self; not only can glimmerings of the inner self be glimpsed through the subconscious, but also the diverse characteristics of the ego touch this personal subconscious. When the ego, therefore, becomes too overbearing it attempts to impede the flow of action. It <u>cannot</u> so impede action directly, for the very act of forming such impediments involves action. Nevertheless such impediments often set up actions that block the overall movement or direction of the action that composes the whole personality.

The delicate inner mechanisms by which inner reality should be constructed into physical reality therefore become seriously affected. Distortions occur almost like mutant mental genes, which are then faithfully and duly reproduced.

What you call negative suggestions represent discordant actions. Unless the main reasons are discovered, the distortive actions will keep reoccurring. In many cases quite a simple exercise will almost immediately begin to make an improvement. With these exercises you are familiar, for in your psychological time the self is momentarily in connection with its more extensive portions.

A clear and undiverted and unbroken electrical circuit and connection is hereby made. Growth within the physical system is the result of suggestion. Without it there would be no growth. You will see here that we are beginning our discussion in the simplest of terms, and we will lead further so that eventually suggestion can be understood for what it is.

It goes without saying that each newborn consciousness within your system carries within it the capsule comprehension of which I have previously spoken; and if you recall, each atom and molecule, each and every smallest particle that can by any stretch of the imagination be called physical matter, contains within it its own independent capsule comprehension—inherent suggestions in coded form, in not one but several codes, that give complete instructions for development and growth.

If your fingers tire you may take a break, and we will continue.

(*Break at 10:11. Jane was well dissociated throughout the delivery. Her eyes had been open all the while, but she had no memory of this. Traffic had not bothered her, and her delivery had been rather fast.*

(She resumed with her eyes again open and very large and dark, in a normal voice and with a few pauses, at 10:22.)

There are translations of <u>intent</u> constantly made.

The innate comprehension of which we have spoken is a basic portion of all atoms and molecules, about which the physical matter is formed, and without which the formation of physical matter would be impossible.

You recall, I am sure, the material concerning the gestalt of the physical body. Here suggestion constantly plays its part in the formation of the tissues, and in all other such areas of development and growth. There are various manners in which these inner suggestions are translated from inner pure energy form into the electrical and chemical systems which compose the physical organisms, and it is possible for errors of translation to occur along these lines.

Recall here also the cooperation that exists between the smallest particles and the cells and organs. Each molecule has its own self-image, without which it could not exist as a physical construction. The subconscious has its own self-image, the ego has its own self-image. When action is allowed to flow unimpeded, the cooperation that is necessary to maintain the efficiency of the gestalt is maintained. It is most frequently the error of the ego, who upon many occasions attempts to deny its dependency upon this cooperation, that sets up impediments, and sets up countersuggestions that <u>can</u> be somewhat considered cancerous, in that if it had its way the ego would envelop all other aspects of the whole organism, and run riot.

It will refuse to assimilate certain experiences. This very refusal is in itself an action. It will attempt to construct itself on a physical level, since it is within the physical system of reality. The cooperation is broken down to some greater or lesser degree. This conflicts with the inner data in the case of illnesses, and the illnesses are actually the result of conflicts of data. It is obvious that the body is equipped to handle many such distorted actions, but a conflict is hereby brought into play, where constructive energies or actions are not given full reign, and patterns of distortions are set up within the system.

If they cannot be overwhelmed they are assimilated, and faithfully reproduced. There are methods whereby you can indeed help your own system, and to a large measure determine the constructive nature of action as it operates within the system, and protect the organism from such distortions before they occur.

I will give you instructions along these lines. Ruburt's habit of requesting before he sleeps that his system effortlessly continue its healthful and natural cooperation is a good one. But this is, while helpful, only a very basic and beginning aid.

This whole subject is much more complicated than you may at first suppose.

Until we had discussed action to some degree, a discussion on suggestion would have meant little to you. We will continue along these lines for some time, even while the subject leads us into others.

Since suggestion is used constantly, and by every cell in your body, then it is not a question of whether or not you <u>can</u> use suggestion, but of how to use it more effectively. And this will involve a balanced personality, for in such a personality action will be allowed freedom of expression. The ego will gain and not lose in the process, but we will not have an autocratic and willful ego, but a reasonable and even disciplined ego that is aware of its position, aware of its own dependency, as well as of its own peculiar and unique perceptive apartness. For the apartness is dependent upon its being a part of the whole gestalt.

Are you fingers tired?

("No.")

We find it most frequently that the ego impedes action by refusals. It attempts to maintain a stability that is indeed illusion. The emotions, as you know, are action. When they are <u>allowed</u> their mobility, then they free the personality from resistances. They actually allow for great stability, since their free expression makes it possible for action to be fulfilled in the manner most constructive for the system as a whole.

When the ego impedes such expression, <u>then</u> the emotions are translated into other actions, and can turn into impediments. It is only because the ego blocks freedom of the emotional expression, out of fear, that it <u>appears</u> to the ego that emotions are indeed fearful characteristics. Dammed up, they are indeed.

It is, again, the ego's misguided attempt to stand apart to gain stability, that makes the ego react in such a manner. It fears loss of control and of discipline. But <u>all</u> appearances to the contrary, the emotions are natural controlling devices that in themselves aid discipline, since they allow for the spontaneous flow of energies outward. It is only when they are denied that they become explosive or dangerous to the personality. Then indeed they result in explosive barrages, ranting and shouting, organic and psychological illnesses, and of unfortunate manifestations.

I believe that I have kept you long enough for one evening, and I will here close our session. My fondest regards to you both, and until you master some of the rules for recognizing or ignoring certain portions of action, you can always stuff your ears with cotton.

My frisky friend Joseph, I will now, with due regret, say good evening until our next session.

("Good night, Seth.")

(End at 10:55. Jane was well dissociated. She blinked, then was out of her trance. Her eyes had been open for the whole delivery, and very dark. Her rate of speaking had been rather fast. She had not been aware of traffic, or any other distractions for that matter, since the first delivery of the evening.)

(Sunday night, June 6, I had a vivid dream which was clairvoyant, and came to pass the next morning while I was at work. Complete records are in my dream notebook. Before the session I made sure to hope aloud that Seth would discuss the dream, but as can be seen it was not even mentioned. This is not an unusual happening, however. I may ask definitely about the dream during a future session.)

SESSION 161
JUNE 9, 1965 9 PM WEDNESDAY AS SCHEDULED

(For the record: On June 1, 1965 I mailed to Dr. G. H. Instream a letter explaining something of Jane's ability and the Seth material, plus a list of the inner senses, a list of the basic laws of the universe, and copies of sessions 138, 141, 142, 149, 153 and 154. The letter was sent c/o Colgate University, Hamilton NY.

(On June 8, we received an answer from Dr. Instream, expressing interest, and inviting us to a symposium at State University College, Oswego, NY. Publicity material on the symposium wasn't enclosed with the letter as stated, so on June 9 we wrote asking for this.

(Jane and I wondered whether Seth would mention the letter from Dr. Instream during this session, but he did not; just as he did not discuss my recent clairvoyant dream. See above, this page. As it happened Bill and Peggy Gallagher, who witnessed the first part of the 158th session, were again witnesses.

(Because of the witnesses the session was held in our living room. Again traffic noise was quite audible, yet it did not bother any of us unduly, as it had during the last session. Jane began speaking while sitting down and with her eyes closed, in a voice a little stronger than usual, and at a fairly fast rate. Her manner was quite expressive and she used many gestures.)

I now bid you a most fond good evening.

("Good evening, Seth.")

I see that we have visitors, and I also bid them welcome.

We will not this evening give a broad outline to our friend, concerning his health. We are indeed, instead, going to progress in a very slow manner, and give him tidbits. If we outline a whole program, then he will plunge into it, and we will have him go more slowly. For the problem already has to do with the fact that he plunges into both dilemmas and solutions, with a desperation that is born from anxiety, if not pure panic.

Nor will anything be gained by a patent and speedy program that is not solidly based on understanding, both understanding of the self in particular, and what you may call the mechanics involved in the creation of the illness itself, and in an understanding of those elements which caused the personality to develop the illness.

Nor do we want to rid him of one illness so quickly that he still feels a need for it, for in such a case he would indeed very promptly develop another. So, though he would wish that we go quickly, we shall go slowly, for the nature of his own reactions causes in some degree the necessity for the illness.

We have in the past discussed in full the manner in which physical matter is formed. We have also discussed the ego, and our friend would do well to read the sessions dealing with the ego, and the ego's relationship to action. For one of the basic reasons for the difficulty lies in the fact that the ego of the present personality does strongly attempt to stand apart from action. It attempts to <u>force</u> action, and to fight action which it does not initiate.

Here we have a blockage. The personality, the present ego, will not acquiesce to action, will not go along with it as part of it, but attempts to force it along its own directions. This will become clearer when passages concerning action and the ego are read.

There is an involvement that would seem, <u>would seem</u>, intense. The ego appears to be extremely intense, but to a large degree this is a deception, for the intenseness is caused by the attempt of the ego <u>not to become involved with action, unless the ego can dominate action</u>. There is no basic trust of the inner self. The personality does not basically recognize or trust the ability of the inner self, and this results in an intense inhibited fear.

The ego of the personality does not trust its own inner organisms. It must attempt to stand apart from them, and keep an eye on them. The ego does not believe that they are treating it right. The ego is therefore in its present circumstances because it fears itself so solitary, since it has to a large degree cut itself off from its inner self; yet not entirely, for the intuitive still speaks.

It has not been drowned completely by any means. Attempting to cut itself off, however, from the wholeness of the whole personality, the ego must strain for its reserves of energy; for in a large measure, it refuses to accept the energy of the whole personality that is available to it.

(Traffic noise had been increasing past the front of our house. Jane's voice rose to some degree of loudness for the rest of this delivery. Her eyes remained closed.)

It will be our concern here, therefore, to aid the personality to discover and use these resources. I will have more to say concerning the manner in which the organic illness has been accepted by the ego, as a part of the ego's self-image. This acceptance does indeed take place in that area of the personal subconscious that is closely allied to the ego.

But this illness is not so accepted by the whole self, or by the deeper layers of the personality, although certain general tendencies from past lives have aided the personality to strike out physically against his own organism in such a manner.

I will now suggest your first break, and as I have said many times, do not break up, for then I should have to pick up the pieces.

(Break at 9:18. Jane reported that she was quite a bit more dissociated than usual for a first delivery. She did not remember being bothered by traffic noise. Bill Gallagher said he agreed in general with what Jane was saying about his case, as far as he could follow the involved sentences in dictation.)

(Still with her eyes closed, Jane resumed at a good rate and in a good voice at 9:25.)

It is precisely because the inner vitality is not accepted by the ego, that when it is acknowledged by the ego it seems so explosive. The ego attempts, this ego attempts, to stand aside and to deny the inevitability of change. The ego in this case, as in many cases, attempts to maintain stability and permanence at all costs.

This ego in particular, and many egos, consider that the self is the ego alone. The ego considers that therefore it must maintain stability and permanence. It therefore attempts to become rigid, because it considers itself the main representative of the self. It attempts to deny the inner emotions because the changeability of these emotions would seem to threaten its own permanence. It does not want to change. Therefore any seemingly small incident will tend to bring forth the explosion of these emotions quite against the ego's inclination, precisely because the ego denies them so vehemently.

The harder the ego attempts to hold down the emotions, the more explosively will they show themselves upon the least provocation, and the more the ego will attempt to hold them down, and the worse the ulcer becomes. This need not be.

This is why there appears to be two such diverse tendencies that show themselves. The personality is indeed divided. The ego fights the inner self, which means of course that the self fights against itself.

Reactions will therefore appear to be intensified. Nevertheless this intensification is a pretense that one part of the self plays upon the other part, for the very intensity of the emotional reaction on the part of the ego to even small stimuli, allows the ego to say to itself "I feel deeply, therefore I know the depths of myself." And this sham allows the ego to continue denying those inner emotions in an effort to maintain its permanence.

What the personality must be led to see is that any real permanence would indeed be the death of the ego and the personality. For as we know, the ego is not the same today, in your terms, as it was yesterday, nor yet as it will be tomorrow. That "I" continually changes.

(Jane's manner had been active even with her eyes closed, and her voice strong. It now became somewhat stronger. She gestured often toward Bill.)

The ego is indeed but one part of the self that speaks for the other portions of the self, but when it tries to speak for itself only, then indeed its words become meaningless, and the words become threats to the rest of the self. The discipline required in following our program as it develops, that discipline will itself represent the first steps to recovery.

In other words the apparent intensity of the egotistical reactions is a sham on the part of the ego, to hide the fact that it refuses to become involved with action as a <u>whole</u>, because it fears for its permanence. When the ego understands, and it will, that it is a portion of the whole self, and itself a part of action, then indeed it will not fear for its own permanence, for it will realize that being a part of action, its very nature is dependent upon change, and vitality, and value fulfillment.

The passages will become clear as the personality becomes better acquainted with other portions of our sessions. There are here indeed other psychological and surface reasons for the illness, and also deeper reasons for the <u>tendency</u> toward this particular type of illness.

I now suggest your break, and I do myself indeed enjoy your pleasant summer evening. I would like to make it plain here, however, that on a surface psychological level, the personality plunges into activity, and it is for the present this portion of the personality with whom we must deal. Nevertheless, <u>beneath</u> there is a denial of involvement, and a strong desire for permanency, both of which are repressed, and the stronger the efforts put forth by the ego to <u>repress these tendencies</u>, then these tendencies will explode with inadequate stimuli. There will be an overaction on the part of the ego to compensate for the refusal to accept involvement on deeper levels.

Now indeed take your breaks.

One more point. The ulcer for example has reality upon many levels, and must be dealt with in a like manner, for it is not enough to handle it even from the viewpoint of the present ego; for indeed causes are involved of which the present ego must necessarily be mainly ignorant. The inner self however has at its command all these reasonings, and all these causes.

(*Break at 9:51. Jane was very well dissociated, she said. Her eyes had remained closed. Toward the end of this delivery her voice had increased in volume, and at times almost boomed out.*

(*She resumed in the same active manner, still with her eyes closed, and in a somewhat quieter voice, at 10:05.*)

If the illness did not exist on so many layers, then indeed it would not be so tenacious.

The very journey involved in self-discovery, the very self-questioning involved, is indeed part of the process of recovery. The energy being used in the maintenance of the ulcer will already begin to take new channels. The thoughts and anticipations of the personality have already begun to stray from the all-important ulcer to the causes behind it, for in this case, as in many others, we find a strange phenomenon.

(*Jane now pointed at Bill, her eyes still closed, then made a passing reference to a discussion we had had at break. She smiled and spoke quietly.*)

It is you, not I, who have been speaking of secondary personalities, and I will not here waste your time and mine in a discussion of why I am not one.

(*Now abruptly her voice became strong and loud.*)

However, we have among us this evening indeed a secondary personality, a strong and savage one. We have here this evening a secondary personality that attempts to rule the complete life of the personality of whom we have been speaking, and its name is ulcer. For where lies the difference? The personality literally lives its life about the existence of the ulcer. It is hardly worth it, for the personality must be led to see that it itself has created the ulcer, both psychologically and physically, in most actual terms, and that it itself can indeed cast it out.

The personality can survive well without the ulcer. If this sounds like a foolish statement it is not, for in many such cases the ulcer is so concentrated upon, and so much energy is used in its maintenance, and it is used as such a scapegoat, that the personality is loath to be rid of it.

(*Jane's eyes opened, and she looked directly at Bill. Her voice had been loud and emphatic, and it continued so until break.*)

It is however excess baggage, and can be cast aside, and will be. It is not a part of you like your arm. It is not a part of you like your legs. You can navigate without it, and indeed you shall. It is not (*Jane's voice became even louder*) part of the image that the inner self gave you. It did not come to you in your chromosomes for duplication.

It has been added for the purposes of the ego, and it can be discarded. It did not come to you as an organ like your heart, and your existence is not dependent upon it. The purpose that it served it no longer serves, and it must now be discarded.

I will here suggest a short break. We will then continue the session at your convenience, or if you prefer we will close it.

("*We can continue.*")

(*Break at 10:15. Jane was again "way out," as she puts it. Her eyes closed, she blinked several times, then came out of her trance. She said her eyes felt heavy when break came. Her delivery had been fast toward the end.*)

(*She resumed in a quieter voice, with her eyes closed, at 10:27.*)

When the ego becomes so rigid, it immediately begins an insidious attempt to block off stimuli, to limit the reaches of perception, to enclose itself in what it considers a safe world.

It begins to reject stimuli, because stimuli must be reacted to, and it rejects action because action must be reacted to. Therefore it chooses areas of rejection. The areas it chooses to reject are determined by characteristics that are unique to the particular ego.

It begins to travel down safe paths, and out of fear it continually enlarges the scope of limitations. In the particular personality's case, perception becomes also limited, and rejections occur. In this as in many such cases foods are rejected. In many such cases the ego itself chooses to perceive only within those areas where it feels safe, and it rejects more and more any involvement that it can avoid. And <u>now</u> the ego has the self-created ulcer to blame, and it rejects many foods, for foods are symbolistic of involvement.

(*Jane's eyes again opened briefly and she looked at Bill. Her eyes were large and very dark. As she spoke now they began to open and close periodically. Her delivery was faster, and her voice was becoming more emphatic, and louder at times.*)

When I said earlier that the ulcer was not a part of you, like a leg or an arm, I meant this literally. Because you believe this literally, literally you have allowed the ulcer to become a part of your self-image, in the same manner that an arm or a leg is a part of a self-image. And it is this connection that we must, and we will, cut.

When you see that the ulcer does not belong to you in these terms, then indeed you will have no purpose in using your energies to maintain it. It is not part of your heritage. It is not part of the whole self; <u>and now</u>, we will see the purpose of the ego in all this is to protect what it considers the self, for the ego considers <u>itself</u> as the only self.

But in its overzealous behavior we find that it is instead threatening the self. Secondary personalities are caused by repressed emotions on a psychological basis that attempts to maintain an ascendancy. Your ulcer is indeed <u>the same sort of growth</u>, but on a physical and not on a psychological level.

I am going to suggest, first of all, that the material which we have mentioned be read, and then for a beginning that psychological time experiments be taken. Joseph and Ruburt, I know, will be glad to take the few moments necessary to explain them.

The very involvement of the ego with the inner self will be of great benefit. Nothing would be gained if I told you now that the ego would allow the ulcer to vanish, for there would still be a definite need on your part to understand. And it is indeed the understanding itself which will allow <u>you</u> to let it vanish.

(Jane was speaking most emphatically and quite rapidly. Her eyes were open. She stared directly at Bill.)

I am an educator, and I have been one in various respects for perhaps more centuries than I am willing to admit, and I do not believe in giving easy solutions, for they are worthless. <u>The direct experience in this procedure will indeed be your own</u>, and because it is your own it will bear fruit.

There is more that I will say along these lines, as you wish. You may again at your convenience end the session, or take a break. I am indeed fond of you both, and if I behave in my own fashion it is because my experience directs me, that solutions must come from within, for problems come from within. Very easily, through suggestion, I could cure, so it would seem, your ulcer.

<u>You still would have done the curing</u>. But while the need is there something else would develop, and so we will show you the way out of the need. For the need is a sham.

(Break at 10:45. Jane was well dissociated. She ended the delivery by staring at Bill again, and speaking in a loud and positive voice.

(Her delivery had been fast, and it remained so when she resumed, in a quieter voice and with her eyes closed, at 10:55.)

We will then bring our session to a close.

I will say definitely that if my suggestions are followed faithfully and systematically, both the suggestions which I have given, and those which I <u>will</u> give, then indeed we will find that the problem is no longer a problem.

For in the very quiet and discipline required to follow the problem, those reactions on the part of the personality will set up actions which will of themselves solve the problem; and we will find that also there will be suggestions given, and very important suggestions, whereby a systematic effort will be made on the part of the personality to enlarge the scope of his action, in spite of the ego's anxiety to limit them, and this itself will seem to work a miracle.

(Jane's voice was now louder and softer alternately.)

I will here close what can be an extremely productive session. Whether or not it is an extremely productive session will be determined by the personality involved.

I would suggest for the psychological time experiments, fifteen minutes to begin with, along the lines of the directions which Joseph has given. You will find here an intimacy with portions of yourself which you would tend to ignore, which the ego would tend to ignore. You will find indeed refreshment and release. I would suggest that the directions, Joseph, be more specific. You can do better than you have done.

(Jane looked directly at me. She smiled.)

I find myself once more literally blackmailed by your human limitations, since I could indeed go on much longer. But I am indeed in sympathy with your precious fingers, and the fatigue of the present group. With Ruburt presently, only presently, I have no worries.

I will however, since I presume it is your wish, end the session, though regretfully. My fondest wishes to you all, but you are all indeed like nervous birds perched on a peaked roof, in the midst of a high wind; at least this evening, and if I treat you with less politeness, it is only because I speak with the license of an old and trusted friend.

("Good night, Seth.")

(End at 11:03. Jane was well dissociated again. Her eyes had been closed except for the one instance noted. Bill Gallagher said he thought he had noticed a change in Jane's features, at least in terms of expression, during this last delivery. It was hard for him to describe, he said.

(For her part, Jane said she had been quite aware of Seth's emotions, as her very active, smiling, and at times quite loud delivery had indicated.

(The four of us were discussing the loud voice effects when Seth came through again. The conversation had turned to holding a session at the Gallagher's home in the country, where we would not be concerned with bothering neighbors, as I had been so acutely concerned during the 158th session. Jane resumed at 11:10.)

Joseph. I will not continue this session, as I understand your reasons for ending it. As I believe I suggested over a year ago, the present witnesses are most beneficial, and I would suggest on some evening when the time is available, that we take advantage of their help, and hold a session under circumstances that allow us both larger scope in terms of quality and in terms of time.

(As far back as the 63rd session, Seth had remarked upon the fact that Peg

Gallagher would make an excellent witness, since she had well-developed subconscious abilities. See Volume 2.

(*Jane's voice had again begun to turn loud, and I wondered whether we would have more voice effects like those of the 158th session. She began to speak more rapidly, and upon occasion let her voice boom out. But these periods were brief, and were quite a bit short of the almost deafening volume she obtained in the 158th session. Strangely enough, her eyes remained closed for most of this closing delivery, opening but once or twice.*)

For with such witnesses we can indeed do very well. I remember most regretfully your worries the other evening, and I will therefore endeavor *(louder)* not to give any demonstrations that may be embarrassing to you personally, or indeed that will cause you any uneasiness.

I do however find myself hampered at times, and it is for this reason that I have made my suggestion. I <u>will</u> indeed now close with my heartiest best wishes to you all, and indeed I will endeavor to lower my voice, so that it cannot be said that we are not decorous. But we have been so serious of late, we have dealt with such serious and weighty matters, that I have not had time to make my personality known, or to speak with you as I would wish.

Because I am so sympathetic, I will then leave you as I found you, in peace and quiet, though indeed there are times, after the quiet of our sessions, when I would indeed speak with more spontaneity, for I have grown most fond of you both, and therefore I become more willing to display what I may call my more playful nature.

I am after all more than a fountain of information, forever seeping over with facts for your edification, and I would speak to you in more playful conversation, when and if the opportunity presents itself. And Joseph, oh dear Joseph, I would even now, but for your natural reticence, really speak out.

(*Jane stared at me and grinned broadly; and for a second I thought she really was going to sound out.*)

However, I know too well this serious, and may I say mature, nature of your personality, though it was not so in Denmark. So I will, with my best respects, and with some regrets, close our session.

("*Good night, Seth.*")

(*End at 11:20. Jane was again well dissociated. Once again, Bill Gallagher reiterated that he thought he detected a change in Jane's features, particularly about the mouth.*)

SESSION 162
JUNE 14, 1965 9 PM MONDAY AS SCHEDULED

(*For the session we had three witnesses: Lorraine Shafer, who witnessed the 144th session, and Bill and Peg Gallagher, who have witnessed the 158th and the last session. The last time Jane spoke before three witnesses was during the 89th session. Since then we have had two witnesses at a time often, however.*

(*The session was held in our living room again, and traffic noise was not a problem, nor were there any interruptions. The five of us sat in a circle, with Jane in her favorite Kennedy rocker. Jane said she preferred the circle arrangement, rather than having us scattered about the room. As it turned out her idea was a good one.*

(*Lorraine is an expert at shorthand, whereas Peg and I use an abbreviated longhand. The session was an extremely fast one, and I finally had to ask Jane to slow down her delivery. She began her delivery with her eyes closed, but she spoke in a rather strong voice and in a very active manner. Much of the time she leaned forward in the rocker, her elbows on her knees, her hands clasped. She used many gestures and few pauses.*)

Good evening.

("*Good evening, Seth.*")

May I give heartiest wishes to our guests this evening.

I have endeavored to study rather thoroughly the condition of the other male present in the room, yourself excluded, Joseph, because we find here an almost classic example of the manner in which the individual subconsciously creates physical matter, and the manner in which the psychological and psychic problems of the individual conspire so that the organic perfection becomes disturbed.

The physical organism reflects vividly and with <u>perfection</u> the innermost state of the human personality. Now. As the condition of your planet in its entire political and social structure reflects the innermost neuroses in every individual, so indeed does the physical individual organism reflect the inner condition of each personality.

You create, as you know, physical matter on a subconscious basis, without knowing egotistically that you do so. You create physical matter as <u>effortlessly</u> and as <u>smoothly</u> and as <u>automatically</u>, and as unknowingly as you create your own dreams.

The ego is not aware of the manner in which dreams are created. Neither is it aware of the manner in which the inner self creates physical matter. Neither, therefore, is it aware of those distortions that cause it to construct faults within physical matter, for in all cases the physical matter of the human body will be subconsciously created in line with inner conditions.

This can work, and should work, to your advantage. However when there is a distortion, as when an ulcer is created, then we begin what can indeed be a vicious circle, for the idea and the reality of the ulcer is then accepted as part of the self-image. And as such it is then more or less automatically recreated.

(Seth now made a reference to Lorraine by her entity name.)

We have here this evening, also, Marleno, who when she arrived was troubled with a stiff neck. Now here we see a temporary distortion, not an organic one. You can see however how such a temporary distortion could become, under certain conditions (that do not operate in your case) permanent.

It may indeed sound like an oversimplification. However, you are exactly what you think you are, and every thought is mirrored in the physical matter of the human organism. This does not happen by some sort of occult magic. It is not the result of some mumbo jumbo. Since each individual <u>creates</u> subconsciously the physical matter of his own image, then it follows that the condition of this image is his own responsibility.

Those present may not as yet be familiar with some very important background material that would be helpful. I have discussed in some detail the electrical makeup of the physical body, and of the atoms and molecules, and cells and organs, that compose it.

I have also discussed the electrical components that make up each thought. These thoughts, then, are automatically translated <u>into</u> physical matter by certain areas of the subconscious. If certain long-standing distorted concepts are held, therefore, then they must be faced and struck out. For otherwise there is an automatic flow of this energy into a false disruptive pattern.

The inner self does indeed have an overall conception of the goals and strengths of the personality. It is then this inner self that must be searched for the answers. I mentioned earlier in another session that the very attempt to seek for an answer to the basic problem will indeed automatically release some of that energy for a constructive purpose.

You will begin to starve the ulcer of its energy. The manner in which the subconscious translates energy into construction of physical matter, again, has been covered in our sessions previously. However it is imperative that the idea be understood thoroughly, for here we have no vague and nebulous theory indeed, but a most practical and definite explanation of the manner in which you yourselves construct not only your own physical image, but indeed your own physical environment.

(Among others, see the 60th-73rd sessions in Volume 2.)

And that which you have constructed, you then respond to through the outer senses, and you react to what you have subconsciously created. It is important that these matters be understood when you are concerned with how to change or alter a physical condition, for the change will come from within or it will not come.

I now suggest your first break.

(*Break at 9:20. Jane was much more dissociated than usual for a first delivery. She thought this was because of the presence of witnesses. She came out of the trance quickly however.*

(*Lorraine's neck felt much better, she said, and Bill's ulcer had quieted down. The conversation turned to the meaning of dreams during break. Jane's delivery was again fast and her eyes were still closed, although her voice was quieter, when she resumed at 9:34.*)

When the time is available, a class of sorts would be advantageous.

The fact remains that much basic material should be comprehended in order for us to continue in the line of suitable explanations. You construct the dream universe in the same manner that you construct the physical universe. For various reasons that have been discussed there is no need, <u>in</u> the dream universe, for the permanence of image, or the <u>apparent</u> permanence of image that occurs in the physical universe.

You construct the dream universe, again, on a subconscious basis. The dream universe is as permanent in its way as the physical universe. You construct dreams whether you wake or you sleep. You are only <u>familiar</u> with your dreams when you sleep, for then your perception and your energy is focused in that direction.

I will here repeat an old definition of many sessions back: <u>Consciousness is the direction in which the self looks</u>.

In sleep, when the ego is quieted, then the self looks in other directions. In sleep the self becomes conscious of its dreams, but this does not mean that the dreams have not existed while you were not conscious of them. Nor does it mean that they cease to exist when you are no longer conscious of them, for they have their own sort of molecular and electrical construction. But the ego cannot tune into that perceptive range.

(*For some material on the electrical field, including ranges, dreams, mass, intensities, weight, etc., see the following sessions: 122, 123, 125, 126, 128, 131, 135, among others. All in Volume 3.*)

As you create physical matter constantly without knowing that you do so, so also you create constantly a dream universe, and this dream universe is as individual as your environment in the physical world. There is also a chemical reaction here, for without dreaming the physical organism could not exist.

With your outer senses, you perceive but the camouflage physical reality which the physical senses are equipped to perceive. In the dream universe you are however free, and familiar, with both space and time in a manner which is denied you in the waking state. Where indeed are your dream locations? Where in space is the street upon which you walk in a dream?

(Among others, see the 44th session for material on dream locations. Volume 2.)

(Among others, Seth talked about the direction of focus of consciousness in the 94th session. Volume 3.)

The location does not exist <u>within your physical system</u>, but the dream location is a reality. It is a superimposed value which you have created, and which is valid and vivid. A dream unfolds. Miles may appear before your inner vision. Are then these miles contained within your head? Are these miles contained within the small skull? Obviously not. But here we are closer to that reality which is beyond space as you know it.

(Jane's eyes opened briefly, for emphasis. Her voice was fairly loud and strong, with an edge in it, her delivery very active. For the most part she was still leaning forward in her rocker, her elbows resting upon her knees, her head tilted down somewhat as she spoke.)

You may in a dream experience two or three hours in a flash of physical time. You have not aged two or three hours. The experience of space and time within the dream universe comes very close to the pure expression of the inner self. For <u>here</u>, free from the ego, the self is relieved of the <u>necessity</u> of constructing ideas into physical reality.

It constructs ideas instead within another electrical system. Yet because of the nature of the personality, no dream exists in a vacuum, and every dream is recorded by the inner self. I am making an attempt here this evening, since we have three present, to give a very brief, and I am afraid inadequate explanation, that will however serve as a basis so that these three, at least, will be able to have some sort of a standing ground for other discussions.

Think if you will then of the manner in which an idea expands. It expands and grows and you feel its vitality gather, yet when you say it grows and expands, it does not grow and expand, again, somewhere in the space between your ears, to burst apart the bones of the skull. It expands in a way that has nothing to do with space.

This we have called the value climate of psychological reality. It is what you may consider your counterpart of physical space. After a short break, we will discuss then your misconceptions concerning space, for you will see that your idea of space is the result of your own physical perceptions. Where <u>you</u> can perceive nothing, you presume to call empty space, but where you perceive nothing there is much.

I now suggest your break, and I thank all of you for both your help and your attention.

(Break at 9:55. Jane was again well dissociated. She said she felt as though the Seth voice was pulling her along. Her trance was deep, she felt very free, she said. She remarked that the feeling was similar to the two Father Trainor episodes, of February 11, 1965 and May 30, 1965; I too had had the thought that there was a similarity here, and thought I detected a hint of a brogue in Jane's delivery at times. She had exhibited a rather marked brogue during the Father Trainor episodes.

(The value climate of psychological reality has been designated by Seth as the first of the basic laws of the inner universe, and was first discussed in the 44th session, in Volume 2.

(Jane's delivery had been fast, almost too fast for comfort, although Lorraine had no trouble keeping up with her shorthand. I asked my wife to slow down a bit. Her eyes had been closed for most of the delivery, and they were closed during a good part of the next one. She resumed at a fast pace and in a strong voice at 10:05.)

My thought here was merely that in perhaps four or five sessions we could deliver a basic, if not thoroughly adequate, explanation that would then serve as a basis for those who attended the four or five sessions, so that any problems could then be discussed in such a manner that the witnesses would be familiar with basic precepts and terminology.

(Jane's voice now became most amused and full of mock fear.)

I was, I was not here suggesting—far be it from me—to suggest that Ruburt give three sessions a week. I would not dare be so presumptuous. I would, literally, shiver in my boots, for he would pursue me with endless protests.

However, with his consent you could do as you pleased. Either have witnesses attend, for example, a Monday or a Wednesday session. Or if you prefer that our own material also progress at its usual rate, then we could perhaps hold an extra, perhaps shorter, session a week.

I am merely making suggestions to be of a help. It goes without saying that many explanations I could give, I can't give in my usual manner, simply because the witnesses do not have a familiarity with our material. A basic requirement here is a thorough understanding of the precise manner in which physical matter is constructed.

(If anything, Jane was now speaking at an even faster rate. Already it was the fastest session I could recall.)

For you look now at Ruburt. There are indeed, now, in this room there are five physical Ruburts. For each of you, including Ruburt, create and project your own image of him, and each of you perceive with your physical senses only that image of him which you have individually created.

(Jane's eyes opened, then closed. In particular, see the 66th session of the series on the creation of matter. In that session also, Seth stated the above statement can be verified mathematically. Volume 2.)

There are perspectives of reality which you yet do not understand. You should understand clearly the ways in which you create these physical images, for they need not imprison you as they often do.

There is a necessity to discover and understand the inner self. There is much material concerning the construction of atoms and molecules that will enable you to understand not only the physical world, but also the dream universe.

Speaking earlier concerning the dream universe, there are many things I left of necessity unsaid. I was saying that any dream location exists in actuality, when you experience it in a perspective which has nothing to do with your idea of space, but which has a depth and a reality at least as valid.

Nor is the dream itself a chaotic action, but a complicated and unique action by which symbols are chosen with such precise and careful attention that they have meaning to all levels of the inner self, and various levels of the subconscious. Here you will find clues as to many of your own conscious problems. Here with study and attention you will find information concerning your own previous lives, which the ego is not familiar with.

Through dreams the self communicates with the self, and with all layers of the self. For the self is not one concrete thing. The self has no boundaries, the self is not limited. Consciousness is the direction in which the self looks, again, but the ego is not aware of the whole self. The ego is not even familiar with the context or the meaning of your own dreams.

(There is much dream material scattered throughout the sessions. See the 87th, 88th, 92nd, 93rd, 94th, etc. in just Volume 3, for example.)

The ego cannot make your heart beat. Why then do you find it difficult to believe that you are more than the ego, for in dreams you meet portions of yourself. You construct realities, and you are indeed familiar with the dream universe that consciously you ignore. And your experience within the dream universe is as vivid and as valid and as <u>real</u>, in every respect, as your waking experience.

Nor are <u>you indeed fully conscious</u>, in your terms, even in your waking state.

You shut off stimuli to concentrate on other stimuli. This is a simplified example of how in the dream state you shut out stimuli usually accepted by the ego, and become conscious of other realities that you usually ignore in the waking state.

You create the dream world continuously. You are familiar with it and intimate with it, and you know it well. In this discussion there should be some remarks made concerning the existence of the inner ego, of which I believe you are not familiar.

I do not want to give you too many details too quickly. The inner ego, however, you may think of as another face that looks inward. We are using an analogy, and an analogy that is for simplicity's sake only. We may say therefore, starting from the outer environment, that you would have first of all what you consider the ego, which I will call the outer ego.

Then, according to our analogy, you will find the subconscious areas; and these areas may be, briefly, differentiated in the following manner.

The foremost or exterior layers or areas deal with the personal selves. Beyond these you will find areas dealing with previous experiences having to do with your own past lives. Within the next area you will find material dealing with the [species] as a whole.

Each of these areas are separated, and between the memories of each past life, experiments will show a layer that we call undifferentiated.

At the furthest or innermost area then, we come to the inner ego, which would then be separated from the outer ego by the buffer of the subconscious. Now it goes without saying that we speak here merely for convenience's sake, for all these areas are not indeed so neatly divided; but to explain their various purposes we must therefore speak of them in this manner.

I will now suggest a break. Or if your hand is not tired, Joseph, we can continue.

("We'll take the break.")

I rather supposed that you would.

(Break at 10:25. Jane was well dissociated. She ended the delivery on a humorous note. Her eyes had been mostly closed. She again had no idea that she had been speaking so rapidly; even Lorraine wondered if Seth was trying to find out just how fast she could take shorthand. I would say that Jane's delivery was faster than ever before, her voice loud.

(During this next delivery Jane spoke at a somewhat slower rate, at my request. Her eyes were closed for the most part. Here again, as noted on page 89, I would say that Jane spoke in quite a brogue for part of the delivery. This was more pronounced than before, and more than a little reminiscent of the two Father Trainor episodes.

(Jane grew up in an Irish neighborhood in Saratoga Springs, NY, and Father Trainor was an Irish priest of the old school. He exerted considerable influence on Jane in her formative years. His girth was extensive, and he read poetry to Jane and her mother, Marie, every Sunday after dinner, with a booming voice and a dramatic

flourish. Jane herself is one-quarter Irish, although as she has often said, she grew up thinking she was Irish, period.

(She resumed in a strong voice and with her eyes closed at 10:35.)

The following basic subjects are necessary for an understanding of what we are trying to say, particularly for any practical application: the construction of physical matter; the psychological and electrical gestalt that results in the formation of a self; the nature of the dream universe; the electrical system, as it is related to both the physical universe and the inner psychic gestalt; the nature of action; mental enclosures; mental genes; and again, all of these subjects in relationship to their reality as action.

It will also be advantageous if an understanding is achieved concerning the manner in which physical material first materialized within your system.

It is imperative, first of all, that the following be understood. We are dealing with words. Words involve us necessarily with symbols, and symbols are merely terms for what you do not understand. Everything, whether—

("Not too fast."

(Jane's speed of delivery was picking up again.)

—you perceive it or not, is action.

A thought is an action. A dream is as much an action as a breath is an action. Although we speak in terms of separation, all reality is a part of action. When we divide action in order to discuss it, we in no way change the reality of action, nor alter its nature.

Actions have an electrical reality. Your outer senses do not perceive electrical realities of this nature. Nevertheless, you are a gestalt of electrical actions. Within the physical matter of your chromosomes there are electrically coded systems. These are not the chromosomes themselves. The chromosomes are the physical materialization of the inner electrical data.

Action (you may if you prefer use the term vitality; I prefer the term action) action continually attempts to express itself in endless formations. It therefore materializes itself in various forms. I term these forms camouflage. Within your system the camouflage is physical matter. It is impossible for action to completely express itself in any medium.

There is, in no circumstance, any closed system. Action therefore flows within all systems and realities. Your physical senses are therefore adapted to deal with a particular camouflage system. They are therefore only equipped to perceive the realities within the physical camouflage field.

(Jane's voice, already loud, acquired more strength and volume. Her delivery was now very emphatic, but her eyes remained closed.)

This does not, however, mean that this is the only reality. It is simply the only reality that you perceive with the physical senses. In order to perceive other realities, you must therefore switch from your outer senses to the inner senses, for the inner senses are clearer, and are equipped to perceive action and reality as it exists independently of the distortions given to it by the physical senses.

For, because you perceive reality in a limited fashion only, this in no way affects the basic nature of reality itself. The ego attempts to stand apart from action, to view action as the <u>result of ego</u>. However, again, the ego's attempt to stand apart from action in no way changes the basic nature of action itself, and the ego merely limits its own perception.

There are no limitations to the self, for the self as a part of action has no boundaries except those imaginary boundaries given to it by the ego.

Joseph, I am endeavoring to go slowly. Am I going too swiftly despite my efforts?

("No.")

(Although Jane was speaking at a rapid rate.)

We find therefore no, <u>no</u> limitations to the self, neither top nor bottom. The self is not enclosed within the bony skull. You call your thoughts your own, and yet how do you hold them?

You do not hold them. They are indeed transmitted without your conscious knowledge, and the self expands. Nor is the self limited physically. Again, this idea is the result of your own habit of perception, for chemicals and air and nutrients that you consider <u>not your self, enter</u> the self constantly from the physical environment; and that which you consider yourself, leaves through the pores of the body.

Nor is the self limited by either space nor time, for in dreams you have an actuality that has nothing to do with space nor time, and these dream experiences change and alter your personality, for action must of itself always change. You are only familiar with a small portion of the self. You are more than you know you are, and your journeys range further.

The self is indeed a more complicated and a more delicate construction than any of you know.

You may now, as you desire, take a break or end the session.

("We'll end it then.")

I will then give you my best regards, and my very best wishes to you all. I will also add that this session is then itself action, and since it is action, it changes both those who attend it, Ruburt who delivers it, and I who give it.

("Good night, Seth.")

(End at 11:00. Jane was well dissociated. It took her a little while to open her eyes. Her delivery had been very active, her eyes opened briefly occasionally, and her

voice had been fairly strong. Both Bill Gallagher and I remarked on the pronounced brogue she had used. Bill said his ulcer had not bothered him, and Lorraine said that her neck felt much better.

(Lorraine and the Gallaghers left soon after the session. Jane, I noticed, seemed to be still wound up and did not immediately retire as she usually does after a session. We talked about the high peak of psychic activity she had reached recently, and she said she felt that Seth was "still around."

(I do not encourage her to give extra sessions as a rule, and did not encourage her to continue now. I was caught between feeling that she could herself choose the amount of psychic activity she wanted to indulge in, and feeling that it was better that she not overdo it. The pace had been active recently.

(Finally, we sat in the living room and Jane once more began to speak for Seth. I had put my notebook away and did not get it. Jane sat on the couch and I leaned back in a comfortable chair. Her eyes were closed, her voice quiet. The short session was somewhat like a conversation between Seth and me, although I did not ask too many questions. What follows is a summary, made up from memory immediately after the session ended. Resume at 11:45 PM.)

SUMMARY

(Speaking for Seth, Jane began by saying that we could forego Wednesday's session if we chose to, in view of the extra work involved recently in the longer sessions. Jane was indeed at a peak of psychic activity now, her highest to date; he liked to take advantage of such periods when he could.

(Seth repeated several times that we wouldn't regret this burst of psychic energy, or the time involved, because it meant an increase in Jane's ability to focus energy. The witnesses tonight had been extremely valuable; for different reasons [which he did not go into]. Seth stated that such gatherings increased Jane's ability to utilize energy on different levels. This ability is still increasing. Seth uses witnesses as "practice" for Jane. Her ability to draw upon others would be very valuable in the "near future." I believe he implied here that Jane would be speaking before larger groups, perhaps soon, and that possibly many in such groups would be strangers.

(Seth took care to see that Jane did not overdo it. He understood my concerns along these lines, and I had nothing to worry about. Any time we wanted to, we could obtain information from him. There would also be times when Jane's energies would be at a lower ebb. There is much about energy and cycles and Jane's abilities that he hasn't explained to us yet. He is fond of us, and we have learned much.

(Seth answered my question by saying it was a good idea for Jane and me to attend the hypnosis symposium at Oswego next month, and to meet Dr. Instream, the director. *The visit would have far-reaching effects, for us and for the material. I had rapport with Dr. Instream from reading his books. This is why I wrote to him in the first place. Jane and I would feel this rapport when we met him, also.*

(Seth enjoyed such casual get-togethers as this, and I mentioned using our tape recorder for more of these, keeping the sessions somewhat shorter to make up for the extra time involved in replaying the tapes for transcription. Seth understood the problems we faced in our daily lives, and didn't want the sessions to take up any more of our time.

(Nor did he recommend that we spend any Saturday nights, either alone or with friends, trying seances or other psychic activity. We needed instead outgoing activity such as our dancing, and being with others. Seth closed by saying we could have time off whenever we wanted to, that we had but to ask, and that I could end any session whenever I wanted to.

(End at 11:59 PM. Jane's eyes opened slowly. She said she felt relaxed, that Seth was gone now and the session was over.)

SESSION 163
JUNE 21, 1965 9 PM MONDAY AS SCHEDULED

(On Sunday evening, June 20th, I again experienced the feeling of sound, as Seth has described it. Jane and I attended a jazz mass presented by Joe Masters in the Presbyterian Church, in Horseheads, just north of Elmira, NY, where we live. This was a very thrilling experience for us, and I believe for everyone else there. The music at times was literally deafening in volume, combined as it was with a large choir and a jazz band. In addition Jane and I, with the Gallaghers, sat in the second row and thus felt the full force of the performance.

(Shortly after the mass began, I became aware of what seemed to be solid but invisible waves that beat against both ears externally. An analogy would be cupped hands clapping against my ears. An extremely rich thrilling suffused my head, then quickly spread to various parts of my body, not evenly by any means. I tried to increase the sensation by concentrating, for instance, on hearing the sound with my left knee when the sensation was strong there, but did not succeed especially. I was reminded of this by the 154th session, dealing with the body's generalized ability to receive stimuli.

(In Volume 1 of The Early Sessions *this sensation, as I call it, is dealt with following Session 23, in Session 24, and following Session 25, among others. I have experienced it frequently during psychological time since then. It is much richer and more varied than the more usual thrilling one notes upon a moving occasion.*

In the above instance, the initial source of the sensation appeared to stem from outside the body, and the waves against my ears had a tangible, solid quality that is difficult to describe.

(Joe Masters is the husband of Dee, who was director of the art gallery where Jane worked for several years. The Masters are discussed by Seth in the 63rd session among occasional others. See Volume 2.

(Jane also felt strong thrilling sensations at the jazz mass, saying they were like the sensations she attains during psy-time, that she calls her good state, and occasionally ecstasy.

(Last Saturday, June 19, Jane received a brief communication from Seth while going about her household chores. Her thoughts had touched upon the sessions dealing recently with Bill Gallagher's ulcer. Jane thought, idly, that some foods would not be practical for Bill to eat. She then received the brief message from Seth, to the effect that our ideas of practicality are often hardly practical.

(Last Wednesday's session, scheduled for June 16, was not held. This was Seth's idea to compensate for the longer recent sessions and the extra typing involved.

(Tonight's session was again held in our living room. It was an extremely hot and humid evening. Traffic noise was more audible than usual but Jane appeared unaffected. She spoke while sitting down and with her eyes closed, in a voice strong enough to penetrate the background noise, and at a good rate with very few pauses. As she has done often lately, she spoke a good deal of the time while sitting forward in her rocker, her elbows resting on her knees, her head tipped down to some degree.)

Good evening.

("Good evening, Seth.")

I see that we will have a private session once again. This is to our advantage; and it is also to our advantage, when witnesses are present, when those witnesses have the peculiar qualities which are of benefit.

There is one small point I wanted to mention this evening, merely for future reference: We have hardly begun any thorough study of the dream universe, and have dealt with it mainly in connection with other discussions. We will however discuss it in detail, and we will use dreams from your own notebooks as examples in this study.

The dreams that you are accumulating therefore will be of great benefit to us, and I have not discussed them in our regular sessions because I prefer to use them as the basis for another body of material.

(Jane's notebook now contains over 300 dreams, and mine somewhat less. The above information may explain why Seth did not discuss my recent clairvoyant dream, which I mentioned in the 160th session.)

What you call suggestion, to return to our present subject matter, is but a projection into the physical universe of data that operates constantly, as a basis for, and within, action. It is basically a psychic manifestation that gives direction to action, and to the various manifestations which action may take.

Suggestion is therefore one of the characteristics of action. The term suggestion is a poor one. As it operates within your system, and within the human personality, the word expectation is a much better term. Nevertheless, expectation is only one phase, for the same kind of inner directive activity is pertinent within all forms of action.

What you call suggestion then is but a small aspect of a larger directive characteristic that is ever part of action itself. It is indeed in the nature of an impetus, an inner impetus that belongs to action, and is not some force separated from action, and acting upon it. This impetus is a natural and spontaneous <u>movement</u> that springs from within action itself. It can even be termed the direction, or the various spontaneous directions, in which action itself moves.

These directions are not forced upon action by any laws. They are merely the resultant patterns with which energy expresses itself. You are only familiar as a rule with this impetus, or these directions, in rather shallow manners, for the ego prefers not to perceive them. These <u>motions</u> are merely the flow which action takes. What you term negative suggestions are usually impeding actions, or directions of action which impede the main directive inner flow. They operate then in much the same manner as crosscurrents, setting up blockages, and impeding main energies by dividing them in several diverse directions.

It is important that it be understood that suggestion, as <u>you</u> know it, is but the manifestation of inner flows and inner directions. Without the inward flows and directions, it goes without saying that action would indeed involve itself in chaotic disorders, without constructive patterns or materializations. It would instead entangle itself within the power of its own energy, and be unable to form any long-lasting patterns or frameworks within which fulfillments and fairly permanent constructions could be formed.

When you speak of negative suggestions, you are actually referring to a situation where such crosscurrents entangle action within itself, and therefore impede the main constructive impetus that unrestricted action allows. Until the energy, once again, becomes disentangled, action will therefore flow also in the crosscurrents, and the <u>main trunk</u> of energy that gives overall integrity and identity to any given unit could therefore be severely threatened.

On the part of any human personality, therefore, it is extremely important that methods be learned to let action follow its normal directive bent within the personality, therefore avoiding these abortive offshoots that impede main directives and purposes of the unit as a whole.

The integration of the whole personality as a psychological unit, and as an effective psychic gestalt, is obviously dependent upon the free and unimpeded flow of action. Any impediments here can be most threatening to the integrity of the personality itself, for one aspect of the personality would benefit at the expense of other aspects.

The personality itself, as you know, is a gestalt of action, and as such it is necessary that the flow of action within it follow the overall directives of the entity and the inner self. When for example the ego is allowed to apply too tightly and too rigorously its inhibitory functions, then this freedom of action within the personality is seriously divided and impeded.

I suggest your first break.

(*Break at 9:26. Jane was fairly well dissociated for a first delivery. Her delivery had been fast, her eyes closed all the time. During this delivery a very heavy rain began to fall; it was noisy, but her voice surmounted the additional noise without trouble. She was vaguely aware of the rain, she said, and of the content of the material.*

(*Jane began to speak again in the same fast manner, with her eyes closed, and in a somewhat quieter voice. Resume at 9:34.*)

I will, Joseph, slow down at your request, whenever it is more convenient for you.

Now. As far as our discussion is concerned, we have in the past mentioned that there are no exact duplicates in any circumstances. There are however, obviously, patterns which are set up by action, that may be thought of as pathways composed of action, through which action then flows.

Once such a pathway has been constructed, we have what you may call an action pattern or habit. Therefore, when cross currents of action are constructed, action will continue in those directions unless it is diverted back to other channels. Then the secondary or impeding channel will automatically be closed off. But all action must be withdrawn from it, for as long as the channel remains, then the possibility remains that the impeding action will reoccur.

There is indeed no hard and fast rule to tell you which actions are basically impeding actions, and which are not. For what may appear an impeding action may indeed turn out to be the burst of a new and constructive direction, which may eventually represent a new and stronger pattern of identity and integrity, that will completely refresh the original unit and add to its vitality and strength.

The inner self here, through intuitive insight, can usually recognize whether an action is an impeding or a constructive one for the purposes of the personality involved. Even an action which appears blatantly as an impeding action, may <u>temporarily</u> serve as a constructive one. It may then <u>turn into</u> an impeding action.

An illness, as an impeding action for example, may nevertheless be a constructive action at any given time, in that it may prevent action within the personality from following more destructive actions. When this destructive possibility has passed however, an illness that is still maintained would therefore become a definite impeding action; for any seemingly impeding action cannot be judged alone, but in the context of other action elements of which any given personality is involved.

It is extremely difficult, but it is possible for the human system to close off, for all practical purposes, a channel that has been used for the flow of such an impeding action. The channel may automatically disappear, but the action itself can never be withdrawn.

We will discuss what you call suggestion in more practical terms, for your particular uses. Nevertheless it is necessary that its basic nature be understood. The ego simply cannot judge, as a rule, whether an action is a constructive or an impeding one, for the personality as a whole.

It <u>can</u> judge whether an action is a constructive or an impeding one for <u>itself</u>. Upon many occasions the purposes of the ego coincide with the purposes of the whole personality, but upon many occasions the purposes of the ego do not coincide with the best purposes of the whole personality. And in such cases the ego is not equipped to judge, except for itself.

It can however be taught a very valuable function here. The first prerequisite is that the ego understand both the nature of its <u>dependence</u> upon the whole personality, and the nature of its peculiar directive abilities in relation with the physical universe. When there is good communication between all areas of the self, and this is a big when, then the judgment of the ego can be trusted to some greater extent.

Suggestions given by an individual on any kind of a conscious basis have to be given with the cooperation of the ego. Many suggestions bypass the ego entirely. Suggestion however, as you think of it, operates both ways. This is not usually understood. Suggestions may come therefore from the physical world, to act upon the personality. Suggestions may also come from <u>within</u> the personality to act upon the physical environment.

You can indeed to a large measure train yourself to react to constructive rather than impeding suggestions. This merely means that you will, or may to some extent, choose the direction in which action within you will move. This also implies that some part of the personality <u>does</u> the choosing, and is capable of distinguishing a constructive suggestion from an impeding one. And here it is necessary that we discuss more thoroughly the nature or characteristics of constructive suggestions versus impeding ones, for one may turn into the other.

No one portion of the personality should be allowed to block the free flow of energy or action. Impeding actions are easily recognized by their effects, psychological or physical, upon the human system. An illness is the result of an impeding action, generally speaking, but there are exceptions to this case, as others.

There are indeed methods by which the flow of action can be turned back, away from the impeding channels, and we will discuss that matter in some detail.

I now suggest your break.

(*Break at 10:07. Jane was well dissociated. She had spoken at a fast pace and with a good voice, with few pauses and with her eyes closed. The rain had stopped, and the humidity was high and uncomfortable. That is, I was uncomfortable, my writing hand moist and clammy. Jane was perfectly at ease, her skin quite dry and fresh. She was not at all aware of heat or humidity while delivering the material, she said, but was well aware of the conditions at break time.*

(*She resumed with her eyes closed, and with a quieter voice, but with the same fast rate of delivery, at 10:16.*)

Again, we will have many sessions indeed, dealing with the gestalt that is the human personality, and at that time much of this material will fall into place.

We are dealing here, again, merely with the various aspects of action. As a personality itself is an action gestalt, within the inner self there is a capsule comprehension of the purposes and intents of the whole personality. These are indeed within the very structure, both psychic and physical, of the personality itself. The ego, <u>on its own</u> as a separate unit, does not have such data, although since it is after all a portion of the whole self, it does have such information available. But when it acts as a unit it does not <u>use</u> such information.

The information is not closed to it. It simply does not use it, and there are several quite sufficient reasons for this, reasons that have to do with the necessary apart manner in which the ego, when it operates as a separate unit, views the physical universe.

When the personality is well integrated, then even when it operates as a separate unit the ego still fulfills the basic purposes of the personality as a whole. It is the communication between the very areas of the self which is so important here, as in many other matters. It is possible for the ego to realize its position as but one part of the whole personality, while it still behaves in a directive manner toward physical manipulation.

This is the ideal circumstance, for when this is the case then the ego listens to the inner self, and then directs its energy outward in a way that is beneficial for the whole gestalt framework. What you call negative suggestions are often judgments of the ego, for suggestion works from the ego <u>to</u> the subconscious, as well as it works the other way around. Such suggestions made by the ego can indeed be caught, and positive or constructive suggestions given to replace them.

However, automatic responses can also be set up, so that only constructive suggestions are reacted to. In such instances however, the inner self should be allowed to make the judgment ultimately, as to which suggestions are constructive and which are not.

There are certain manners that are more advantageous than others in the giving of such suggestions, and we will go into these at another session. We may also, indeed, begin at least a partial study of the framework of the personality as it is related to action, for such a discussion will follow along well with our material on suggestion.

It must be understood that the personality is indeed an action within action, and that it is therefore never stationary. Indeed suggestions, being the directions in which action moves, represent the very impetus that constantly changes the action of any given personality. It goes without saying, once more, that all of these designations imply a separation which does not exist in fact, and imply definite boundaries which are not present.

For all actions merge one into the other, and none are truly independent; and all units merge one into the other, and all boundaries shift, and are arbitrarily chosen. Boundaries are the results of the limitations of perception, for a unit seems to end where perception of it ceases.

This has been a most constructive session, and its flow has been unimpeded. I wish you both a fond good evening, and as always I enjoy our sessions. I feel quite benign this evening, and enjoy our solitude. There are, however, other important elements. I bid you good evening.

("Good night, Seth.")

(End at 10:40. Jane was more dissociated for this last delivery, she said. Her eyes were closed for the whole session, her delivery fast for the most part, her voice strong.)

SESSION 164
JUNE 23, 1965 9 PM WEDNESDAY AS SCHEDULED

(Tuesday night, June 22, 1965, I had another clairvoyant dream which came to pass the next morning on my way to work. I believe it is a case of suggestion, given by a dream, then influencing my behavior, unwittingly, the next day. I hoped aloud

that Seth would discuss it tonight, but as in my dream mentioned in the 160th session, he did not. I record all dreams I recall, as does my wife.

(Jane has been using her twenty-minute psychological time period recently for health purposes, with excellent results. For a related specific incident, see the description of her dentist episode in the 152nd session. She has also been attaining excellent "states" during her psy-time periods. Again, she keeps records.

(It rained this evening, and in the cooler weather we held the session in our small back room. Using this room increases our sense of privacy, being sheltered from most noise as it is, and the risk of interruptions. Jane was quite restless during the session, changing position in her rocker frequently. She spoke with her eyes closed for the entire session; at times her delivery was quite fast, other times it was broken by pauses. Her voice was about average for the most part.)

Good evening.

("Good evening, Seth.")

Impeding actions represent actual blockages of energy or of action, dead-end accumulations. In one manner of speaking this does not mean that the action is terminated, however.

It does mean that action is turned into channels that are not to the best interests of the whole personality. The energies appear concentrated and turn inward, affecting the whole system. They represent offshoots, again not necessarily detrimental in themselves, but only when viewed from the standpoint of the other actions that form the personality framework.

Such actions naturally possess all the characteristics of action in general, and therefore will seek other methods of materialization and expression. An attempt at discipline will be made. The structure will seem, that is the impeding structure will seem, to maintain itself. The whole personality at any given time, because of its own nature and characteristics, has only a given amount of energy available to it in practical terms, though ideally speaking its energy is not limited.

However, a certain portion of the energy practically available to it is therefore spent in the maintenance of this impeding action. It is obvious therefore that less energy is available to the personality for actions more beneficial to the personality system as a whole.

This situation can be serious in varying degrees, according to the impetus and intensity of the original propelling cause behind the impeding action. If the impetus is a powerful one, then the impeding action will be of more serious nature, blocking up large reserves of energy for its own purposes. It obviously becomes part of the personality-psychological structure, the physical structure, the electrical and chemical structure, invading to some extent even the dream universe.

It is, momentarily, literally accepted by the personality as a part of the self, and here lies its danger. It is not just <u>symbolically</u> accepted, and I am not speaking in symbolic terms. The impeding action, as seen in an illness for example, is quite literally accepted by the personality structure, and by all corresponding systems, as a portion of the self. Once this occurs, a conflict instantly develops. The self does not want to give up a portion of itself, even while that portion may be painful or disadvantageous. There are many psychological reasons behind such a psychological truth.

For one thing, while pain is unpleasant it is also a method of familiarizing the self against the edges of quickened consciousness. Any heightened sensation, pleasant or unpleasant, has a stimulating effect upon a consciousness to some degree. It is a strong awareness of activity and life. Where the stimulus may be extremely annoying, and humiliatingly unpleasant, certain portions of the psychological framework accept it indiscriminatingly because it is a sensation, and a vivid one. This acquiescence to even painful stimuli is a basic part of the nature of consciousness, and a necessary one.

(Jane now took a very long pause, sitting motionless with her eyes closed.)

Even a quick and automatic rejection or withdrawal from such stimulus is in itself a way by which consciousness knows itself. The ego may attempt to ignore or escape from such experiences, but the basic nature of action itself is the knowing of itself in all aspects; and in a basic manner, in a very basic and deep manner, action does not differentiate between pleasant, painful or enjoyable actions.

These differentiations come much later and on another level, and in a later evolutionary development. But because the personality is composed of action, the personality also contains within it this characteristic of action, in that it accepts all sensations as expressions of itself, and does not discriminate between stimuli.

Action accepts all stimuli in an affirmative manner. It is only when action becomes compartmented, so to speak, in the development of highly differentiated consciousness, that such refinement occurs. I am not here saying that unpleasant stimuli will not be <u>felt</u> as unpleasant, and reacted against, by less self-conscious organisms. I <u>am</u> saying that less self-conscious organisms will rejoice even in their automatic reaction against such stimuli, because any stimuli and reaction represents sensation, and sensation is another method by which such action knows and expresses itself.

I suggest your first break.

(Break at 9:31. Jane was well dissociated for a first break. She had been restless,

her voice quite expressive.

(Jane said she had experienced another "concept feeling" while speaking, as she had in the 149th, 151st and 153rd sessions. Unlike the others however this involved more of a feeling rather than any visual images, and made describing it difficult. It involved, Jane said, some kind of inner comprehension that she was learning something in a new way, as though some kind of undifferentiated sense was operating and soaking up information. The feeling of being inside a concept, she said finally, was as good a description as any. As she has mentioned before, she believes she becomes aware of such concepts when Seth is dealing with material that is difficult to put into words.

(Jane resumed in the same rather fast manner, in a good voice and with her eyes closed, at 9:44.)

On a very basic level, as consciousness with a self (but no conscious "I" exists in the most minute division of consciousness), all action and all sensations and all stimuli are instantly and automatically and joyfully accepted, regardless of their nature. At this level no knowledge of threat exists.

Action at this level is conscious of itself, but the "I" differentiation is not <u>definite enough</u> to fear destruction or painful stimuli. Here we merely have action knowing itself. And knowing itself, it knows its basic indestructibility, knows its own oneness, and has no fear of destruction, for it is also part of destruction itself, from which further action will evolve.

The complicated organism which is the human personality with its physical structure, has evolved, along with many other structures, a highly differentiated "I" consciousness, whose very nature is such that it attempts to preserve the apparent boundaries of identity. To do so it chooses between actions, for the very choice, or act of choosing, and ability to do so, represents the nature of identity. But beneath this sophisticated gestalt are the simpler foundations of its being, and indeed the very acceptance of all stimuli without which identity would be impossible.

Without any acceptance of painful stimuli the structure could never maintain itself, for the atoms and molecules within the structure constantly accept painful stimuli, and suffer even joyfully, their own destruction; being aware of their own separateness <u>within</u> action, and aware of their reality within all action, and not having complicated "I" structures to maintain, there is no reason for them to fear destruction.

They are aware of themselves as a part of action, and therefore through capsule comprehension, which we have discussed, the simple atoms and molecules are aware of their own basic immortality. All this is basic knowledge, if you would understand why the personality accepts even an impeding action, or pain or illness, as a part of itself, despite the ego's resistance to pain.

We have yet to discuss pain and pleasure. However the subject will be covered thoroughly, in sessions dealing with the nature of the human personality.

Now, however, you understand the reason why even an impeding action is literally accepted by the personality as a portion of the self, and why therefore efforts must be made that will coax the personality to give up any portion of itself, if progress is to be made. Once the personality can understand that an illness has been accepted as a portion of the self, then even the ego will be an aid.

(Jane now took another long pause.)

We are also helped here by several characteristics of the personality, in that it is forever changing, and its flexibility will be of benefit. We merely want to change the direction in which it moves, or rather the direction in which some of its energy moves. It must be seen by the personality that the impeding action is a hardship on the part of the whole structure, and that this particular portion of the self is not basic to the original personality structure, but only adopted.

The longer the impeding action is accepted as a part of the self, the more serious the problem. The impeding action or illness however is *not* a part of the basic personality structure, or action gestalt, which is composed of action patterns formed since birth. Compared to this truly astounding structure, that is the result of the memory of every atom and molecule, this impeding action is relatively unimportant, and when correct methods are used, it can be dislodged without too much difficulty.

The peculiar nature of the impeding action or illness has much to do with its persistence. The whole focus of the personality can shift from constructive areas *to* a concentration of main energies in the area of the impeding action or illness. In such a case the illness actually represents a new unifying system. Now, if the old unifying system of the personality has broken down, the illness, serving as a makeshift, temporary emergency measure, may hold the integrity of the personality intact until a new constructive unifying principle replaces the original.

In this case the illness could not be called an impeding action, unless it persisted long after its purpose was served. Even then, without knowing all the facts surrounding the personality, you could make no judgment, for the illness could *still* serve by giving the personality a sense of security, being kept on hand, so to speak, as an ever-present emergency device in case the new unifying principle should fail.

This discussion will necessarily involve us with the structure of personality, and with the nature of what you call suggestibility.

I suggest your break.

(Break at 10:12. Jane was well dissociated. Her eyes had remained closed, her pace had been mostly rather fast, her voice a little stronger than usual. She used a few pauses. She resumed in the same fast manner at 10:20.)

It is therefore impossible to consider an impeding action, such as an illness, without taking into consideration the particular structure-unifying devices, subconscious and conscious personality tendencies.

In other words, an action cannot be judged as an impeding one without a thorough knowledge of the other actions that result in the makeup of any given personality. This is extremely important. To overlook this point is to risk the adoption on the part of the personality of a more serious illness.

Unifying principles are groups of actions about which the whole personality forms itself at any given time. These unifying principles may change, and do change, usually in a relatively smooth fashion, when action is allowed to flow unimpeded.

When it is not allowed to flow unimpeded, following the patterns or channels for its expression that have been evolved by the personality, then various blockages of energy occur; with such blockups of inhibited action, small blockages occur frequently, and the blockages or impediments themselves must be understood, not as something apart from the personality, but a part of the changing personality.

Indeed, oftentimes they serve to preserve the integrity of the whole psychological system, and to point out the existence of inner problems. Often they serve temporary functions, leading the personality from other more severe areas of difficulty. I am not here saying that all illness is good. I am saying that illness is a portion of the action of which any personality is composed, and therefore it is purposeful, and cannot be considered as an alien force that attacks the personality from without.

This is an extremely fascinating area of study, and one that we shall pursue rather vigorously. The whole personality must be led to choose those actions which are of the most benefit to itself as a whole, and its integrity as a unit is determined by its choices in this matter.

I will at various times use as an example your friend's ulcer, simply because the ulcer represents an excellent example of an impeding action or illness. It must therefore be clearly understood that an impeding illness is a creation of the personality itself. The very effectiveness and nature of the personality, and health of the personality, is dependent upon the manner in which it handles its ability to choose between various kinds of action.

Without the choice there would be no personality. The exaltations and triumphs of the personality are as much a result of this ability to choose between actions, as are its illnesses and disasters. In <u>almost</u> all cases, impeding actions are the result of a refusal to allow action to flow unhampered in certain directions. It seeks other outlets, and these outlets are caused by fear.

I suggest a brief break, and then I will continue unless you prefer that we end the session.

("We'll take a short break then.")

(Break at 10:39. Jane was fully dissociated, she said. Her eyes had been closed, her voice good, her delivery fast. She resumed at the same fast rate at 10:44.)

Now, while it is basically true that the personality is composed of action, and that its very awareness and identity is a result of action—

("Not too fast.")

—this is not meant to imply any negation of psychological or psychic values, although these are also actions.

The personality structure can be studied from many viewpoints. We are now studying it in relation to its basic reality as action. While it may seem that the personality would be a result of a <u>series</u> of actions, this is not basically the case. The personality in actuality is simultaneous action, that is composed of actions within actions. Portions of it are conscious of its awareness as a part of action, and portions of it attempt to stand aside from action.

This attempt forms the ego, and is itself action. If illness were thrust upon action, or upon the personality from the outside, then the personality would be at the mercy of outside agencies.

Now, in so far as everything is basically action, the personality is affected by outside agencies, but in a most basic manner it <u>chooses</u> those actions which it will accept or reject.

An illness can be rejected by the personality. The <u>habit</u> of illness can be rejected. Illness is sometimes in the overall, however, beneficial. A given illness, that is, may be beneficial. When action is allowed to flow freely, then <u>neurotic</u> rejections of action will not occur; and it is neurotic rejections of action that often cause unnecessary illnesses.

For we will be involved here with a definite classification as to <u>when</u> an illness is beneficial and when it is detrimental. This will be most important. An illness is almost always the result of another action that cannot be carried through.

When the lines to the original action are released and the channels opened to it, the illness will vanish. In some cases however, you see, the thwarted action may be one with disastrous consequences, which the illness may prevent. The personality has a logic of its own. We will be involved for many sessions to come with these problems, for they are of basic value, and practical value.

We will, then, later discuss the manner in which the difference can be seen between a beneficial illness, and a severely detrimental one. We will see how a temporarily necessary illness can be greatly lessened, and the symptoms minimized, while the illness is <u>still</u> retained as a temporary emergency measure, and then gradually allowed to disappear when its presence becomes unnecessary.

We will also see how an unnecessary and detrimental illness, that does not serve such a purpose, can be dismissed.

I will now end the session, but it will indeed serve as a basis for many discussions, concerning the relationship between action, suggestion, personality, illness and health.

My fondest regards to you both.

("Good night, Seth.")

(End at 11:00. Jane was again well dissociated. Her delivery had been fast, her eyes closed all the time, her voice good.)

SESSION 165
JUNE 28, 1965 9 PM MONDAY AS SCHEDULED

(It was a very hot and humid night, but in order to avoid interruptions we held the session in our small back room. I was affected by the heat much more than Jane was; as usual, she seemed almost impervious to such distractions while she was in trance.

(Jane's eyes remained closed for the whole session. Her voice was quiet, her delivery rather fast. She used a few pauses, none of them very long.)

Good evening.

("Good evening, Seth.")

I would like to continue with our discussion concerning the nature of the human personality in its relationship to action, and in connection with the matter of illness and health in general.

This will be, I trust, a quiet and peaceful session.

It must be thoroughly understood that under no circumstances is the personality a static or motionless construction. It is, instead, a collection of spontaneous actions. Only when it is viewed in this perspective can you begin to understand how it forms its own health. All basic adjustments to the personality, in a basic manner, must come from within, through regroupings of characteristic actions about unifying principles.

The personality itself exists in many dimensions, as you know, and it has its reality within many other fields than the physical field, and is indeed basically not nearly as allied with the physical field as you may imagine. These unifying principles of which I spoke are themselves main, dominating groups of actions, about which the main energies of the personality group themselves.

These unifying principles themselves, however, constantly and imperceptibly change. Upon another occasion we will consider the ways in which these unifying principles may shift. In many cases it may appear as if exterior circumstances formed such inner shifts, changing the whole unifying structure of the personality, and shifting the personality into what would appear to be entirely uncharacteristic activities.

In such a case, however, the shiftings still come from within. The active gestalt of the personality is indeed so complex, the actions that compose it are so intertwined, that only the deep, interior intuitions of the personality involved will ever come close to a complete understanding of the workings of the particular personality system.

Such understanding simply cannot follow logical lines. The intellect may indeed grasp some of this understanding from the intuitions, but the intellect itself is aware of only minute portions of the whole personality. Again, this is not meant to minimize the value of the intellect. The fact remains that answers sought by a personality can only be found through a traveling within the actions that compose the self. Within our last session, I explained some of the basic psychological heritage that resides within the action makeup of the personality. There is no escaping this heritage, and it is so important that without it the personality system could not be built up.

I spoke, for example, of the acquiescence of action at certain levels to any kind of stimuli, indiscriminately, whether painful or pleasurable. Without this basic acquiescence, actions would not have been given the freedom to break patterns down and evolve new ones of them. This is not necessarily a more primitive aspect. It is simply a basic characteristic of action at certain levels, and the human personality, with its complicated ego structure, is nevertheless composed of many actions that operate at this level.

In a most basic manner, a denial of stimuli is a negative action, if any action could be called negative. I do not, of course, speak in human terms, where every stimuli for example should then be followed or sought out indiscriminately. This is not my meaning. I am talking of deeper biological levels, and indeed of levels that are buried within tissue itself.

The very nature of the ego and of the personality is formed by the ability to choose between actions or stimuli; but life as it is not connected to a highly differentiated ego, rejoices in all stimuli, as sensation, whether it is pleasurable or painful, for these distinctions do not exist in your terms. In the beginning of our sessions I spoke in a general manner, for example, saying that trees and plant life had a consciousness, but not a developed ego system. The tree, therefore, is conscious of the pain connected with, say, the severing of a limb.

(See the 18th session, in Volume 1.)

It does not fear destruction however, as the ego does. It still fights for survival, of course; but the consciousness of plant life involves a consciousness of self as it operates within action. It sees or feels itself as a part of continuing action, and because of this inner atomic knowledge it does not fear destruction, basically, knowing that it will be changed into other kinds of action.

Its identity is within action. To say that its identity and its continuity or sense of continuity is within action, is not too far off, although the word continuity in this instance would be misleading.

I suggest your break.

(Break at 9:26. Jane was dissociated more than usual for a first delivery. She had been quite comfortable on this hot and humid evening. She resumed in the same quiet and fast manner, with her eyes closed, at 9:36.)

It is only lately that your psychologists have even begun to understand the connection between biology and personality, and they understand it in only the most simple of terms.

To begin with, not enough is understood about the biological structure, for the nature of the atoms and molecules that form the biological structure is still largely misunderstood, and very little has been done in this field.

("Not too fast.")

The personality exists in a diffused fashion within the physical system, and it therefore is most basically composed of those biological heritages, and those heritages that are a property of cellular structure, long preceding multicellular existence.

We have to some extent explained the reality of the personality within the electrical system. We have to some extent explained its basic origin within inner reality. We have explained the fact that the potentialities of the personality and of the self are basically unlimited. But during its alliance within the physical system, it is diffused within the cellular structure, and interrelating actions between the biological system, the electrical system, and the personality structure actually form the reality of the human individual.

(See the following sessions in Volume 3 for material on the electrical system: 122 to 128, 131, 135, among others, and 162, 164 in Volume 4.)

You cannot probe into the one system without affecting the others. It is basically meaningless to consider the personality as separate from the simultaneous actions of which it is composed. The personality, as you know, has also a reality within the dream universe. It should be obvious that in a most basic and practical manner the personality however is not involved with physical time to any degree. Only a part of the personality, the ego, is so involved. It is obvious of course that the personality system will react to stimuli that seem, to the ego, to be far divorced in time. That is, the personality may react to a stimuli in the present that occurred originally twenty years ago, to the <u>ego's</u> understanding of time.

But past, present and future as such simply do not have meaning to the other aspects of the personality. The idea and reality of physical time parallels the development of the ego. Consciousness <u>of self</u>, alone, is unaware of your physical time. The physical time idea is a product of the ego's tendency to make finer distinctions in order that it can classify and categorize, and therefore identify and give permanence to its own sensations.

In most circumstances the arrangement is an excellent working operation. However, when the ego carries its categorizing tendency too far, it may reject whole areas of significant action which has been experienced by the whole personality. It may choose to reject whole areas for various reasons, usually out of a mistaken fear that the actions involved threaten the permanence of itself.

Such a rejection is definitely an impeding action. It is this rejection on the ego's part that is the basis for so-called neurosis in many cases. The fault is not that a particular action has been buried <u>by the subconscious</u>. The fault is that the ego has refused to <u>accept</u> the action from the subconscious, therefore impeding the natural flow of energy. Naturally, all actions are not recognized by the ego, nor is it necessary in any case.

It is when <u>significant</u> actions, important to the whole personality, are so rejected that the difficulties arise. It is also true however that these refusals to assimilate action on the ego's part are also an integral part of the characteristics of the personality as a whole action. In each individual, certain categories of action <u>may be</u> habitually denied. As the characteristics of a personality may be somewhat deduced from those actions which the ego accepts, so also much may be learned about any given personality by a study of those actions which the ego habitually denies.

As a rule, secondary personalities are given their energy as a <u>direct</u> result, so to speak, of a too-rigorous and rejecting ego. In many, though not all instances, such a secondary personality may represent simply the whole personality's quite healthy attempts at expression that have been too long denied. You get a regrouping of unifying principle actions, and a division of energies about two different ego systems.

It should be obvious that in Ruburt's case no such habitual rejections by his ego have backed up in this manner. The secondary personality, however, is of course a reality in many circumstances. It can be considered as an impeding action in the same manner that an illness can be considered, but its overall value, or detrimental effects must be judged, again, as with an illness, on the overall service or disservice which it performs for the whole personality.

Without such a secondary regrouping of actions for example, a much more serious open breakage, a deep personality cleavage, might in some cases result. In some cases the secondary personality is, again, an emergency measure that will eventually tide the whole personality over, allow for the expression of actions before their explosion completely disrupts the personality system; and then the secondary personality structure may be dispensed with for all practical purposes, to be recalled however upon another emergency.

In such a case the secondary personality may represent the best of the available alternatives that can be practically taken by the personality to maintain itself. The impeding action, then, would have a survival value.

In some cases of course the secondary personality would be a severely impeding one, stealing away the main energies. However, it must be understood that from the whole personality's viewpoint, a strong ego, that is a <u>dependable</u> one, and one that will also allow necessary expression, is a necessity. Therefore from the standpoint of the whole personality, the adoption of a new ego, <u>so to speak</u>, with a more practical grouping of unifying principles, could be the best solution of the previous ego, the previously dominant ego, (if it) had been an incapable one.

In this case the so-called secondary personality would express the whole personality to better advantage, and actually reinforce its permanence and identity. After your break, we will discuss the purposes of the ego to some degree.

I suggest your break.

(*Break at 10:11. Jane was well dissociated. She had thought she was speaking slowly, whereas in reality her delivery had been rather fast and quiet.*

(*The parentheses near the end of the second paragraph above indicate that the two enclosed words are missing from my notes, for whatever reason. Jane was speaking quite rapidly at the time; I could have missed them.*

(*Jane resumed in the same quiet manner, with her eyes closed, at 10:21.*)

The personality must be understood from all these viewpoints, and it must be understood as an action gestalt.

The ego must be understood as having certain general necessary characteristics. Again, it <u>must</u> attempt to see itself as apart from action, even though basically the attempt to do so must fail. The attempt however allows the ego to act as a front man, so to speak, an organized and disciplined agent to deal with physical environment for the whole personality.

A very delicate network of imbalances is here maintained. The ego must not be too rigid, or too much a disciplinarian, or it ceases to speak for the whole personality, and becomes a warden, imprisoning the main expressive urges of the deeper self. It must not on the other hand be composed of too disorganized a system of actions, for in this case it is not capable of maintaining a consistent sense of identity or purpose, and is not strong enough to act in a magnetic manner, that will attract or hold the basic energies of the personality.

As far as Ruburt's personality structure is concerned, we are extremely fortunate. The ego is secure enough, and strong enough, as an organizing agent, for the basic personality energies, so that it can allow me to communicate without fear that the personality structure will be in any way disrupted.

Indeed as you may have observed, the personality continues in a rather unruffled fashion, considering the circumstances. This is why valid communications can occur between us, and it is also the reason why such communications rarely occur, generally speaking. In the case of an insecure ego you have two immediate problems, and are involved instantly with difficulties:

The basic personality would be fearful of such communications, knowing instinctively the weakness of the ego. The ego would be extremely insecure. On the other hand, the personality would almost welcome a strong organizing force, regardless of its source, and could tend to latch onto it as much as possible. A study of secondary personalities is most fascinating, since such a study would give you an excellent idea of the manner in which the ego in general is formed, for it is but a unity of energy under auspices of the strongest actions characteristic within the given personality system.

These energies are naturally drawn from within the whole personality. What is not generally recognized is the fact that the ego itself constantly changes. It is only when the change is unusually vivid, and definitely perceivable, that you speak of secondary personalities. But the main characteristic drives of any given personality shift continually; for all its attempts in the opposite direction, the ego must change just to exist, and its very permanence is dependent upon its flexibility.

The ego, then, is as much characterized by those types of action which it habitually denies, as by those types of actions which it habitually accepts. It is not the <u>only</u> organizing aspect of the personality, however. It is simply the organizing aspect of the personality in its dealings with the physical environment. The inner ego is another organizing feature of the personality in its dealings with inner environment.

You may take a break, or you may end the session.

("I guess we'll end it then.")

I will then bid you a fond good evening, and we will for a time be concerned with the various aspects of human personality. You should find these discussions of great benefit. I enjoyed our quiet session.

("Good night, Seth.")

(End at 10:43. Jane was well dissociated, as she had been for most of the session. It took her several moments to open her eyes. My writing hand was tired from the fast pace. Apropos of this, Jane said that subjectively the session had seemed about fifteen minutes long to her.)

SESSION 166
JUNE 30, 1965   9 PM WEDNESDAY AS SCHEDULED

(John Bradley, of Williamsport, PA, was a witness to the session. John has witnessed quite a few sessions and read much of the Seth material. Indeed, John was the first to witness a session, on February 18, 1964. The last session he witnessed was on February 24, 1965. See Volumes 1 and 3. John was in an excellent mood tonight.

(The session was held in our front room, and was free from interruptions. Once again Jane spoke at a fast rate; several times I had to ask her to slow down. As is often the case with witnesses, her delivery was much more active. Although her eyes remained closed for the whole session, her voice was loud and at times quite a bit deeper than usual. She was very restless in her chair, changing position often. It will be remembered that John's entity name is Philip.)

Good evening.

("Good evening, Seth.")

([John:] "Good evening, Seth.")

My heartiest regards to our friend Philip, irregardless of his own rather frivolous good evening.

I would here like to continue our discussion concerning the nature of the personality. Joseph, if I speak too quickly, I hope I can rest assured that you will ask me to slow down.

("All right.")

As we mentioned in our last session, the personality cannot be considered alone, but it must be thought of in its relationship to action and to all those aspects of reality of which it is a part.

When it accepts an illness as a part of its own self-image, then the illness becomes an actual <u>part</u> of the reality that is the self. The personality must therefore be considered as a <u>biological</u> reality. It must also be considered as an electrical reality, as a psychological reality, for any experience is automatically translated into all these systems.

I would suggest that our friend with the ulcer read our last two previous sessions, for this will bring home to him the fact that he does indeed, literally, consider his ulcer as much a part of himself as an arm or a leg. He considers the ulcer, in fact, <u>more</u> real and necessary than an arm or a leg, since his whole life now revolves about this illness.

In such a case the whole personality structure adopts such an illness as a new unifying principle, about which life activities are then centered. That man, for all his seeming outwardness, fears to relate himself in a basic manner toward the outside environment.

(Jane smiled, and pointed to John. Her eyes were still closed. Her voice was now loud and active, with a strong edge.)

We do not have that trouble here, for here, if we may use Philip as another example, we find better balance. Philip relates himself well in an outward manner, insisting to some extent that he maintain <u>also</u> his inward integrity. I am here mentioning the two personalities and bringing them together in our discussion because they are both salesmen.

As such their positions demand outgoing natures. But one of our salesman has an ulcer and the other man does not. There are obvious reasons for this, and reasons that will allow us to delve more deeply into the nature of the human personality in general.

We will for the purposes of our discussion <u>ignore</u>, for now, certain aspects in Philip's personality, such as a deep secrecy which is indeed based on fear, because this characteristic and others will not help us progress in our particular subject matter. We will instead content ourselves with a comparison of the two personalities in regard to certain characteristic reactions, which <u>tend</u> to lead the personalities toward health or illness.

What is required of them both in their daily working lives is in many respects precisely the same. They are both excellent salesmen. They are both intimately familiar with the use of energy, in that they are able to use their own energy to affect the minds of other individuals. But their reactions are entirely different, and Philip's past life experiences prepared him for the nature of his present occupation, where he is dealing with medicinal matters.

(Seth dealt with one of John's past lives and his connection with medicine in an amusing way during the 21st session, of February 3, 1964. John knocked on our door during the session, but since we had not yet begun having witnesses, we asked him to return later. As soon as the door closed behind John, Seth went into a rather lengthy rundown on him, much to our surprise. At that time, neither Jane or I had

seen John very many times.)

He is, <u>in</u> a more basic manner than he may realize, deeply committed here. He is quite content with his ability to affect the minds of others. Our other friend, to the contrary, is afraid of this ability, and distrusts it, and is not at all committed to the product that he sells.

But this is not the only reason that one man has an ulcer and the other man has none, for we are involved here with characteristic reactions and with habits that have been engraved within each personality since last physical birth, and before. I will now suggest your break, and we will continue with this particular discussion.

The matter of the surveys will be in due time discussed, Philip. I will be glad to tell you the little that I know. I now suggest your break.

(Break at 9:20. Jane was well dissociated, far-out, she said. Her delivery had been very active, her voice loud at times, her pace fast, her eyes closed.

(She ended the session with a smile, referring to the survey discussed by John before the session began. This was a detailed psychological questionnaire that John had recently completed for his drug company, Searle. John felt that the questions were loaded, that his answers, which were very frank, would be used in considering him for advancement.

(Jane resumed in the same active manner, her eyes still closed, her voice strong, at 9:33.)

I am, as always, fascinated by your discussions with guests during your break periods.

There is much I will say at a later date, having to do with Ruburt's truly <u>idiotic</u> performance in visiting the supposed medium in your town.

It would seem to me that his nature would be somewhat above deliberately leading the poor deluded woman astray by lies. She is at best deluded and neurotic, and embarrassingly sincere.

Since when does Ruburt stoop <u>so low</u> as to make fun of fools? If anything, the woman deserves pity, and hardly scorn. I was not pleased with that performance.

(Jane smiled and frowned. Her voice now became more amused and less scornful, but not much quieter.)

On the other hand, I did watch with some amusement as the scene was enacted in a small room, and as the ghosts were supposed to materialize in the doorway. I do therefore on the one hand somewhat appreciate Ruburt's reaction. In one of my more friendly moods, I might indeed have tried a materialization of my own that would have frightened the poor woman out of her wits.

Nevertheless, I did <u>not</u> do so, and I feel duty bound to mention the fact that Ruburt's performance was dishonest, and there was no good reason for it. It would be much better for him also if he stayed <u>out</u> of the investigation that he so gleefully entered into with Peggy Gallagher, concerning the so-called mediums in your town.

In all cases that I know of, these women are indeed neurotic and misled and self-deluded. Nevertheless they harm no one. They listen where no one else will listen. They are well-meaning, and occasionally they are able to use their inner abilities.

There is nothing wrong with the idea of an investigation. Ruburt simply should not be involved in it. It is <u>not</u> his place. It is not his area, and because of his conscientiousness, and <u>hardheadedness</u>, he would be much harder on these women than is necessary. But the thought of him baiting an elderly 72-year-old self-deluded woman is too much.

(*Jane's voice grew to a near shout, briefly. She said later that she did not know the age of the woman medium being discussed here, but that she had taken it for granted it would be in the seventies.*)

We will now return to our previous discussion.

We find that Philip believes, basically, in the products that he sells. We find that the general nature of the products is related to experiences in past lives. We find that he has endless energies <u>when he wants them</u>, at his disposal.

(*Her eyes still closed, her voice again louder, Jane pointed at John Bradley.*)

We find that he relates well to the outside environment. And then we have this secrecy of which I said I would not speak. We also find, in your other friend, boundless energies and a genuine <u>ability</u> to relate to others. But the personality is torn against itself. It does not believe in what it is doing, and here we will find a comparison between this tendency toward secrecy on Philip's part, and this divided nature on the part of your other friend.

(*The other friend being Bill Gallagher. Bill and his wife Peggy have witnessed the 158th, 161st and 162nd sessions.*)

For when your other friend is relating to the exterior environment, he does something that Philip does not do. He closes himself off <u>entirely</u>, as much as possible, from the inside environment. Philip insists, in a rather cocky manner, in taking his own inner integrity along. Your other friend <u>cannot</u>, so far, relate the inner and the outer selves. He can relate to the inner self or the outer self, but he has not learned to unite the two, nor allowed for any understanding or communication between them.

When he is at work he thinks "This is not me, this is not myself." The inner self has not so far recognized this other portion of the personality. When our friend Philip sells he is thinking "This is me. You can like it or not, but <u>buy</u>

what I am selling." But he <u>believes</u> in what he is selling.

Your other friend sends a part of himself into the marketplace, and leaves the essential part of himself at home. He is an expert salesman. He enjoys selling. But he will not <u>admit</u> that he enjoys it to his own inner self. The ulcer is caused by many things, and we have discussed some of them.

It is nevertheless the <u>physical</u> materialization of this lack of communication. Its purpose is basically a <u>good</u> one. The results are obviously poor. The ulcer is an attempt to force a recognition of unity from the various levels of the self. It is, literally, a physical bridge. At this time it is an impeding action, but it can be dissolved and resolved, according to our previous discussions.

The <u>dependent</u> portion of the personality is literally appalled at the more aggressive aspects of the whole personality. In the case of Philip, we find these aggressive tendencies welcomed. But <u>because</u> basically Philip is able to unite the various levels of the self, there is no such deep and persistent physical problem. The aggressiveness is given reign and acceptance. The tendency toward division in Philip's personality shows itself in this tendency toward secrecy, which affects most deeply the nature of his home life.

You may take a break if you prefer, or I will continue with the session.

("We'll take the break.")

As you wish.

(Break at 10:00. Jane was again well dissociated. Her pace had been fast, and my writing hand was tiring. I had already asked Seth to slow down several times, and now at break asked Jane, as Jane, to see what she could do about the problem. In recent sessions her rate of speaking has pushed my writing ability to the limit, even with the rather elaborate system of symbols and abbreviations I have evolved for taking down the sessions.

(Jane began at a pace slightly slower, in the same strong and active voice, with her eyes again closed, at 10:15.)

As Philip suspected, his questionnaire is indeed loaded.

However, the fact that it <u>is</u> so set up does not change the earlier predictions which I have made. There will be a definite demand that changes be made because of the financial losses that are being suffered.

This will not happen overnight, but it has already begun; and the forces that are now working toward such a reorganization will suffer, within six months, a seeming downfall from which, however, they will indeed recover.

The recovery process will take a year but the forces then will be very strong, and the reorganization is inevitable.

("Not too fast.")

Within five years there will be a definite change in Philip's place of employment and living area, when he will accept a much better position, and wholeheartedly.

The reorganization however will occur <u>before</u> this time, and there will be talk of changes for him, as there have been, and some minor changes will occur. But the main change in Philip's condition with the company will not occur until after the inevitable reorganization.

It will occur within six months to one year after the reorganization. My idea of time is obviously not your own, and I cannot at this moment pinpoint the particular date. Also, there are some variables which cannot be adequately predicted because of conditions that will change drastically the attitudes of two men within the organization, and also a death which will occur in the higher organizational realm.

At the time of the reorganization those who have spoken out will be sought out, and <u>those</u> who did not speak out will be on the firing line. Again, I am not sure of the date of the death that will be involved here. It will occur within a year and a half, and perhaps within six months. The repercussions will not be immediately felt, but they will be one of the basic causes that will lead officials to decide upon such a reorganization.

(*John Bradley has witnessed the following sessions: 37, 54, 63, 70, 95, 135, and 166, the present one. In most of these Seth has dealt with John's connection with Searle to at least some degree, making the type of predictions he makes in this session. To sort out the rather complicated pattern of these predictions would require a study of the above sessions. To date John has agreed with their content, but most of them are of such long range that little has yet developed against which to check.*)

Philip's connection with the conservative groups, politically speaking, will strangely enough have something to do with the promotion which can be later expected. This connection will not have to do with the fact that his group is conservative, necessarily, but will have to do with the fact that he exerts leadership in that area.

His political movements are being closely watched by one man in particular, but the interest is being caused by his ability to organize, rather than because the political movement involved is a conservative one.

Oddly enough, the fact that the movement is conservative will work to his advantage in very strange ways. Though they may not agree with his political beliefs, they will on the other hand trust his integrity because the movement <u>is</u> conservative. They do not believe that he would follow an unpopular cause unless he believed in it. They will want a man who is sincere. They will also want a man who can lead. They will be afraid of a liberal. I hope that this is sufficient. After our next break I will give you what additional information I have. You may take a break, or we will continue with our session.

("We'll take the break.")

I should from here on call you "I will take a break Joseph." I do, however, appreciate the work that you give to our sessions, and if you will forgive my humor I will forgive yours, as I sometimes am acquainted with it on those few occasions when I look in on you between sessions. By all means take your break, and if you prefer I will then continue.

(Break at 10:32. Jane was again well dissociated. She ended the delivery with a smile. Her pace of dictation had been so fast recently that I took a break whenever I could.

(It might be noted that I again detected traces of what I call a brogue in Jane's manner of speaking this evening, and thought it more pronounced as the session wore on. She does not have this characteristic usually. This brogue had been quite pronounced at times during the 162nd session, witnessed by Lorraine Shafer and Bill and Peggy Gallagher, and I have noted traces of it during subsequent sessions.

(This accent has been apparent in other sessions in a minor way at times. Perhaps I am more conscious of it recently because of the two Father Trainor episodes. See the 131st and the 158th sessions. During these readings Jane's brogue was unmistakable. Jane grew up in an Irish neighborhood in Saratoga Springs, NY, and is a quarter Irish. She had no father at home, growing up as a child, but Father Trainor, a frequent visitor, was Irish.

(John Bradley said he was thoroughly convinced that a reorganization would have to take place in his company, that great financial losses were being suffered. This theme has run through Seth's predictions concerning John's company for the past year or so. John himself has suffered some paper losses in stock values, and is of course concerned.

(Jane resumed with her eyes again closed, and in a somewhat quieter but still fast voice, at 10:43.)

We will shortly conclude our session.

However I will add a few notes. Philip is now being seriously watched and considered for another position. His immediate superior is basically not his friend, although personally they may get along well. It is others in higher positions who are watching him.

("Not too fast.")

I will endeavor to speak more slowly, and I will be directed in this respect Joseph by you, if you will make your wishes known during the delivery. There is one other company in particular with whom Philip could become involved to his advantage.

It is situated in the Midwest, perhaps in Minneapolis. It is presently a small firm, comparatively speaking, but it will expand drastically within a short time. He will become involved with this company I believe irregardless, either as a competitor or as a member of the organization.

(Jane's brogue was now becoming more pronounced again.)

If he uses his patience it will be for his best advantage, <u>everything</u> taken into consideration, to remain with his present company, and his impatience will not serve him well if he leaps too fast.

The stock of his present company will drop still further. This will be another reason for the inevitable reorganization. The stock will go very low, and it will be this financial loss that will make the reorganization itself come about. The head man within the company will suffer a loss of power, although he may retain his title.

(As of July 3rd, G. D. Searle stock closed at 54 1/2. John told us that a few months ago it had been in the low 60's.)

Philip should not stray from the medical field, although for various reasons he would not function well as a physician. He will always be able to deal with physicians however, to his advantage and theirs. If he puts his efforts <u>into</u> the company, and his energy, he can go as far within it as he desires.

I will not give any further information this evening concerning these matters, but he may check with me from time to time if he so desires. There is a short man of whom he should beware. I will now conclude our session.

My heartiest and best wishes to you all. If you prefer you may take a break and continue it as you wish. I am always at your beck and call.

("We'll say good night.

(End at 10:50. Jane was well dissociated—far-out, again. Her eyes had remained closed, her voice had been a little quieter.

(John did not know of any smaller drug company near Minneapolis, he said, but could check that area in a directory in the library of his hometown, Williamsport, PA. We usually see him every month or six weeks; if he unearths some pertinent information he will let us know by a card or letter so that it can be inserted in the record.

(John agreed with Seth's statement, concerning his immediate superior not being, basically, his friend. He had not told Jane and I this, although we had met the individual in question once, briefly, here in Elmira at an art show. John had no idea of a short man of whom he should beware.

(The three of us were discussing the session and related matters when Seth abruptly came through again. Resume at 11:10.)

The fact that Philip has become involved with a political movement will indeed, of itself, have much to do with the promotion that will follow <u>if</u> he waits for it.

There was in the past disagreement as to his capability in the field of human relationships, as far as the ordinary person is concerned. The impetus that allowed him to become involved is only too well now recognized within the company.

There is an individual within the political organization who, all unwittingly, gives information to Philip's superiors through a family in-law relationship. If Philip for any reason allows his enthusiasm for this political group to wane, this will reduce his chances for advancement within the company, for it will be taken as a mark of fleeting interests.

Philip would do well in his home relationships to be more open, for there is a possibility that his secretiveness could here cause serious difficulties. The home relationship is a strong basis for his inner security, and if he threatens it this will be seriously reflected in his other areas of activity.

(End at 11:14. Jane was fully dissociated. She had no idea of the material. The delivery was totally unexpected, she said, a complete surprise to her. I was also surprised. Jane's eyes had remained closed; her voice had been rather loud and fast.

(John agreed with Seth. He said that as far back as last January his suspicions had become aroused, when one of his superiors had mentioned John's involvement with a political organization. John had not told anyone in the company about his activities in politics at that time. From what Seth said in the above delivery, John now believes he knows who the individual is who might be passing along information about him.)

SESSION 167
JULY 5, 1965 9 PM MONDAY AS SCHEDULED

(The session was held in our quiet back room. Jane spoke while sitting down and with her eyes closed for the entire session. Her voice was quiet, picking up a little volume as the session progressed. Her speed of dictation was slow, with pauses, in the beginning, but by first break had attained its usual rather fast pace.)

Good evening.

("Good evening, Seth.")

The personality must always be considered as motion, for no aspects of it are ever still.

With the exception of the ego, the various parts of the personality do not react to time as a series of moments. All is experienced as present. The child therefore within the adult personality is not dead, nor are his reactions considered, basically, as reactions which are part of a past behavior pattern; but these reactions exist side by side with adult reactions.

This should be clearly understood, yet the personality is far from static. But what it was always changes, but that which was is always taken along.

We are going to have a brief session this evening for several reasons, but there were a few points considering the personality which I did want to make clear.

That which was is constantly taken into what you call the present. The ego may choose to use or not use various reactions. It may reject various reactions as a part of the past, for it is the ego alone who is concerned with past, present and future. The ego's denial of a reaction however does not cause the reaction to disappear from within the personality, at least as part of possible pattern reaction.

Many reactions, many patterns of reactions, are rejected by the ego upon some occasions and accepted upon other occasions, but as a rule such alternate behavior is annoying to the ego itself. The ego deals with cause and effect, and often denies particular reactions because it decides that they are not effective. The ego is fairly rigid, comparatively speaking. Rationalization is one method by which the ego justifies its acceptance of a reaction which it once rejected as ineffective.

Such alternative reactions frighten the ego because they seem to injure the ego's self-image. Yet all characteristic reactions, whether denied by the ego or not, are kept for use as alternative actions. In many cases actions unacceptable to the ego may be precisely those actions that are necessary for whole other areas of the personality. When too many actions are restricted by the ego, they may begin to form impulse patterns or groupings of various rejected impulses. These then adhere through attraction, and attempt to find expression regardless of the ego's attempts to restrict expression.

The ego must act therefore as a director of activity in the personality's relationships with the physical environment. The ego is concerned with purposeful action. However when the ego is too restrictive its conception of purposeful action becomes so narrow that many legitimate and necessary impulses are dammed up, forming these rejected action patterns.

As the number of rejected impulses grows, more and more energy is of course concentrated in this area, the energy that is inherent within the impulses themselves. This sort of grouping together of rejected impulses will occur mainly when the ego's restrictions are too severe, so hampering that very deep and basic needs of the whole personality are being denied expression. It is therefore for the benefit of the whole personality that these impulses be given expression.

I suggest your break.

(Break at 9:16. Jane was well dissociated for a first break. Her eyes had remained closed and her delivery had speeded up considerably. She resumed in the same manner at 9:23.)

In many instances the ego then feels a lessening of available energy and a definite shortage of energy may occur, so that the ego finds it more difficult to handle its relationships with the outside environment.

It feels the concentration of energy that has collected to form the rejected action patterns, and indeed it may feel that this unified rejection pattern is then even an enemy to its own superiority. It may, with more force than ever, attempt to hold back the expression of these impulses, and its fear of them grows.

The rejected action patterns, however, will find outlet. The nature of the outlet will be the result of the nature of the particular patterns themselves. The quality of the outlet will depend upon the intensity of these patterns, and the necessity or the degree of necessity, for their expression. Unless some adjustments are made at this point, the ego will have nothing to say with the direction that these patterns may take, simply because it will not accept their legitimacy.

The strength of the ego of course is also a factor here. If the ego is not a particularly strong one to begin with however, the conflict will seldom reach these proportions. Instead the ego will merely be slightly surprised at behavior which it does not condone, but eventually will accept because it has been forced to recognize its reality.

When the ego is a very rigid one however, it will not accept the reality of these rejected patterns so easily, and according to the nature of its rigidity it may restrict so many areas of activity that the inside action, or the inside impetus for expression, almost equally balances the ego force itself.

As this point is reached the ego obviously becomes more disturbed. In very few cases however does the conflict reach this sort of proportion. A lack of communication between the ego and the inner self is obviously one of the main causes for such difficulties.

We will use tonight's material as a basis for some other discussions. This evening's session will be a brief one. We will hold Wednesday's session as usual. I am interested here with a regeneration of energies at this time. I am indeed pleased that this was a quiet session, and I prefer that sessions this week be fairly brief. You can both use the rest, and regenerate your energies. You may need them.

("Why?"

(Jane smiled, her eyes still closed.)

I anticipated you would ask the question when I made the statement.

It was no coincidence that you both took today off. The freedom was excellent for you both, and I am simply giving you the opportunity to regenerate your energies. They are not at low ebb, but an excess of energy will serve you both well during your symposium.

We will hold Wednesday's session, however. I will now bid you a fond good evening, and my best wishes to you both. We have had quite intensive sessions for some time now, and I simply prefer that you are allowed a rest before your trip.

There is something here we will discuss at a later date, concerning the rhythms within these sessions, for they follow certain inner rhythms of activity, and I am always concerned that we use these to advantage. In some cases this entails longer and more intensive sessions. At other times it involves shorter sessions, particularly when I have *some* eye out for future events. My best regards now, and good evening.

("Good night, Seth.")

(End at 9:44. Jane was again well dissociated.

(I was tempted to try to obtain more information from Seth about immediately future events, following up his own hints, but did not do so because he called for a short session. Jane and I leave Elmira this Friday, July 9, to attend the Hypnosis Symposium at New York's Oswego State University College on July 9, 10 and 11.)

SESSION 168
JULY 7, 1965 9 PM WEDNESDAY AS SCHEDULED

(Lorraine Shafer and Bill and Peggy Gallagher were witnesses for the session. Lorraine has witnessed the 144th and 162nd sessions, the Gallaghers the 158th, 161st and 162nd sessions.

(The session was again held in our front room, with all of us sitting in a circle. Jane's eyes remained closed for the whole session. She spoke while sitting down, and in a voice a bit stronger than usual. Her manner was quite active and much of the time she leaned forward, elbows on her knees. We anticipated a short session. Jane actually began speaking at 8:56.)

May I now wish you all the heartiest of greetings.

I am pleased with our group. However this will be a short session. It is not because I grow weary. It is merely, again, that I must watch for your human limitations, and it will be best that you have all available energy at your beck and call later on for your trip.

Whenever it is possible, I would suggest that our gentleman with the ulcer read our last sessions. Indeed, I believe that he has somewhat *less* of an ulcer now, although the degree is slight. I will also, if I may, congratulate the writer of the newspaper article, even though my own name was nowhere mentioned, for it goes without saying that I am indeed truly humble.

(*Jane's voice was quite amused. The reference here is to the story Peggy Gallagher wrote for the Elmira Star-Gazette concerning Jane's ESP book. It was excellently done, and was printed on July 6.*)

We will not involve ourselves with any deep and weighty matters this evening, and you may slow me down, Joseph, when you prefer. You will find, incidentally, that within a fairly short time that the stock of which we have spoken will take a quite severe drop, after which it will slowly rise.

(*See the 166th session, which John Bradley witnessed. Seth discussed John's drug-company employer, G. D. Searle, during the session, and stated then that Searle stock was due to fall still more. As of today, July 7, 1965, the stock closed at 55.*)

There will be three people in particular with whom you will be involved at your meeting, three men. One of these will be younger than the others. There is, I believe, a book which you will be asked to read, and there will be an appointment made. As you suspect, there was no coincidence involved when you chose your Dr. Instream. The affair will work out much better now, for in the past circumstances would have prevented not his interest, but his availability. There will indeed be a change that is only now beginning, in the daily <u>ways</u> of your lives, and you are both subconsciously preparing yourselves.

The changes <u>will not</u> suddenly show themselves. This is merely a slow beginning, but the initial steps have been made, and the first and initial program has been completed. It is developing even better than I had hoped, and our own material will now begin to really develop, for we have enough background to enable us to cover subject matter that would have been impossible at an earlier time. But the first portion of our program has been completed in many other ways, having to do with the development of abilities, and with the development of that gestalt which we now form.

I will suggest your break, and we will then at least briefly continue. I would here add however that those others in this room have <u>also</u> helped us in at least one phase of our program. Take your break, and we will then continue.

(*Break at 9:11. Jane reported that she was fairly well dissociated for a first delivery. Her voice had again acquired a touch of that peculiar accent, or brogue as I call it. She resumed in the same active manner, with a bit louder voice, at 9:19.*)

It was from the beginning necessary not only that Ruburt's abilities be developed, but also that Ruburt's <u>ego</u> not be left in the dark.

His ego is indeed a healthy and vigorous one, but of a <u>stubborn</u> bent. For our purposes however this is actually excellent, for he is learning effectively to operate <u>well</u> in the physical environment while at the same time he is manipulating within that inner reality.

This is a difficult procedure, and in all cases and in all developments of this nature, there must be no attempt made to browbeat the ego, for in this way lies schizophrenia and disorientation. Ruburt's abilities now are <u>beginning</u> to develop. We are sure of our foundation, and this was most necessary.

We can now begin shortly on other aspects of our program, the second. You are not unfamiliar with this program, Joseph, nor indeed is Ruburt. Your own inner knowledge is most adequate. It is Ruburt's independent ego that is here a <u>strong</u> helpmate to us, for since we have taken it into consideration it allows us leeway while automatically keeping the whole personality in good balance.

His abilities will indeed improve to a large degree. Your own strength and balance and inner abilities provide a large part of the psychological climate in which we can operate. You also act, in that you provide both added energy and help Ruburt to receive these communications. I have promised you that I would explain more clearly the nature both of your abilities and their part in our venture, and so I will.

I mentioned if you recall Peggy Gallagher last year; and the couple, I knew, had peculiar abilities that would help us here.

(See the 63rd session in Volume 2. Jane now smiled and turned toward Lorraine Shafer. Her eyes were still closed.)

There will be not, <u>not</u> answers, but questions, shortly for our other guest. We shall provide the questions, and <u>she</u> shall provide the answers. She is asking the wrong questions, and the answers to them will not help her.

We will also have more to say concerning the ways in which such a gestalt as this is composed. Again, I will let you take a break, for I am dealing relatively easily with you this evening, and then we will again continue.

(Break at 9:30. Jane was fairly well dissociated. Her voice had acquired a strong edge and had been fairly loud. Concerning her accent, which I have called a brogue, Lorraine and Bill Gallagher said they thought of it as a cultivated, well-educated accent acquired perhaps by one who had spent some time in Ireland, for instance, then moved on to live in another country—England, for instance.

(Lorraine was not consciously aware of the questions she has evidently been considering, according to Seth, although she said she is aware of the ideas she has about the Seth material.

(Jane resumed in the same manner, leaning forward in her chair and with her eyes closed, at 9:40.)

I was not speaking of specific questions. I did not think that our guest had a list of questions from one to ten, which I was being asked to consider.

I was speaking of those questions which our guest asks herself, and these are the questions that she subconsciously would like me to answer. We will go into these matters again upon another occasion.

There are a few other remarks that I would make concerning your journey. First of all, although I said earlier that Ruburt should not take a vacation, in many respects he will not be taking a vacation. He will have much to do.

(Here Jane smiled broadly, then sat quietly for a moment.)

You can also be of aid, both of you, as far as your brother Bill is concerned, Joseph, and I suggest that you take steps to speak with him, and if necessary we will hold a session, <u>if</u> the circumstances are correct for our purposes.

I see you also in a group of four. <u>If</u> there are five, the fifth will be a woman, and one man in this group will later be of benefit to us. I am pleased indeed that we have come so far in such a brief time. We have done well, particularly since the foundations for this sort of venture are so important. We can now go forward, fairly certain that Ruburt is strong enough to carry the burden. It is more than worth his while.

I regret that you yourself have been so necessarily preoccupied of late, in preparation for your journey. And yet Joseph, this is also well worth your while.

I am taking the opportunity to speak concerning these matters, since I had already decided not to cover any complicated material for our session. I am also giving you more frequent breaks, since I am again aware that your energies will be needed. Our material in general however can now expand; and indeed, though not always, some extra dimensions and perspectives may be added to our sessions.

I anticipate meeting the distinguished company.

I here suggest your break, for I am not going to give you a preview. You have much to look forward to. By all means take your break. And you will see, Joseph, that I am not overworking your fingers.

(Break at 9:55. Jane was well dissociated as usual. The discussion that followed during break was very lively. Jane's voice had been loud last delivery, and active; and she resumed in the same manner, smiling often, at 10:05.)

As always, I find myself amazed at your discussions, and I always seem to be lurking somewhere in their shadows.

I am as you know a rather humorous gentleman. But <u>someday</u> we will have jokes that are not on me. You have not heard me laugh yet. It can however be arranged, according to the circumstances; for I do not laugh unless there is something worth laughing at, and we can arrange a good-natured harmless but <u>amusing</u> joke, at no one's expense.

SESSION 168   129

(Jane's voice had been climbing the scale somewhat as far as volume went, and her rather fast delivery became even faster. Seth/Jane was highly amused while delivering the above paragraph. Strangely, as far as I recall no one had ever mentioned the possibility of Seth laughing, myself included.)

It is only when I am not concerned with our weighty material that I can afford thinking in these directions. The second phase of our program will include definite expansions in the scope of our general material. It will show expansions in the manner in which we allow ourselves to operate. We will have greater leeway, and this is to the good.

To a large measure Ruburt's confidence has been won. It was most necessary that we go slowly, particularly in the beginning, for if our foundation was not strong we would have never progressed. The whole venture would have been lost. There is no fate in these matters. Our venture was not fated to be. Our venture represents gestalts of energy coming together in quite natural manners. It was necessary however that we meet in such a manner without clashing.

Many sessions ago we spoke of transparency, and I said that <u>true</u> transparency was <u>not</u> the ability to see through, but to <u>move</u> through.

(See the 12th session in Volume 1.)

Energy moves through all fields and all systems. You are enabling the energy which is yourself to realize its existence within other systems; and speaking merely in terms of energy and action, we are here involved with transparent motion as energy moves from one system to another.

This is not done at <u>all</u> times, but the ego is not usually aware either of the motion nor of the other systems involved. Through your own abilities, and partially through circumstances that happen to be favorable, you are able with my help, to some degree, to add this experience of mobility to your natures and transfer the knowledge to the conscious ego.

We will later be concerned more deeply with this transparent mobility, for it operates within all systems. And without it your own physical system would not exist. When the nature and behavior of energy as it is seen in action is understood, and when it is applied to the mobility of the human personality, then such sessions as ours will be taken for granted, though this I admit will take a while.

I will now let you take a break, or as you prefer you may close the session.

("We'll close it then.")

(Seth/Jane smiled.)

I will then meet with you shortly. My best regards and heartiest good wishes to you all.

("Good night, Seth.")

(*End at 10:20. Jane had been well dissociated as usual. A lively discussion now developed among us as to the nature and possible origin of the brogue or accent Jane had displayed during most of the session.*

(*The discussion was sparked because of Seth/Jane's pronunciation of the words "fate" and "stock" in particular, and others similar. Bill and Lorraine did not believe the accent to be Irish, even considering Jane's early years in an Irish neighborhood and her association with Irish priests.*

(*Bill Gallagher knows something about languages. He made so many good points that I asked him to write them down for the record. He had just begun when Seth came through again, loud and clear. Jane's voice was strong but not close to matching the rather spectacular 158th session, for example. It was obvious that she and Seth enjoyed the proceedings immensely. She spoke rapidly and used many gestures, but her eyes remained closed throughout. Resume at 10:44.*)

I am not going to hold you up. However, I see that our group will have its Jesuit member.

(*Bill Gallagher's head went back in a soundless laugh.*)

I shall be discussed from all angles, and scrutinized, and like the monks in the Middle Ages we will wonder if I can fit on the head of a pin, but I will not get stuck. I am indeed flattered, and as Ruburt mentioned a change of perspective is good.

The inquiring mind of our Jesuit member is indeed refreshing, and the very inquiry does him good. He hit upon several excellent points, and he will discover more. I enjoy this Jesuit; and for Ruburt's benefit I will indeed tell you that the likeness that you have painted of me, Joseph, is excellent.

(*Her eyes still closed, Jane pointed to a portrait I had just hung. It was of a short heavyset bald man, beckoning to the viewer to come closer. I had been working on it for some weeks.*

(*The idea for it had come to me one day and I had begun work on it at once. In view of some rather odd sensations it had engendered within me I had thought it might refer to Seth, or myself in a previous life. Jane had admired it at once, even from the first drawing, and insisted all along that it pictured Seth.*

(*It is of interest here to note that in the 134th session Seth also announced that I had painted a likeness of him. This painting shows a much younger blond man, bearing no resemblance to the other portrait. I have not asked Seth about the discrepancy yet of course, but Jane feels they both represent different facets of the Seth entity or personality.*)

I knew that Ruburt would recognize me, and the word fate is pronounced fate.

(*This play upon words, in Seth/Jane's peculiar accent, brought forth laughter from the group.)*

I will now, with my true dignity, bring this fateful session to a close. I would continue but for my innate good manners. I will at another occasion give our Jesuit some rather fateful measures to contemplate, and perhaps we will ask him how many ulcers can sit on the head of a pin. My best and most sincere wishes to you all. I will sign myself <u>fatefully</u> yours.

("Good night, Seth."

(End at 10:55. Jane was well dissociated. She took quite a few moments to open her eyes. She said a word Bill had used had started her off again, to her own surprise. Bill said Seth used the Jesuit simile to make his point very well. He also said his ulcer had been much improved lately; it had bothered him a little earlier today, for instance, but hardly at all this evening.

(Jane was keenly aware of Seth's emotions during the above delivery, she said, and as always it made the delivery most enjoyable. When this involvement takes place, she feels reserves of energy sweeping her along, welling up from Seth, even when she might feel tired to begin with.)

(My sensation of Friday night, July 9, 1965.

(Sometime during the night while sleeping in Johnson Hall, a residence hall at Oswego State University College, I was awakened by some noisy students in a nearby hall. It was raining and I lay in a pleasant drowsy state.

(I then began to feel an enlargement in both of my hands, and in the left side of my face as it lay upon the pillow. The sensation progressed to a remarkable degree, lasted for well over five minutes by my estimation, and was unmistakable. The feeling grew until each of my fingers felt themselves to be <u>several inches</u> in diameter. I could literally feel or sense their greatly-enlarged diameters.

(At the same time, I would get the feeling that the fingers of each hand were united or combined into thick clublike paws, as though I was wearing great baseball gloves. The two sensations were sometimes apparent together. Either or both were very pleasant after the strangeness disappeared, and I lay quietly and deliberately did my best to analyze and remember each sensation. The sensation finally dwindled slowly away.

(I recalled, also, that as I was drifting off to sleep upon retiring that evening, I had been aware of a slight sensation of tingling or thrilling in my hands. This mild sensation has been a rather standard one for me during psychological time, when presumably I was in a light state of dissociation. This was by far the most pronounced feeling of enlargement that I have experienced, and is separate from the other strong bodily sensations of thrilling, or the feeling of sound as Seth describes it, that I have known upon a few occasions.

(For data on my other sensations and some visions, see the following sessions:

22, 24, 26, 27, 65, 145, 146, 163. These would not include, either, the "fat hands" sensations that Jane and I experienced during sessions.)

SESSION 169
JULY 12, 1965 1:37 PM MONDAY UNSCHEDULED

(Jane and I attended the Hypnosis Symposium at Oswego State University College at Oswego, NY, on Friday evening, July 9th, and on Saturday and Sunday, July 10 and 11, at the invitation of Dr. Instream, codirector. I had written to Dr. Instream on June 1, 1965 and sent him sessions 138, 141, 142, 149, 153 and 154, plus lists of the inner senses and the basic laws of the inner universe as defined by Seth. [Jane calls the good doctor Instream in The Seth Material, © 1970.]

(We had no real opportunity to talk with Dr. Instream until Sunday evening at his home, after the symposium was over. During our discussion Dr. Instream revealed that he had mailed the sessions listed above to his friend Dr. Gardner Murphy, at the Menninger Clinic in Topeka, Kansas, and asked for his opinion. Jane and I answered Dr. Instream's questions as well as we could, and made an appointment to attend his Monday morning class at the college. This was to be followed by lunch with him before we left to visit my brother Bill in Rochester.

(To digress a moment: As predicted by Seth in the 168th session of July 7, Jane and I did find ourselves involved with three men in particular, one of whom is younger, at the symposium. Two of these men are physicians in their fifties, with whom we became rather well acquainted at lunches, etc., and exchanged addresses. The third man is a psychology instructor at the college, perhaps in his late thirties. On Saturday evening he leafed through some of the Seth material briefly, then pronounced it the work of a clever schizophrenic. This upset Jane briefly but she recovered well. During our Sunday evening visit, Dr. Instream demolished the young psychologist's diagnosis rather easily.

(Seth also said in the 168th session that we would make an appointment, as we obviously did to see Dr. Instream privately. Over coffee Monday, Dr. Instream asked if we had read F. W. H. Myers' Human Personality. Seth had said we would be asked to read a book, but Dr. Instream did not insist that we read this work. We also bought two books by Dr. Instream at the college bookstore Monday noon.

(We lunched with Dr. Instream at Howard Johnson's, adjacent to the campus. This interlude was longer than we had anticipated, and after the talk had dealt with matters psychic for some little time Jane announced that she felt uneasy. She thought Seth could give a session. Dr. Instream then suggested that we go to his office where it would be private and quiet.

SESSION 169

(This is but the second session we have held outside of Elmira, the other being the 89th, of September 19, 1964, held at my brother's home in Rochester, NY, before three witnesses. Jane was now a little concerned at having a session away from home and in daylight. At the same time she had wanted to hold a session for Dr. Instream, feeling this would explain more about the sessions than any other method could.

(Jane began speaking while sitting down and with her eyes closed. Her eyes remained closed for the entire session. Her voice was stronger than normal, and echoed somewhat in the crowded office. At times it became louder, but never approached the volume of the 158th session, for example. Her pace was rather fast, and she used many gestures while speaking as Seth. I had to ask Seth to slow down several times during the first part of the session.

(This first part of the session is verbatim as usual, until the interchange between Seth and Dr. Instream began at 1:59. Here the pace began to speed up as the two talked back and forth, and in the interests of spontaneity, and because this was a new development in the sessions, I made no attempt to slow Seth down, nor to record every word Seth or Dr. Instream spoke.

(Instead I took down the gist of their conversation, key words and phrases, and thus captured most of what they said. No major topics of conversation, for instance, were lost. Jane and I also left with Dr. Instream at his home on Sunday evening, copies of sessions 150, 151, 158, 160, 162, 164 and 165.)

I would like to give my greetings to Doctor Instream.

We are working here indeed with human limitations. However, within the range of human limitations there is indeed much that can be done.

My field is indeed education, and my particular interest is that these abilities of human personality be understood and investigated. For these are <u>not</u>, dear Doctor, these are not sudden unnatural occurrences.

We are dealing with inherent abilities of human personality, whether or not the personality is focused within physical matter, but I am indeed aware of the difficulties which shall be encountered. I appreciate your interest and concern. I have some difficulties with Ruburt's own rather stubborn attitude at times; but we must also take this into consideration, and so we shall.

I will indeed see what experiments can be made, working within the limitations that are, unfortunately, what we now have to deal with. At a future regular session, I will endeavor in a more specific manner to discuss what <u>can</u> be done here, and what cannot be done. We can do much, much we cannot do. But since we do understand both the potentialities and the limitations, then we can indeed make the best of what we have.

I have said this often, but I meet you for the first time: I am indeed no misty-eyed ghostly spirit, materializing in the middle of the night. I am simply an intelligent personality no longer bound by your physical laws. Nevertheless these are limitations, when I must accept these physical laws in order to prove to pompous nincompoops that what we, you and I, know exist does in fact exist.

I will seriously endeavor to do what I can do, considering our circumstances. We need have no worries concerning the personality with whom I work, since there is by now some sort of a rapport that will work for us. My cooperation can be counted upon. It goes without saying that all of this cannot happen overnight, but we shall begin.

I am very happy that I have been allowed to speak directly to you. There is in our material, if you will forgive my lack of humility, some hints and some specific remarks that will show the direction in which we can operate. I will be more than happy to work for our common goal when I am dealing with a personality who is not stupid, who is open-minded.

For Ruburt's and Joseph's sakes, I stayed well within the bounds of propriety. I do not overtly speak out against men who have no imagination, and little concept of any reality but their own. But if we work together, I will reserve for myself the privilege of saying to them what I choose. Otherwise I shall work well within the bounds of propriety. But if they will deal with me, so shall I deal with them.

I will not keep you. Like myself, you are a busy man. But I will see what can be done, and we shall work along those lines, taking into consideration the potential, and quite human, limitations.

I now bid you a most fond good afternoon, and thank all for the opportunity for this small discussion. I have endeavored to keep the voice somewhat under control because of the proximity of other offices. My heartiest regards to all.

(*End at 1:50. Jane had been fairly well dissociated, she said. Her eyes had been closed, her voice good but nothing exceptional.*

(*Dr. Instream asked Jane how much of the delivery she could remember, and Jane replied that she retained a generalized memory of what had been said. Dr. Instream said the voice effect was somewhat unusual, and questioned us about Jane showing fatigue afterwards. We told him that Jane had little if any fatigue after such displays, no matter how long they might last, and referred him to the 158th session as an example. This session was among those I had left with him Sunday evening.*

(*Dr. Instream said that Jane was in a light trance during her delivery, and that automatic speech was involved. Our conversation then turned to the matter of scientific proofs and related subjects. This was also one of the subjects we had discussed at lunch, leading of course to Seth's subject matter in the delivery just concluded.*

(*Up until this point I had made a verbatim record as usual, and had thought the little session in Dr. Instream's office ended. An exchange now developed however,* that was new to us in the sessions, involving Jane, Seth, Dr. Instream and myself. The pace quickened to some degree, and as stated before I made no effort to interfere with the spontaneity of the session. Unless otherwise noted what follows is the exchange between Dr. Instream and Seth only, and reports the gist of their conversation as taken from the notes and quotes I made on the spot. Nothing is included here which depends on my memory alone.

(Times noted indicate when Jane was in trance and when she came out of the state. When she remained in trance while Dr. Instream was speaking she listened to him intently, sitting with her eyes closed and her head cocked forward. Her voice was fairly strong as before, and very briefly at times it hit a stronger volume. She resumed as Seth at 1:59.)

I will not keep us. Nevertheless spontaneity must be allowed for primarily. Then the sort of evidence with which you are concerned, Doctor, can be obtained. However, if we are overly concerned for effects then the spontaneity disappears. The ego comes in and we are lost....

([Dr. Instream:] "Exactly... we must proceed carefully, without pushing....")

Correct. For that will give us our effects.

([Dr. Instream:] "I'm out of my depth here, Seth... spontaneity is important....")

It is our doorway... If objects come through, if evidence comes through, it comes through that doorway.

([Dr. Instream:] "Yes... the trouble is our human limitations... our methodology is important to us here... if we are to get others to listen to us....")

We will in a regular session take this into consideration... it would be of great benefit if you and others would understand that these limitations exist only because you accept them.

([Dr. Instream:] "Yes....")

I will not endeavor to go into this in any detail at this time. We will work within these limitations and see what we can do. The human is not innately limited... the waking state, as I have said often, is as much a trance state as any other state. Here we merely switch the focus of attention to other channels. All that is required is that we switch the attention... consider merely that all types of awareness are trance states... consciousness is the direction in which the self looks.

(At 2:03 Jane came out of the trance state and opened her eyes. A discussion followed involving the sessions in general, the field of psychic investigation, proofs, etc. Jane went back into trance and resumed as Seth at 2:25.)

Irregardless of our particular interests, I look forward to long conversations with you on less formal topics... like yourself, I am independent. We have many fields of common interests... the personality should always be considered in an elemental way as patterns of action. It is never stable. When you attempt to tamper with various levels you change it. When you crack an egg to discover what is inside you ruin the egg. There are other ways to get inside the egg, and they are not too difficult to do... you have the sort of mind, Dr. Instream, that will be of great benefit to us here. We do not need a hammer to crack the eggshell. I am an egghead, but I do not need a hammer to be cracked.

(*Jane ended this delivery on a strong note of humor, and in a good voice. She remained in trance.*

([Dr. Instream:] " We'll get insight on this... I'm human, I need to learn... we need proof.")

Your attitude may enable us to get some proofs. But others who say this does not exist will <u>never</u> get proof. All of our evidence will not be of a nebulous sort. If we succeed, some of it will be definite.

([Dr. Instream:] "Some evidence we already have is difficult to deny... we must conduct a methodical investigation of these things.")

This is one of the main reasons why I have not tended toward the seance atmosphere, why I have avoided blatant superstitious displays... we have some factors that will work for us, and we will have more.

([Dr. Instream:] "I'm in over my depth... need time to consider what we can do, what your ideas are.")

We will make definite efforts in that direction. There will be a time lag while I build up Ruburt's acceptability in this direction, but I anticipate no difficulty. My boundaries are different than yours...we will attempt to discover what we can.

(*Jane came out of her trance at 2:32, discussed her voice effects during sessions briefly with Dr. Instream, then went back into trance as Seth at 2:33.*)

In the past I saw no reason to dominate these sessions with any particular effects. That was not my main concern. I will however at our sessions try to manage a greater variety of effects. The particular voice effect, for example: This is nothing difficult, it proves nothing. What would it prove?

(*Briefly, Jane's voice became stronger.*

([Dr. Instream:] "You're quite right.")

For my own enjoyment I use such tricks at times. Such effects have served to increase the confidence of Ruburt...I am not a pompous ass. The voice can occur at any time, but it is hardly the kind of evidence with which, Doctor, you are concerned.

(*Jane came out of her trance at 2:35. Since we do not have a phone we gave Dr. Instream the number of our neighbor across the hall, Leonard Yaudes.*

(*Dr. Instream talked of bringing a couple of others into the sessions but did not* mention them to us by name. He stressed that it was best to be very careful about inviting others to participate. Also he mentioned that he would like an example of voice effects on tape, as long as we had a recorder, and we discussed mailing the tapes to him from Elmira. Jane then went back into trance as Seth again at 2:48.)

We will, as a gesture of good will, see that you will have a voice display on tape. I realize that this is but a gesture on my part. Then we will consider more serious possibilities, as far as evidence is concerned.

([Dr. Intream:] "Okay, as far as it doesn't interfere with your plans, Seth.")

We will consider ways in which we can work within the physical circumstances. I want to also use the potentials in which I can work. I am somewhat sly... I am used to getting around corners. We will indeed try, within our scope of action, to do what we can. I am used to opening eggs without cracking them.

(Jane came out of her trance at 2:53, ending on a humorous note. Dr. Instream said that the impression he had of Seth was of a very mature and capable mind. He was interested in getting this impression on tape because the Seth voice itself reinforced this feeling. Seth, he said, possessed tremendous insight.

(The conversation then turned to the psychic societies, and to the director of the American Society. Jane and I received two brief letters from the director, concerning the Seth material, on March 23, 1964 and April 23, 1964. Jane then went into trance again, and began speaking as Seth in a strong and assured voice at 3:00.)

I am an excellent debater. I can hold my own in any conversation. Forgive my lack of humility. I can hold my own with your good doctor in New York, I can take him for you... I also know my own limitations, but I do respond to human relationships.

([Dr. Instream:] "That tickles me, Seth.")

I have to admit that I am most pleased at our discussion. I am amused at your reactions, and my own... this is my first opportunity to talk with you... I have not pushed in the past for any kind of arrangement where proofs can be obtained....

([Dr. Instream:] "You can take care of yourself.")

We must all take care of ourselves; and I know with whom I am dealing.

([Dr. Instream:] "We'll get better acquainted.")

We shall indeed, and make arrangements for future sessions.

(Dr. Instream now commented upon the fact that Jane had no apparent fatigue while using the Seth voice.)

The increase in voice will not produce fatigue. It never does. Also, there is no invasion of Ruburt. The personality with whom I am working is intelligent. For reasons that I will explain much later, it was necessary that I align myself with a personality who is both intelligent and intuitional. I do not want to shove the ego aside. I have no need or wish to shove the existing personality aside. We get along well.

There is much here to be studied about personality. From your viewpoint the information available to you can be practically endless. There is much to be learned about perceiving other realities. Trance states are only a beginning. The self is made of action. Teaching the self to expand is most important, and the ways are not difficult... this is what makes the experiment interesting. This is <u>not</u> beyond human abilities. The structure of the personality makes this possible.

The peoples of the East know more about this, but they have closed their eyes to the human conditions of existence... they live in poverty and filth, and there is no real reason for this. Experiments in expansion can be carried on that I will be glad to discuss with you... they can be for the use of any intelligent personality.

([Dr. Instream:] "Some very interesting possibilities here....")

I deal with possibilities, and so do you.

(Dr. Instream now asked Seth about the possibility of bringing some other people in on the sessions.)

We must not deal with the overly gullible or skeptical. The mean will work for us very well.

([Dr. Instream:] "Yes, I agree....")

I have no objection, except that we must not deal with the gullible or skeptical. The gullible can do us more harm than the skeptical.

(Dr. Instream agreed again; and Seth/Jane's voice, strong to begin with, took on a note of mock horror.)

I <u>quail</u> before such a possibility. I can to some extent deal with the skeptic. With the gullible I cannot deal. We will indeed at all times try to be as reasonable as possible. I do become impatient. This is a characteristic of my own. I try not to let it direct my relationships.

([Dr. Instream:] "I will try to be most careful... it can be a matter of gradual unfolding.")

There is no great rush. We will proceed... I have built up the foundations well.

([Dr. Instream:] "It's too bad Elmira is 120 miles away... you have no telephone....")

We may see that this is of no great difficulty. It may work for us.

(Dr. Instream said that he had been thinking of the possible damage that publicity could do to the sessions.)

I am somewhat concerned. When Ruburt's book is published the fact of the sessions will be known. We have not had to deal with this in the past. I make no effort to direct Ruburt's writings in any manner. What Ruburt has said in his book has been up to him, and therefore we have to deal with the results.

([Dr. Instream:] "I can help Ruburt meet such problems... some people get steamed up over this subject. The criticisms could hurt if you weren't prepared... but we can ignore such critics.")

Your attitude is very much like my own.

(Dr. Instream said it was best to pursue a policy of denying nothing, to ignore the criticisms and go our own way. We should avoid personal polemics in the field and not get involved; just as he has always gone his own way. Jane, as Seth, sat listening intently. She nodded.)

Yes, but you have had to put up with very much. This is indeed unfortunate. Your own potentials should have been given much greater reign. The human personality continually both amazes me, amuses me, and completely appalls me. Charlatans are often more deeply rewarded... I ask you to forgive my extended monologue.

([Dr. Instream:] "No, that's all right, it gives me insight... tells me who I'm dealing with. The book will be criticized... a barrage of criticism. It can't be helped... but Ruburt must be rendered unsusceptible....")

(A case in point, Dr. Instream continued, was our meeting with the young psychologist on Saturday evening. See my notes on page 132. Dr. Instream said to forget such encounters. Jane again nodded in agreement, and her voice again became stronger briefly.)

The meeting between the two was indeed upsetting to him.

Nevertheless, he recovered rather quickly. The experience did him much good... a practical example... had it not happened now, a much more vicious attack would have occurred at a later date.

([Dr. Instream:] "Yes... we'll act as a buffer.")

I am particularly grateful for your interest and concern.

(Dr. Instream said that people often do get hurt, when instead they should be protected. He knows Dr. Rhine and another director personally, and voiced suspicions about their methods.)

[The other director] is too much concerned with his own personal image. He does not want to be involved with anything that may fail... this is a personal concern of his. His ego is such that it makes him, in a strange manner, often <u>prevent</u> the sort of effects that he seeks. He asks too much, and receives too little. He will always be that way.

(Dr. Instream agreed.)

There is a sweetness in the nature of your Dr. Rhine.

(Again Dr. Instream agreed.)

That sweetness allows for spontaneity, and explains why many of his cases succeeded. But for entirely different reasons Dr. Rhine also gets too involved, and the end result is the same... we can get effects, but the laboratory atmosphere will not help us.

([Dr. Instream:] "Yes.")

I will now let my friend Ruburt have his cigarette. I would myself prefer a cigar.

(End at 3:28. Jane had been dissociated as usual. Her voice had been good up until the end, and she now displayed no unusual fatigue. Her eyes had remained closed for the entire session.

(Dr. Instream agreed with Seth's brief sketches of Dr. Rhine and the other director. He said that Dr. Rhine's sweetness had led him into traps where his controls were not rigid enough during experiments, that his disposition was of the type that would not make him crack down. On the other hand, the other director was too strict. Dr. Instream used these examples to point out how important the correct methodology was in trying to obtain proofs in psychic investigations.

(As we said good-bye, I offered to send Dr. Instream a copy of the session.)

SESSION 170
JULY 19, 1965 9 PM MONDAY AS SCHEDULED

(The regularly scheduled session for last Wednesday, July 14, was not held because Jane and I were on vacation.

(We had indicated to Dr. Instream last week that we would record a session upon returning home, and ship him the tape for his own use. Jane and I had not used our recorder much lately, so we practiced with it last night, establishing proper distances from the microphone, and volume settings. The session was recorded with the Gallaghers as witnesses, at their home, and turned out well. There follows the little talk Jane gave on tape before the actual session began:

("This is Jane Butts, speaking in my usual voice. My husband, Robert Butts, and I live at 458 West Water St., Elmira, NY. The date is July 19, 1965, the time is about 8:30 PM. The following Seth session, number 170, is being recorded at the home of Bill and Peggy Gallagher, Pine City, NY, with them as witnesses.

("The recorder is operated by my husband. It is a Sears Silvertone. The Tone and Volume One controls are set as far to the left as possible during recording. The Volume Two control has been set at 4, and unless otherwise noted this setting will not be changed for the rest of the evening, whether I am speaking as Seth or myself. I am

SESSION 170

sitting between five and six feet from the microphone, and will keep this position throughout the session. The entire recording is being made on Monaural One, Side One and Side Two.

("Breaks during the session will be indicated by my husband announcing the time. The next time you hear my voice it will be 9 PM, and I will be speaking as Seth."

(Note that Jane did not include the speed, 3 3/4, in the above announcement.

(Jane had felt for several days that Seth would address the session to Dr. Instream, and so he did. Jane's eyes remained closed for the entire session. She began the session while sitting down. More or less as I had anticipated, she began speaking too rapidly for me to take notes effectively, although at times during the session I was able to keep up with her. Peggy Gallagher also took notes. Thus this session is taken from the tape itself, largely, and necessitated replaying it several times.

(Jane actually began speaking at 8:57. Her voice was stronger than usual from the beginning, her manner active. The recording was begun with the footage set at 000 prior to Jane's introduction, on Monaural One, Side One.)

Good evening.

("Good evening, Seth.")

I will address my remarks this evening to Dr. Instream, with whom I am at least now somewhat acquainted. I will speak fairly slowly, since Ruburt is taking his time in order that Joseph may take his notes. Notes in our circumstances are fairly important.

There are some matters which I would discuss with you, Dr. Instream. They are matters in which we both have some deep concern, and some considerable interest.

Let us first consider the trance state. Let us for example consider the following circumstances, which are happening only in our imagination. We will therefore consider this imaginary circumstance: an individual is in a trance state. His focus of attention is rather severely limited in some aspects, and yet in other ways it is very strongly focused.

The individual involved is aware of very little as far as physical objects are concerned. There is, for example, a table in front of him. The table is real, it is physical. Under ordinary circumstances it could be seen and touched. Objects could be placed upon it; and yet, Doctor Instream, our entranced individual is not conscious of that table. In his state he is concentrating upon some object which we cannot see. Now, consider: we will attempt to <u>prove</u> the existence of this material table to this individual who is not aware of it. How, therefore, could we prove to <u>him</u> that this table exists, when he is not aware of it in any manner whatsoever? His attentions are focused elsewhere. For him the table does not exist. We have indeed a rather delightful dilemma; and yet, is this not what you require of me? I speak of "you" simply because I have come in contact with you. I recognize only too well your sympathy and your understanding. Nevertheless the situation in which you put me is exactly like the situation which I have only now described.

Your attentions are indeed focused elsewhere. <u>You</u> are in a trance as well as Ruburt is in a trance state now. This is far from unusual. I use you, dear Doctor Instream, only as an example. Consciousness of any kind is merely the direction in which the self looks. I told you this at our brief meeting. Consciousness is the <u>focus</u>, the direction of focus. Your ordinary consciousness is as much a trance state as any trance state induced through hypnotism. Therefore it is nearly impossible to convince a subject in trance that something he does not see exists.

If you have already suggested that the table does not exist for him, he will never see the table. The table will not seem to exist. The table will <u>not</u> exist in actuality for this subject in the trance state. It ceases to have any meaning for him at all. Nor will he recall or remember any meaning for him that that table might once have had.

Though objects upon the table be dearly familiar to him, in his trance state he will not recall them. Any sentiment involved with the objects on the table, such sentiment will disappear and have no meaning. The ordinary state of consciousness is no different from that trance state. You have merely turned the focus of your attention into different realities. <u>My</u> attention, and <u>my</u> reality, is mainly focused in another direction.

Adequate scientific proofs, such as science so surely needs, requires the enlargement of consciousness; <u>not</u>, my dear doctor, on <u>my</u> part, but on the part of science. There are some things that I can indeed do, and I will do what I can. Nevertheless the fact remains that I am indeed extending myself, and my dear doctor it is <u>science</u> which is not extending itself, and it is <u>science</u> that will not meet reality halfway.

I am as I told you an educator, and as such my main concern is <u>with</u> education, is <u>with</u> ideas. I want to tell you exactly what you want to know, and if you will hear me then to a large measure you will have to accept some of my terms, for I am quite willing to accept some of yours. Much of this has to do with your idea of the theory of suggestion. If you would read some of our material, it would then become obvious to you that mental suggestion is indeed the basis upon which <u>all</u> reality is founded.

Therefore it is not <u>overplaying</u> the point to say that <u>all</u> psychic phenomena is caused by suggestion. For my dear doctor, without suggestion, without automatic and continuous suggestion, no human being would breathe one breath. I am indeed happy to be able to speak to you in this manner. There are several points that I would like to cover this evening, for I have you here now, you see, where you cannot talk back to me.

I shall of course take advantage of the opportunity, but then you will have time to speak to me at your leisure. There are many points to be considered, and these matters certainly cannot be covered in one evening such as this. I hinted at our last discussion that it is indeed within the ability of the human personality to become aware of other realities while still keeping contact with physical reality. Manipulation in the physical universe is of course a necessity, but there are ways by which the human individual can become aware of other quite valid realities, and still maintain balance and control within his own <u>more usual</u> field of activity.

I now suggest a brief break, and we will shortly resume with our discussion.

(*Break at 9:12. Jane had been dissociated as usual. Her eyes had been closed and she had remained seated for the entire delivery. Her voice had been stronger than usual, and she had spoken at such a rapid pace that I had not been able to keep up with her in my notes. The bulk of the above delivery is thus taken from the tape. The delivery ended with the footage registering 333 on the recorder, Mono One, Side One.*)

(*Jane resumed in a slightly slower manner, but still too fast for my notes, at 9:20.*)

My dear Doctor Instream, I will speak slower, since my friends are having trouble keeping up their notes. We must also take this into consideration.

Now. In the dream state it would be impossible for the dreamer to prove the existence of the familiar street outside of his familiar door. His attention is momentarily directed toward a different sort of reality. The ordinary trees outside of his window do not exist for him. It would be highly difficult to ask a man while he dreamed to prove the physical reality of the bed in which he slept, or the bedside table which was at his head, or to prove the existence of the wooden floor upon which the bed rested. Highly difficult indeed, for such objects do not exist for our dreamer.

Therefore it is also highly difficult for <u>me</u> to prove my own existence to you, for you are not focused within my field of attention. You are focused within the physical universe. I will indeed go along with this endeavor. It is nevertheless a difficult one. I understand most thoroughly, my dear Doctor Instream; I know, again, with whom I am dealing. You, at this point in our acquaintanceship, have little to lose by being so kind to me, and so permissive and sympathetic in your attitude. I say this because we understand each other very well.

There is indeed no reason for you, in your position, to jump in with both feet and wild erratic enthusiasm. Nor, my dear doctor, is there any reason at this point why I should leap in with both feet, and with wild unrestrained enthusiasm. I am working through and with Ruburt. Ruburt is a writer by profession and I am, again, a rather sly individual, for Ruburt will express my views for me, and this is what I am interested in.

I am interested in education. You, my dear doctor, are interested in visual aids. This is all right. We are in a very basic manner interested in the same matters. It occurs to me once more that I am speaking too swiftly for our notetakers, and I will once again endeavor to slow down. As far, incidentally, as automatic speech is concerned, let me say that there is nothing compulsive in Ruburt's speaking. He allows me to speak indeed. I have his politeness to thank that he does not interrupt me, but his speaking is not compulsive in that he is so driven.

Joseph, may I ask you if I am again speaking too swiftly?

("Not at the moment.")

(Jane had slowed her pace somewhat, and I was now having some success in keeping up with her. Peggy Gallagher evidently was having better luck; she had been writing steadily ever since the beginning of the session.)

All right now. You may be interested to some degree, dear Doctor Instream, in the sort of personality through whom I speak. I wanted a personality who was at the same time both intelligent and intuitional. I wanted an ego which was well balanced, healthy and strong. Yet I also wanted a personality which would allow itself the spontaneity necessary, and the inner freedom, so that such communications could take place. A personality without basic stability would not serve my purposes, and a personality that was too rigid in its beliefs and abilities would not serve my purposes well.

If you will read the Seth material you will also find that there are other reasons why I speak through Ruburt.

I realize only too well that reincarnation is a shady subject by far, most unpopular. I assure you however that in any discussion with your psychologists on this matter, I shall hold my own. Again, the attention, the energy of all human personalities, as a rule, are severely focused in one scope of reality only. They are indeed in a trance.

This is necessary. I have no qualms with this, but it is possible, and in this stage of your evolution it is necessary, that the human personality learn to become flexible, to change the focus of awareness so that other realities can be perceived. There are indeed as I have said, effects that I can show you, and I will.

Effects that will at least be of some import; but you must remember the table in our analogy of the man in the trance state.

Those who will not see, <u>they will not see</u>. I will do my best. However, such effects will appear in the middle of quite ordinary sessions. For again, only spontaneity will give us any results at all.

I know that our notetakers are by now weary, and I am indeed most appreciative of their efforts in my behalf. I will ask you to bear with me, dear Doctor Instream, and we will shortly return to our small chat.

(Break at 9:35. Jane was well dissociated as usual. Her eyes had remained closed, she had remained seated. Her voice had been strong and expressive, if somewhat on the same keel throughout the session so far. The voice effects began to show themselves after this break. Footage at break was 552, Mono One, Side One.

(Jane resumed at a good pace and in a good voice, still seated and with her eyes closed, at 9:46.)

I can indeed give you, and quite easily, evidence of clairvoyance, and I will in future sessions. But my dear Doctor Instream, what will this prove? It will not prove my existence to those who will not accept it. It will simply be said that Ruburt is clairvoyant.

I will, and can, give you evidence of telepathy, and what will this prove? It will not prove my existence, not to those who will not accept it. They will say merely that Ruburt is clairvoyant, and Ruburt has telepathic powers. If I materialized in <u>full sight</u> of twenty good and weighty witnesses, what indeed would this prove to those who would not accept the proof?

(With the above paragraph Jane rose to her feet and her voice grew stronger. She did not move from her position before her chair, and thus the distance from her face to the microphone did not vary a great deal. I believe it increased a little. I know the angle changed somewhat, since we had set the mike on the table so it directly faced her when she was sitting down. Now she spoke from above it, but we believe the stronger voice more than made up for the increased distance, and was still able to show the variation in the volume of Jane's voice as the session progressed. She took to her feet at about 9:50.)

It would prove nothing to them. They would indeed insist that twenty good and worthy witnesses were under the influence of suggestion.

Therefore what proofs can you require? And in all honesty's sake, what proofs do you think that they will require? What good will it do if through Ruburt <u>I literally shout from the rooftops</u>, and <u>raise</u> my voice, and shout that I am indeed who and what I say I am. What will this prove?

(During this paragraph Jane's voice really grew in strength and volume, although it was to become stronger later on. She began to approach the volume of the

voice used in the 158th session. When these effects came on, Jane usually stood upright, with her head back to some degree; this made me think of a trumpet. Strangely enough however her mouth did not open more than an inch. And of course during these effects she displayed no evidence of strain. This voice is not a shouting voice, but simply an innately stronger voice.

(*The massive voice effects continued from now on in greater or lesser degree; they will not all be listed. One will have to listen to the tape of this session to really achieve any idea of the voice range Jane displayed.*)

You are not so gullible, nor am I, to suppose that those who do not want to accept evidence will ever accept the strongest evidence imaginable. Those who will not see, will not see. And those who will not listen, they will not listen. You wanted a voice display, and so indeed shall you have it. And what indeed will such a display show? That Ruburt has lungs?

You know, and I know, that it is literally impossible for a woman such as she to speak in tones as loud and deep as those which I am now using. But you speak of proof, and your psychologists speak of proof. Though I have Ruburt speak in tones as deep and ungodly as a frog's, this will mean nothing.

(*Jane's voice had been very strong, very loud. Now it began to diminish.*)

Again, if I stood clear as day in the middle of a meeting room, with twenty fine and sturdy, respectable fuddy-duddies, what would this prove? They would swear that they were under the effects of suggestion. I <u>will</u>, I will for my own amusement, give you in the future <u>many</u>—not one but many—clairvoyant effects. Again, for my own amusement.

Now. I trust your integrity, and I am quite certain of my own. Between us, what do you think we can accomplish? We can accomplish much despite my sarcastic remarks, but it will not be easy and it will not be quick. You will indeed <u>live</u> many years yet, before <u>we</u> meet face to face. And when we <u>do</u> meet face to face then indeed, if you will most respectfully forgive me, there will be <u>hell</u> to pay.

For though we do have the same interests there are many areas in which we do not <u>now</u> agree. But I will see if I cannot bring you around; and if you will forgive me my dear doctor, this humility of yours is indeed overdone. There is nothing of what I have said that you do not understand, your comments to the contrary. You pretend with yourself. If you will forgive me, for I am speaking to you as one old crony to another, you are too sly to stand up straight and <u>say</u> who you are, and <u>what</u> you are, and accept the responsibility for your own abilities. You do not want the world mad at you.

I do not blame you. My own inclinations may not exactly be the same. You stand up well for yourself within certain limits, and then you become humble.

Your abilities are much greater than this. Your achievements are much greater than this. You may interpret the following statement as you wish: however, this engagement is important to both of us. You know it and so do I. I say once more: I know <u>with whom</u> I am dealing, and by now <u>you</u> know with whom you are dealing.

You see now, I forget. I become involved with the very personal relationship between us both, but I have been asked to give voice effects, and so indeed I shall comply *(louder, briefly)* out of the goodness of my heart, and because of the amusement which it affords me. However I take this encounter with utmost seriousness, and I may presume that your attitude is the same.

I will now suggest that a break be taken, if you will bear with me once again; I look forward to the more friendly conversations which will occur between us in the future. For such formality indeed, and such mechanical limitations, do not allow me to achieve that friendly informal attitude that I would prefer, and I enjoy answering your questions, for in many ways you are indeed a man such as I was.

(Break at 10:06. Jane was dissociated as usual. She remained standing until break, with her eyes closed. Her voice was strong, quite loud at times, somewhat slower, and at times had humorous overtones. Footage 762, Mono One, Side One.

(I now had to resume the session on Mono One, Side <u>Two</u>. I made a brief announcement of this on the tape. I also announced the times of breaks on the tape. Jane resumed while sitting down and with her eyes closed, and in a good voice, at 10:18.)

Ruburt and Joseph also to some extent, and for <u>good</u> reasons, hold back. I do not resent this. They find it difficult to imagine that they are dealing with a case which will be indeed well investigated.

There are many reasons why adequate proofs for immortality have not been received in the past. These reasons have to do, among other things, with the laboratory experiments and atmosphere, which do not allow for spontaneity.

They also have to do with the idiotic and gullible attitudes of those who have been involved with many notorious seance cases. For here we find self-deluded well-meaning nincompoops, ready and willing to accept any fraud, and cry <u>hallelujah</u>! *(Much louder.)*

What you have needed, and if you have the sense to perceive it, and I think you have, was a situation where both logic and intuitions were allowed full play. We will have much to do with each other, my dear doctor, and you know already that this case is one for which you have long waited.

(Jane now stood up again. As usual she remained just in front of her chair, her eyes closed, her hands thrust into the pockets of her slacks.)

I myself have indeed long awaited some circumstances which we now can take advantage of for our own benefits. However, I am not mainly concerned with proving for you the fact of my own existence. *(Strong voice.)* Let us now be honest. Are you concerned with proving your existence to me? Hardly. You take it for granted that I am aware of your existence, and I assure you so I am. But neither am I concerned with proving my existence to you. I am however very interested in education. If I have to pull a few tricks out of the bag to get my ideas across, then so I shall.

However, we return again to the fact which neither of us can afford to ignore. We are each in a trance, you and I, *(louder)* but the focus of attention is within different fields. We speak with distortions. The material which I have already given will explain most clearly many ideas which are absolutely basic, for unless these ideas are clearly understood, then *(louder)* you will have no logical reason to accept anything that I say.

You will not have the framework within which I exist. My existence is not dependent upon your recognition of it, any more than your existence is dependent upon my recognition of you. You will exist whether or not I admit that you are real. And so my dear friend, I shall exist whether or not you accept my reality.

Indeed, I should not be harsh, and I do not mean to be. This voice which I adopt forces a certain meaning upon me, through inflection, which sometimes is not intended. Ruburt, who cooperates with me so well, still is not certain that I am I. So indeed, how shall I blame others? I am hampered indeed, for whenever I speak in tones of ordinary conversation, then indeed I cause these poor people hours of notetaking. You may not know it, but you will help us out in these matters in the future.

If I speak to you personally in what may seem to you a frivolous manner, it is because I am concerned with the personal contact between us this evening; for the personal contact between us will insure that you read what I have said, and I will indeed get my way.

(Jane's voice again climbed the scale in volume. It became very loud and strong, rising and falling. During some passages, up until break time, the volume of sound she produced made my ears ring. I would say that in these passages she exceeded the effects produced in the last part of the 158th session. It will be remembered that the Gallaghers were witnesses to the first part of that session.

(As before, Jane, on her feet again, stood just before her chair, threw her head back, and let the sound pour out. Much of the time the great voice was humorous. She smiled often while speaking, gesturing freely. She was obviously enjoying herself.)

And may I also say that if voice effects are necessary in order that you read my material, then my dear doctor voice effects galore shall you receive. *(Very loud.)* For I am above all things, once again, an educator, and as such like all educators I am sly, and you shall receive whatever effects you require in my good time. And you will therefore be intrigued enough to read the material which I have presented, and I will get my point across.

(Continuing loud, with the high spots underlined:)

I do not imagine that this information will save the world. It will take more than myself <u>and twenty gods beside</u> to handle that problem. I do however insist that in my not too humble way, I can do <u>something</u> to set you right. And by <u>right</u> and by <u>you</u> I do not refer to you, Doctor Instream, but to humanity at large. I do not pretend, either, to know definitely what is right and what is wrong for your universe.

I may not know what is <u>right</u> for it, but I certainly know what is wrong. What is wrong is your limited perception. What is <u>wrong</u> are the arbitrary limitations which you have set upon reality; and these limitations, while set by you, nevertheless operate as if they were absolute. I say again, if any small and simple treats of voice *(louder again)* will serve to make supposedly sane men stand up and listen *(louder, strong, very strong; Jane's head was thrown back as though to let the great voice out unimpeded)* then so I will speak out in <u>loud and hearty tones</u>. *(If possible, even stronger here. Then the voice began to soften. Jane displayed no strain or fatigue.)*

It is however most unfortunate that intelligent men will not listen to intelligent and sane and illuminating data without requiring such magician's tricks as this. I am however and always have been quite practical. And as a practical personality *(loud)* I am as sly as any psychologist ever thought of being. I will therefore manage.

I now suggest a break, out of due respect for our notetakers. And for our Jesuit here, who so studiously examines my every move and gesture, I am indeed quite flattered in my own way. You may all take a break, and I will then continue.

(Break at 10:40. Jane was dissociated as usual, she said. She had remained standing until break, with her eyes closed. She felt no fatigue from the voice effects. Her pace of dictation had been somewhat slower and I had been able to keep up with her. Footage at 412, Mono One, Side Two.

(Jane resumed while sitting down, with her eyes closed and in a good voice, at 10:56.)

I am myself quite happy, and somewhat amused by our relationship, my dear doctor, for in many areas we are indeed very much alike. I know and I appreciate the fact that you are not a young man. I know indeed that you lean toward a belief in immortality, while at the same time you cannot entirely accept the possibility without some sort of scientific proof.

I am also quite aware of the cruelty that would be involved if I led you on in this endeavor without due consideration. I can only tell you that I appreciate both your objectivity and your beliefs. I will do my best, my dear doctor, to satisfy you in both respects. You may call it chance. You may call it if you choose coincidence. You may name it in whatever way pleases you: nevertheless, it is because of my personal rapport with you that I will bother with any displays at all.

If I did not _feel_ such a rapport with you I would not bother, for it is nothing to me one way or another if my existence be accepted or rejected. My concern is with the material I am presenting.

(*Jane stood up once more before her chair. Her eyes were closed. She was smiling and gesturing. Now as she spoke she leaned forward some of the time, as though getting restless at merely standing upright in one spot. And again her voice began to display pyrotechnics, first loud, then soft; partially indicated in the following paragraphs.*)

And here you see an example of my sly nature, for Ruburt (*louder*) will present my material for me. Regardless of its source, the material speaks _loud_ and clear. It is largely disregarded, the sort of personality which is required in this endeavor. It simply happens that because of past relationships I know Ruburt well, and Ruburt knows me _far_ better than he imagines.

He knows well who I am, and _I_ know who he is. All this studied reluctance on his part is a game, quite an amusing ruse. (*Louder.*) He knows I am who I say I am. Nor should Joseph's part in this endeavor be forgotten. It is more complicated than you may suppose.

Now. I have trained Ruburt and taught Ruburt so that his valid clairvoyant experiences can be put on some sort of scientific basis. He keeps records, which will be invaluable. He is an intelligent and intuitional personality, and should be given credit. He is _not_ however some demigod walking the face of the physical earth; and your word "medium" leaves much to be desired. Again I say as I have said before, all human beings are _breathers_, and in this respect all human beings are mediums.

Your terms mean nothing. If I sound aggressive, you must indeed read between the lines. I have said often that I am not humble, in your terms. Yet in many ways I recognize only too well the limits of my own knowledge and potentialities. _You_ know what I mean, my dear Dr. Instream, when I say that this case will give you what you want.

Again, I apologize if this session embarrasses you, if I am too personal. But regardless of our scopes of activity _we_ are not young men. We know what we want. You have more time than you suppose, not only in your present life but in others.

Now. Quite practically your personal and practical interest in immortality will give the <u>impetus</u>, the emotional impetus that will indeed allow me to deliver what you want. This is perhaps one of the most important statements of this evening's session. Emotions are more important than you suppose. There is no fraud in me. There is no fraud in Ruburt or Joseph. They are not stupid and they are not gullible. <u>You</u> are not stupid nor gullible. They are not caught up in pseudoreligious nonsense. This will serve us well.

At another time, at another occasion when we have an afternoon together, you and I can discuss the God concept, for it continually fascinates me, and it continually fascinates you.

(Seth has discussed the God concept and related subjects in the following sessions, among others: 31, 51, 62, 66, 81, 95, 97, 115, 135, 147, 149, 146, 151.)

You must be aware that the next move is up to you. <u>If</u> you do not make a next move then neither of us is out a thing, and it will have been a most delightful encounter.

However I do not sincerely believe that such will be the case, and I can assure you that I am not one to dillydally. I am deeply aware of my responsibilities to Ruburt, through whom I speak, and I will endeavor to protect this personality from <u>undue</u> or <u>unnecessary</u> bother. But I will in <u>all</u> manners cooperate in any sincere effort that will add to the knowledge of the human [species] in general.

It would be unfair of me to back upon an elderly gentleman's desire for immortality, and I would never stoop to such a practice. <u>I was myself</u> an elderly gentleman, and I understand too well the soul-searching aspects of such a reality. You may therefore be assured that I will not play on such human limitations. I will under all circumstances never take advantage in <u>any</u> such manner.

I say this only to let you know that I understand any innermost doubts that you might have concerning the possibility that others would so take such advantage. I thoroughly enjoyed our brief meeting. Our conversation indeed was most beneficial. I appreciated the give and take. This may not sound like a very scientific document, yet in many ways it may be more scientific than you imagine, for its effects <u>will indeed</u> be felt.

I will now suggest a brief break, and we will then conclude our brief session. I regret, my dear doctor, that it remains a monologue.

(Break at 11:18. Jane was dissociated as usual, and was not displaying any undue fatigue from the long session. She remained standing until break, her eyes closed all the while. Her voice had been good, yet quieter than the really strong display of the earlier delivery, and I had been able to keep up in my notetaking. Peggy

had no trouble either. Footage at 686, Mono One, Side Two.

(I did not know exactly how many feet of tape were left on our recorder, due to inexperience, yet saw that the session would have to end before too long or we would run out of tape first. Although Seth/Jane started out in a relatively quiet manner on this last delivery, another voice display, perhaps even better, began to develop. Jane resumed the session while sitting down and with her eyes closed. Her pace was faster, and after a few sentences she rose to her feet once more. Resume at 11:29.)

Ruburt and Joseph are, again, in many ways reluctant. They are more humble than is necessary also.

They are *not* humble where their own work is concerned, but they find it difficult to accept the possibility that they are involved in such a venture as this one. We have here merely a conglomeration of excellent circumstances, and we shall take advantage of them, Dr. Instream, you and I. Our purposes somewhat complement each other. *(Loud, very loud and strong.)*

I am concerned because I want the theoretical material to be widely distributed. I am not primarily concerned with giving effects or proofs of my existence. I know that <u>I</u> exist as you know that <u>you</u> exist. How would you feel if someone asked you to prove your existence? If you answer this question honestly, then you will see that I am far from being as irascible as it may appear. I bend over backward to understand. I bend over backward, and this is most difficult for me. *(Strong.)*

You must also understand that I work to some extent within the human limitations of Ruburt's own personality, and you have underestimated that personality. You have not underestimated <u>my</u> personality.

I am no secondary personality. There is no case of multiple personality here. What you have if you take advantage of it, is Ruburt's personality, which with Joseph's help is capable and willing to perceive more than one reality at once. You will not, my dear doctor, get a second chance in this endeavor.

There is very much concerning the characteristics of the trance state which you do not yet understand, and I can help you here. Hypnotism may seem very strange. It involves no more, however, than a study of human personality, for it involves nothing more than a switching of focus. It is imperative, if we are to speak easily, that you read the material having to do with the specific ways in which the human individual creates physical matter on a subconscious basis.

I have not left this in general terms. Your mathematicians can verify much of it.

(Jane's voice had been slowly growing in volume since last break. Seth now pulled out more stops than ever before, I believe. The voice display now became deafening. My

ears rang, off and on, for the next few paragraphs. I saw Peggy and Bill blinking. Jane merely stood in front of her chair, head thrown back. As stated before she exhibited no strain in producing these stunning effects. The electric eye on the recorder closed, meaning that it was recording, as far as I know, at maximum volume.)

Now. Because I have been called upon to give a voice display, so shall you see that I can do so. *(Very loud and strong.)* You will also find at the end of this session that Ruburt's vocal chords are in no way fatigued; and I can so speak here for hours, nor would this bother Ruburt in the slightest degree. If such a display serves to convince you of my validity then so shall it be. I find it difficult to imagine that you need such childish play to convince you of that which you already know. *(Loud and strong.)*

Let it not be said that I do not cooperate; and before twenty psychologists, my dear friend, we shall be most willing to comply. But we have our conditions, and if your conditions shall be met *(very loud here, to slowly subside)* my dear friend, then so shall mine. *(Loud again.)* We will give and take. I shall not give and give. If you consider this display a childish one, then let me remind you that I consider your requests in the same manner.

If I sound theatrical, if I sound irascible, kindly remember that to make my point I work with disadvantages and distortions which would make you speechless. I do sincerely understand your <u>true</u> sympathy. As I said earlier I <u>feel</u> a rapport. Nevertheless I feel that I must indeed make my position clear.

All those here present may take a break, or end the session as they prefer. This will indeed be a most significant session.

("We'll end the session then.")

I will then give my due respects to Doctor Instream, and also ask for his understanding as I make certain points quite emphatically, in order to make certain that they are made at all. We will, between us, come to an understanding; and those effects which he desires, <u>in time</u> can be given.

We must to some extent consider Ruburt's own personality, and all protection that is possible should be given here. Doctor Instream can act in this behalf, and I will consider such actions as a gesture of his faith; though the word faith is not meant as any alternative to the word science, it is quite possible to have both.

(End at 11:45. Jane had been dissociated as usual. She remained standing in her accustomed spot until the end of the session. Her eyes had remained closed, her voice had been good all the way, with some very strong and vibrant passages. In my opinion these exceeded the loud passages in the 158th session. Jane had cleared her throat a few times toward the end of the session, but now displayed no strain, or

unusual fatigue.

(*This point was abundantly made, for although we did not know it at the time, the session was due to resume at midnight. At the moment the footage scale on the recorder read 860, Mono One, Side Two. We had a little tape left, so I decided to use it to demonstrate for others the fact of Jane's immunity to voice fatigue. The following is taken from the tape verbatim, and includes a statement from Bill Gallagher, who witnessed the session with his wife Peggy. It was made immediately after the end of the session; perhaps a few minutes were lost here when I made a false start on the recorder, due to inexperience, and had to start the exchange between Jane and myself over.*

([RB:] "This is Robert Butts. All right Jane, how do you feel?"

([Jane:] "All right already." [*Voice light and chipper.*]

([RB:] "How was your voice?"

([Jane:] "Same as ever."

([RB:] "Doesn't feel tired?"

([Jane:] "Never does."

([RB:] "You don't feel any unusual fatigue?"

([Jane:] "You know I don't." [*Laughing.*]

([RB:] "Well, that's fine."

([BG:] "This is Bill Gallagher. I want to verify the fact that the 170th Seth session was held in my home on Holden Road, where it was witnessed by my wife and myself on July 19, 1965, from 8:57 to 11:45. What you hear on these tapes has in fact occurred, and Jane was within view at all times; and I don't know what else I can add, other than the fact that it was a very astounding presentation."

([Jane:] "This is Jane Butts. I just wanted to add that Peggy and Bill, in some way we don't understand, seem to be of a great help in our sessions. And whenever they come to our sessions I seem to feel some kind of reinforcement that I don't quite understand either, that appears to be most helpful."

(*Footage at 876. I added the following notes a couple of days later.*

([RB:] "This is Robert Butts again, speaking two days later on July 21st. I would like to add that the 170th session, which you have just heard, and which formally ended at 11:45 PM last Monday, July 19, resumed that night at midnight. It involved an informal exchange between Jane, Seth, Bill and Peggy Gallagher and myself, and lasted until about 1:30 AM. Our tape was almost exhausted and so it was not recorded. Seth also stated he did not care particularly to have it on tape, or have notes taken. During this exchange Seth was in an excellent good humor. I joked with him about the voice display, and he responded with another which was both stronger and longer-lasting than the one on tape here. Our ears rang, really, before it was over. And when it was over at last, and we were all weary, Seth, or Jane, was as capable as ever. Jane had no voice strain or fatigue that we could detect. Seth said he could continue until dawn, and I believe it quite possible. Jane just threw her head back and let the sound come out."

(Footage at 887.)

(The session resumed without preamble at midnight. Our active discussion after I had finished with the tape brought it about, and it involved an exchange between Jane, Seth, Bill and Peggy, and myself, in the manner of the 169th session held in Dr. Instream's office.

(Although Seth said to forget about notes, I found myself making a few after a few minutes, out of habit. Peggy also made some, and what follows is taken from these two sources; nothing is included here that is not touched upon in the notes. Seth talked at a normal rate, and neither Peggy nor I made a serious effort to get it all down. Some of the material was a repeat, in a more informal way, of what Seth had said during the session itself. During this exchange it was obvious that Seth was enjoying himself immensely. More than once he referred to Bill Gallagher as his favorite Jesuit, and this is getting to be something of a standing joke between Bill and Seth.

(None of us asked questions that might lead to totally new, unfamiliar material that we might wish later was recorded. Bill wanted to ask Seth to comment on the God concept, but thought this was a complicated subject. He settled instead for a question pertaining to a large wooden Tibetan statue he and Peg had purchased in Ithaca, NY. To our surprise this subject developed a few complications of its own.

(Seth was rather loathe to discuss the statue at first, but kept throwing out bits of information about it in between his protests. During this time Jane remained seated, her eyes closed. The statue, of a mythological or Godlike being in a sitting position with its arms upraised, did come from Tibet, Seth said—a small area in a southwestern corner of the country. I asked him for the name and he said he did not think Ruburt could pronounce it. The closest he could come via spelling was S-w-a-s-o-o-w-a-n. Swasoowan.

(The statue originated in the 12th century, and its name is not the same now as it was, Seth said. The statue represented the God of the Universe. There is some information on it in a book in the Elmira Library. The word Sense is involved here, Seth said according to my notes, although it may need translation. I do not remember why.

(Seth said that originally the statue was accepted as a gift by a missionary, a Father Hogan, in payment for healing the daughter of a chieftain. Father Hogan was 46 years old. It was carried by him to a shop in Hong Kong and sold. Father Hogan was a Jesuit. Seth said the statue is not an original dating from the 12th century; this one dates from the late 18th century. [Bill Gallagher later verified this, telling us that a professor of Tibetan art at Cornell University, in Ithaca where they had bought the statue, had so stated. Ithaca is some 35 miles northeast of Elmira, NY.]

(The statue was taken by an American from Hong Kong to San Francisco in 1905. Seth was not positive about the date. He mentioned 34th Street, and I believe referred to New York City. A man named Bryant purchased it in San Diego, for his daughter, and transferred the statue from there to New York by nefarious ways. Seth then called Bill a romantic Jesuit.

(I joked with Seth about the great voice effects, and Seth agreed that he had not yet reached the peak in voice effects, at least as far as volume went. Whereupon Jane rose to her feet again and treated us to a voice display that in my opinion exceeded to some small degree the voice effects we had taped this evening. This was a prolonged display that lasted more or less for the balance of the session, and seemingly could have continued until dawn without effort on Jane's part, just as Seth said. The volume of sound hurt my ears at times.

(Seth said again that he considered such effects childish, but that it would be a small sacrifice to make if it helped to get the material across. Again he dwelt upon the difficulty of proving immortality. No matter what he did, people would say it was trickery. He still maintained that he could offer proof that would be sufficient, in time. He repeated again that he could not play on Dr. Instream's desire for immortality in order to arouse his interest in the material.

(What I think could be a very important point now came up when Peggy asked Seth about the question of proofs. Seth said that proofs she would accept would not be accepted by science. One proof to come, he said, would involve very strong facial changes in Jane during sessions. When I asked if these could be photographed he said yes.

(During most of the above dialogue, Seth spoke in a very loud and strong voice; Peggy estimated it could be heard for a city block.

(To recap: Seth also said, referring to photographic proof of facial changes in Jane, that if she took the photographs for instance [Peggy is a reporter for the Elmira Star-Gazette], she would be accused of collusion with Jane and myself.

(Referring again to the question of immortality, Seth said that all of us in the room knew what it was like to be old men, and that some of us had also been old women. He did not get more specific on this last point.

(Our bank account would never go below $700.00.

(Jane's poetry and my paintings were good, and would achieve their own kind of immortality.

(The Seth endeavor is well worth our while. Seth said he would arrange things so that I spent no more time writing up the material than I do now. He also bellowed that he would one day speak in an auditorium filled with psychologists.

(In answer to a question of Bill Gallagher's, Seth said Bill did well to refuse a promotion that would have necessitated his moving to Detroit. [Bill also works for the Elmira paper, in advertising.] Seth said that Bill was on the right track, that once he gets his physical problems straightened out, meaning his ulcer, he will be doing very well.

(There was more to this part of the session, but I believe that between us Peggy and I covered most categories discussed. End between 1:30 and 1:45 AM. Jane seemed as fresh as ever. The rest of us had had it.)

SESSION 171
JULY 21, 1965 9:14 PM WEDNESDAY AS SCHEDULED

(Note the late starting time. Tonight's session was almost not held at all. Both of us were tired from Monday's extralong session, and had decided not to hold a session tonight. I worked until almost 9 PM transcribing notes from Monday's taped session, then upon reconsidering told Jane it was okay with me if she wanted a session. Jane then decided to hold a session, and said she thought it would be brief.

(Jane had been much surprised at hearing her voice, as Seth, as it was taped Monday, July 19, for Dr. Instream. The power of the voice had amazed her, whereas I had taken it for granted because of long hours spent listening to it. She also was uneasy in that she felt Seth was too harsh at times; she worried about the reception Dr. Instream would give the tape, since Seth spoke in no uncertain terms. I thought that Dr. Instream's reception would be perfectly fine, and that in this tape Seth, and Jane, had made their points just as they wanted to.

(The session was quite short. It was held in our quiet back room. Jane spoke while sitting down, with her eyes closed, and in a voice somewhat deeper than usual. Her pace was slow.)

Dear friends. This will be a brief session.

Do not fear that many sessions will pass before we return to our own material. Our last session was indeed an important one. We have all the time available that we need. The material itself will develop to the fullest possible scope.

I knew what I was doing in our last session. The straightforward attitude will save us difficulties in the future. It is natural that Ruburt was startled when he heard the way he sounds when he allows me to speak.

This will pass, but it is all to the good that he was able to hear the voice. We will see to it that you are not too badly inconvenienced in any investigation.

I appreciate the basic inconvenience which the sessions cause, and I will endeavor to help you in whatever way I can, so that you are to some small extent repaid.

I regret that when the voice has a loud volume it does indeed sound quite harsh. I assure you that this is not my intent. For Ruburt's benefit, I have made no promises that I cannot keep. I cannot force, and will not attempt to force, Ruburt to accept my independent structure on a conscious level. He will do so in time.

Do you have any questions, Joseph?

("Nothing in particular, I guess. I'm satisfied with Monday's session.")

I will not keep you, as I realize that your time has been occupied with notetaking. I am always pleased to speak with you, and I regret the technical difficulties involved on your part. That is why, now and then, I enjoy sessions on a less formal basis, without your notes. It allows you some freedom, and it allows me the opportunity to speak with you in a more normal manner.

If you have no questions then I will not keep you. One point first: Doctor Instream is the best man that you could have contacted. If you have no questions I will give you some rest.

("Good night, Seth.")

(End at 9:25. Jane was dissociated as usual. She said Seth enjoyed the little session. Jane also said she retained a general idea of what Seth had said. She always knows what he is saying at the moment; the trick is to retain it after coming out of trance.

(On July 20, Jane and I received a letter from Dr. Instream, in which he mentioned the possibility of a session with another doctor at Oswego State University College; the other doctor also wanted to consider the study, within limits Seth may feel advisable.

(Also on July 20, I mailed copies of the 168th and 169th sessions to Dr. Instream.)

SESSION 172
JULY 26, 1965 9 PM MONDAY AS SCHEDULED

(On July 23, we mailed the tape of the 170th session to Dr. Instream. On July 26 Dr. Instream's letter arrived, acknowledging receipt of the 168th and 169th sessions.

(Tonight's session was witnessed by Lorraine Shafer and Bill Macdonnel. The last session witnessed by Bill was the 133rd, of February 17, 1965. Lorraine

witnessed the 168th, of July 7, 1965. It will be recalled that Bill Macdonnel's entity name is Mark, and Lorraine's is Marleno.

(*The session was held in our front room, with the four of us sitting in a circle, roughly. Jane spoke while sitting down and with her eyes closed. Her pace was rather fast but I had no trouble keeping up with her; nor did Lorraine, using shorthand.*

(*Jane rather surprised us by opening the session in a voice that was surprisingly deep and somewhat loud. I can say that the voice was somewhat deeper than her voice in the 170th session, though lacking of course anything like the sheer volume displayed in that session. At times it was almost a bass voice, quite vibrant, produced without visible strain. Indeed, Seth was in an almost jocular mood.*

(*Jane's voice was fairly deep in the 151st session. There have been some other instances of a voice deeper but not necessarily much louder or stronger; my estimate is that she reached her deepest voice in the 33rd session, of March 9, 1964. In that session her voice was also loud, much louder than in tonight's session.*

(*Jane actually began speaking at 8:59.*)

Good evening.

("*Good evening, Seth.*")

My heartiest greetings to our visitors.

I hardly find it necessary to deliver any massive voice displays this evening, and so we shall largely dispense with such activity.

("*Not too fast.*")

We will make an effort to return to our own material.

There are however a few remarks which I will make concerning other matters.

Now first of all Joseph, when I speak too quickly you simply must tell me so. If you do not speak out then indeed I am not to blame—

(*There came a knock on the door, and Jane stopped speaking. We don't use our front room for sessions anymore unless we have witnesses, in order to avoid the risk of interruptions. In the past such interruptions have been physically painful for Jane. She has compared the shock of an interruption to being doused with ice water.*

(*We all sat quietly for a moment. I was then surprised to note that Jane had come out of her trance with no difficulty, and that her eyes were open. In fact, it was she who answered the door, to speak briefly with someone who was looking for another apartment on our floor.*

(*In the 136th session such an interruption was enough of a shock to Jane to cause Seth to end the session. During the session with Dr. Instream, the 169th, held in his office at Oswego, Jane demonstrated an ability to go into and out of the trance state very easily. This marked the first time she had switched focus so easily, repeatedly. Now, Jane walked back to her chair. Before she was seated she had reentered the trance state, and was speaking. Resume at 9:01. Her voice was still quite deep.)*

We will here encounter no such difficulties as were encountered in the past. Ruburt will find that he is able to return to himself almost automatically. In some circumstances this will serve us both very well.

Now. We will indeed cooperate in any investigation in which we may become involved. We will however progress at our own rate, without due speed, and we will in all cases keep our own sessions as uncomplicated as possible.

Any effects that are demonstrated will appear within ordinary sessions. I will endeavor indeed to see that they are as definite as possible, and as clear-cut as will be desired. But spontaneity will as always remain a prerequisite for any such displays.

You will not be pressured, Joseph, for I shall see to it. Nor will Ruburt be pressured. We are so far dealing, however, with <u>men of good will</u>, and it is for this reason that we shall cooperate. The material itself is my main concern, and I know that it is your own.

There will indeed be a give and take between the <u>three</u> of us, and your good investigators. I thought it best in our recorded session that I speak frankly, <u>now</u>, and so I did.

I am interested in adding now to our own discussions, for it is time that we enlarged both their quality and scope. We will almost immediately embark upon a more concentrated study of the personality as it operates within its dream reality.

We will <u>also</u> discuss a matter which will be of extreme interest in the area of therapy, for we will be concerned with health and its relation to the dream universe. This will be most significant.

I will let you take a break, since I am attempting to take the human limitations that are involved in our situation into consideration. There is no reason why you must take notes until your fingers feel as if they would drop. First however, I wish to give particular greetings to our friend Mark, who has consented to visit our circle. I speak fondly in my own manner. By all means take your break, and we will continue with our session.

(Break at 9:14. Jane was dissociated as usual for a first delivery. Her voice had remained deep until break. She said the knock on the door didn't bother her at all. She thinks the ability to switch in and out of the trance state so easily made itself known during the session with Dr. Instream at Oswego; Jane feels however that she must have been preparing herself for this step forward without being aware of it.

(Jane's manner had been smiling and active during her first delivery, and it became even more so when she resumed speaking. She often leaned forward in her chair, gesturing and pointing even though her eyes remained closed. Her voice, still

deep, hit occasional stronger spots so that it almost boomed out. I began to wonder what our neighbors might hear, since our windows were open. Resume at 9:24.)

In future sessions, in the immediate future, we will deal with the dream universe in relation to many new aspects which we have not considered in the past.

You will then discover that this dream situation can be used for your own advantage. We will go into the ways and means by which such advantages can be obtained. The information will be of a very practical nature, and it will still serve to advance our theoretical material.

We will also be concerned with the framework of the human personality as it exists within several levels of reality. We will conclude our discussion concerning the nature of action, in so far as action is considered by itself. We will <u>always</u> be concerned with a discussion of action, even though other subjects are under consideration however, since it is impossible to divide action into various parts even for the purpose of discussion.

Shortly after, we will take a group of sessions to discuss particular dreams, and interpret them. In no case will we ever <u>leave</u> the basic material. It will serve as the framework from which, and within which, all of our sessions have their existence.

(Here Jane's voice was deep and loud.)

We will also find that it becomes natural and easy for Ruburt to speak in the manner in which he is now speaking, as a matter of course; and full concentration can still be given to the material in which we are interested.

There are questions which were asked in a general manner before your session began this evening.

I have no reason particularly not to answer them. However the questions involve more than you know; I am, Marleno, no guardian angel. I do not flap my wings. I have no wings to flap.

(Lorraine had asked the questions. Now Jane, her eyes still closed, leaned forward in her chair toward Lorraine. Holding her arms outstretched she moved them up and down like wings.)

My interest is concerned with those personalities with whom I am involved, and the circle of my interest includes those who come to these sessions; as indeed your own interest includes those people with whom you are acquainted. I never attempt to meddle into the private lives of those with whom I am concerned. If I am invited to comment, then I do.

I am indeed <u>aware</u>, in a general manner, of the main events in your life and in Mark's. But unless for some reason these are brought forcibly to my attention they remain as a part of my generalized knowledge.

(Jane was very restless in her chair, now leaning forward, then back. Her voice was still deeper than usual. She smiled.)

I find that in black and white my words may sound harsh. Yet I do not so intend them. I am simply concerned with your existence, and with Mark's, in the same manner with which you are concerned with the existence and circumstance of a friend.

I am indeed aware of many of the events in both of your lives, but it is relatively simple for me to so acquaint myself with your situations. I am willing at any time to render whatever services I can so render, but I do not walk ghostily through your rooms; and most certainly I do not peek through the windows.

There are <u>reasons</u> why certain personalities have been drawn to our sessions. This is obvious. Some of you have known each other in past lives. There are other reasons which, if you will excuse me, we shall not consider this evening simply because you do not yet have a basic understanding of certain issues which are involved. You can be assured of my interest and concern. My scope of activity is simply larger than your own.

I am aware of more and yet the <u>reason</u> for my concern could be called a quite <u>human</u> reason. You were drawn to the sessions for various reasons. These have something to do with both my interest and my concern. Mark in his own way is also so drawn.

I will never turn aside from human problems and human relationships in these sessions. The material itself must be oriented toward such relationships. I will for Joseph's benefit here state that the material itself will <u>in</u> the future be closely studied. It will form a basis for an upward thrust of mental activity and understanding.

This session is somewhat in the nature of a transitory session, for we will almost immediately in following sessions return to our main interests.

I will now suggest that you take a break. I will also tell you, Joseph, that with my voice I am like a bird trying out its new wings. *(Jane's voice grew abruptly much louder, briefly.)* And if I grow overenthusiastic I trust that you will forgive me. I will here in your apartment however keep a careful watch.

(Break at 9:47. Jane was dissociated as usual. She remembered some of the subject matter in a general way, and thought that if she tried hard enough she could retain more of it. Her eyes had remained closed, her voice had been a little lighter in timbre at times.

(Jane resumed in a deeper voice, at a good pace and with her eyes again closed, at 9:58.)

We will shortly conclude this evening's session.

I am attempting to take some workload from Joseph now. He needs a rest in this respect. We will however in our next session return to our usual format.

I will answer any questions that any of you might have.

(*I looked at Lorraine and Bill, but neither of them had a question prepared. I too was caught by surprise.*)

Otherwise we will shortly end. I am concerned that we return to our material, for there will be times when it will be necessary for us to focus our energies in other directions. Such circumstances will not arise frequently, but they will arise. I am most sympathetic, Joseph, to the predicament in which you found yourself last weekend, and when we are alone we will discuss efforts that may be taken in the future. You did very well, considering the whole situation.

(*The above passage refers to my parents. Seth has discussed them at various times in the past and his advice has been very helpful. Among others see the following sessions: 17, 18, 21, 27, 53, 93 and 94, ranging through Volumes 1, 2 and 3.*)

As always I regret leaving you. You may rest assured that I will hold my own with your psychologists. I am very fond of your Dr. Instream, however. We shall proceed in a way that will serve us all very well, and *(louder)* you need have no doubts concerning the affair in general.

It is very possible that Ruburt will soon discover that I am who I say I am. He <u>knows</u> this subconsciously, but I am speaking now of a conscious recognition. I now bid my friends a fond *(deeper and louder)* good evening. And if I do not sound like a nightingale, it may be said that I speak in tones not quite as bad as a grandfather frog.

("Good night, Seth."

(*End at 10:05. Jane was dissociated as usual. Her voice maintained its deep tones until the end of the session. Seth closed out on a loud and deep and humorous note. And again, the peculiar accent that Bill Gallagher insists is not an Irish brogue, was in evidence at times during the session.*)

SESSION 173
JULY 28, 1965 9 PM WEDNESDAY AS SCHEDULED

(*Jane has been practicing psychological time regularly, but reports that she has achieved little besides her usual excellent state. She has had no unusual or startling experiences since Seth cut her psy-time periods to 20 minutes, in the 151st session.*

(*Jane has had some striking clairvoyant and telepathic experiences outside of psy-time, however, and is keeping separate records of these. Three such instances in the last two weeks have been especially interesting. One was clairvoyant, two were telepathic. Two of the experiences have been verified so far by the other people involved.*

(*This evening's session was held in our small back room, and was very peaceful and quiet. Jane spoke while sitting down and with her eyes closed. Her voice was quiet and she used pauses for the first time in quite a few sessions.*)

Good evening.

("*Good evening, Seth.*")

We will have a quiet, and all in all a rather brief session.

We have taken advantage, and we will continue to do so, of good circumstances and high periods of psychic activity. It is only fair that I allow you to rest now and then. Very seldom will we have vacations as such, unless of course you request them. For this reason we will go slowly this evening.

I will however begin a discussion concerning the personality and its relationship to those dreams which it creates.

We have discussed this subject to some degree. However we have not begun a study in depth. It is now time for us to do so. The personality as you know is composed of energy gestalts. The dreams created by the personality can be considered therefore as a part of the changing personality. We are speaking here in one context only, for we know that the dream universe is also to some extent independent of personality.

In this particular context however the dream world will be considered in its relationship to the personality. In many ways the dream universe does operate within this context, and is part of the personality framework. As the personality is changed by any experience or any action, so it is changed by its own dreams. Here again we see how energy or action operates within itself. We can even trace the actions and interactions.

As a personality is molded by his exterior circumstances, so is he also molded by the dreams that he creates, and which help to form his interior or psychic environment. To the whole self there is little differentiation made between actions that are of an exterior nature, and actions that are of an interior nature. While the ego makes these distinctions, the basic core of the personality does not do so.

A particularly vivid dream is every bit as real to the inner self as a vivid psychological experience that occurs within the waking state. It is important here that we realize that as far as the basic self is concerned no distinctions are made in this respect. The personality creates its dreams; the dreams are then experienced. The experience is indelibly recorded, and then changes the personality, again, in the same manner that any experience would.

The individual therefore reacts to his interior environment or psychic environment in the same way that he reacts to his physical situation. And as he changes his physical situation through reacting to it, so he changes his interior or psychic situation as he reacts to it.

It goes without saying that the dream universe is every bit as real to the inner self as the physical universe is to the conscious egotistical self. The physical universe is <u>relatively</u> (underline relatively) as unimportant to the inner self as the dream universe appears to be to the egotistical self.

The core of the self is obviously aware of all realities to some extent. If portions of the self did not coincide then it would be impossible for the whole personality to ever operate as a unit. Here we simply have spirals, so to speak, of evermoving actions that compose the whole self. But portions of these spirals coincide, and in this analogy the spirals of action not only have those dimensions which you understand, but other dimensions with which you are not yet familiar.

The designations put upon these units of action are highly artificial, and represent limitations that are quite arbitrary. We mentioned in an earlier session something to this effect, in that you simply perceive a small portion of such action, label it as a unit, can perceive no further, and so suppose that what you see or perceive is all <u>there is</u> to see or perceive.

The self is limitless. Where your perceptions fail, boundaries seem to appear. This has much to do with your conception of the reality of dreams, for it appears to you that dreams cease when you are no longer aware of them. Another portion of the self however <u>is</u> aware of them.

You may take your first break, and we will continue.

(Break at 9:23. Jane was dissociated as usual for a first break. Her pace had been good, even with pauses.

(Seth has discussed dreams to some extent in many sessions; too many to list here. He was discussing nightmares as far back as the 15th session, dream locations in the 44th session among others, the layers of the subconscious and dreams in the 92nd session. For a few examples of the manner in which Seth interprets dreams, see the 85th, 93rd and 94th sessions. See the 151st session for material on dreams, moment points and time, the 162nd for dreams and the electrical field, the 164th for dreams and impeding actions.

(Jane resumed, again with her eyes closed, and sitting down, in a quiet voice, and at a brisk pace, at 9:31.)

On one level the personality does attempt to solve problems through dream construction.

In many cases these problems are not those belonging to the ego, but to other layers of the self. We spoke in a fairly recent session of illnesses as impeding actions.

(See the 163rd and 164th sessions.)

In dreams the personality <u>first</u> attempts to solve many problems, and to give freedom to actions that cannot be adequately expressed within the confines of the physical universe.

If the personality handles his dream activities capably, then the problem action finds release. When the ego is too rigid, it will even attempt to censor dreams. When the personality in general is too rigid, freedom of action is not entirely permitted even in the dream state.

When this solution fails the impeding action will then materialize as a physical illness, or as an undesirable psychological condition. The dream experience however is much more richly varied than you suppose. There are ways which we shall discuss that will enable a personality to deal more effectively with the dream situation, and to use it more effectively with the dream situation, and to use it more effectively.

This is a rather simplified explanation. Consider however a situation in which the personality needs to express dependency, but feels that such an expression is not possible within his waking experience. If he is able to <u>dream</u> in such a manner that he can construct dream dramas in which he plays a dependent part, then the action is satisfied.

In many instances this is exactly what happens. The individual would not of course as a rule remember such a dream on a conscious level. Psychologically however the experience would be completely valid, and the dependency therefore expressed.

(The above paragraph brings to mind the fact that Seth discussed a dream of Bill Macdonnel's during the 84th session; Bill witnessed the session, and afterwards told us he had no conscious memory of the dream, which had taken place a few days before the session according to Seth. Yet Seth analyzed the symbolic content of the dream rather thoroughly, saying it was an important one for Bill since it bore upon his home and professional life. See Volume 1.)

Dreams can be interpreted as you know from many viewpoints, since their reality exists within various aspects of actuality. The dream experience itself, and I cannot stress this too strongly, is as real as <u>any</u> experience to the basic self. It follows that instructions may be given <u>to</u> the self, so that various problems can be solved within the dream situation.

The solution may or may not be given to the consciousness. In many instances this would not be necessary. The inner ego of which we have spoken is the director of such unifying activities, and while the inner ego is mainly concerned with inner reality, it is also aware of physical existence.

(Jane now took a long pause, sitting quietly without moving for perhaps a

minute. It was the first such pause she had used in quite a few sessions.)

The inner ego is indeed the "I" of your dreams, having somewhat the same sort of position within the inner self as the ego itself has to the physical self. Actions however merge within the inner ego. The scope of awareness is more complex. We will at a later time discuss this inner ego in connection with the dream situation and health.

Dream dramas are not nebulous theaterlike productions. Their own dimensions, in <u>their way</u>, are every bit as valid as those of waking life. They are as coherent. They affect the self sometimes to an even greater degree. The dream personalities are indeed fragments, projections of the self, all working out various roles, seeking various experiences, searching for solutions and gratifications.

(The word fragment was first used in the 4th session, Volume 1, page 22, by Frank Watts. Actually the Frank Watts personality was in the process of being superseded by Seth then, and on the next page Seth announced his presence by name. This was on December 8, 1963. The word compartment had been used in the third session, with a similar meaning.)

These dream personalities or fragments indeed have their own consciousness. They are as <u>un</u>aware, and <u>as</u> aware, of you as you are of them. They exist once you have created them. No action can be withdrawn. It must complete its nature according to the dimensions in which it exists, and so the dream personalities or fragments continue to exist whether or not you are aware of them.

The inner ego however is to some degree still familiar with their activities. Solutions found by these dream personalities are automatically picked up by the inner ego, and transmitted to the various levels of the self. The dream world changes as the personality changes, so that it is always a part of the mobile personality framework.

It is always <u>within</u> this framework, but not always does it maintain the same relative position within it. The stability of the personality depends in some degree upon the effectiveness with which it handles and manipulates these dream situations. It is realized that the personality manipulates within the physical universe, but the fact is not generally accepted that similar manipulations must be made within this dream universe.

I suggest your break.

(Break at 10:01. Jane was dissociated as usual. She said she can usually recall what she said when she is dealing with personalities, such as Dr. Instream. She finds the kind of abstract material presented above difficult to retain, however, outside of a very general idea.

(Jane had delivered the above material while sitting down and with her eyes closed. Her voice had been quiet, her manner slow and with pauses. She resumed in

the same fashion at 10:07.)

Much work has been done in the attempt to interpret dreams. None, or very little, has been done to <u>control</u> dreams, or to control the direction of activity within dreams.

Upon proper suggestion the personality will work out specific problems in the dream state, as earlier mentioned. If the solution is not clear to the ego, this does not mean that the solution has not been found, necessarily. There may even be instances where it is not only unnecessary but undesirable that the ego be familiar with such a solution.

This problem-solving aspect of dreams is rather important, and can be utilized with rather impressive practical results. We are merely beginning to scratch the surface here in this discussion, and we will devote a number of sessions to it. We have spoken about the importance of expectation. With practice dream activities can also be directed in this direction.

(For some material on expectation see the following sessions, among others: 79, 135, 157, 158, 159, 160, 163, 164, 169, in Volumes 2, 3, and 4.)

Dreams do <u>express</u> a personality's basic reality. Negative dreams <u>tend to reinforce</u> the negative aspects of the personality, helping to form vicious circles of unfortunate complications. Upon suggestion dream actions can be turned toward fulfilling constructive expectations, which can themselves effect a definite change for the better in the personality involved.

I am speaking now of general circumstances, since there are occasions when negative actions seek expression quite legitimately, and without any danger to the personality involved. We will have much more to say concerning these connections between dream actions and the balanced personality. Again, there are many ways in which dreams can be used beneficially, and with deliberation.

I told you that this would be a fairly brief session, and so I here end it. My best regards to you both. Do you have any questions?

("Do you dream?")

I do dream, but not necessarily while in a sleeping state. I am conscious of these actions that occur within the psychological framework of my personality. Theoretically the human personality <u>can</u>, or could, be conscious of dreams even while he was in a waking state. Practically however this does not appear to be of benefit, nor does it seem to occur.

The human personality within the physical system cannot <u>juggle</u> realities with any ease. If you have no more questions we will end the session.

("How's my old friend, Frank Watts?")

(Jane smiled, a reaction that I expected. It will be remembered that the sessions began when Jane contacted the Frank Watts personality. Frank Watts in turn is a

fragment of the Seth entity. Seth discussed Frank Watts to some degree in the 85th and 88th sessions, promising more data in the future.)

I greatly enjoy your laudable concern with Frank Watts. He is indeed quite well, thank you.

("Is that all you're going to say about him?"

(Jane smiled again.)

He is on his own. I will some evening say more.

("Has Dr. Instream listened to the tape we sent him?"

(We mailed the tape of the 170th session to Dr. Instream on Friday, July 23. This is the session Seth addressed to Dr. Instream.)

He has.

("What did he think of it?")

He was fascinated.

("Did anybody else listen to it with him?")

I do not know.

("Well, I guess that's it, then."

(After a short pause Jane's eyes opened.

("Good night, Seth."

(End at 10:27. Jane was dissociated as usual. Her eyes had remained closed, her voice quiet. She said Seth had felt no apparent urge to elaborate on any of his answers to my questions. He was concerned mainly with the general material. She said she sensed a slight irritation on Seth's part when I asked if anybody else had listened to the tape with Dr. Instream; it was as though Seth could get the information to answer the question, but didn't feel inclined to so exert himself.

(Jane said that after thinking over the recent occasions when strong voice effects were demonstrated, as in the 170th and 172nd sessions, she feels that Seth uses the voice as an insulator for herself and as a projection of himself.)

SESSION 174
AUGUST 2, 1965 9 PM MONDAY AS SCHEDULED

(To our surprise, we received the tape of the 170th session back from Dr. Instream on July 29th, Thursday. We had mailed it to him on July 23rd, Friday, taking it for granted he would want to keep it for a while. No letter accompanied the tape. We noticed the tape had been transferred to a new reel, so took it for granted that Dr. Instream had played the tape, as stated by Seth in the 173rd session of July 28th. See page 169.

(In the 166th session, which John Bradley witnessed, Seth stated that the stock

of John's company, G. D. Searle, would go very low before making a recovery presumably. This was on June 30, 1965. Since we have been watching it Searle stock has fluctuated somewhat. On July 3 it closed at 54 1/2. On July 29 it reached a low of 50 1/2. On August 3 it closed at 53 1/4.

(The session tonight was held in our back room, and was again a quiet one. Jane spoke while sitting down and with her eyes closed. Her voice was quiet, her pace rather slow.)

Good evening.

("Good evening, Seth.")

I cannot stress too strongly the fact that mankind in general is aware of very little outside of physical reality.

He has managed to organize physical reality because he focuses so intensely within it. His knowledge of other realities is limited however to infrequent glimpses. He perceives bits and pieces of other realities. As long as his perception in this manner is so disorganized and so fragmentary he cannot hope to compose any conception of the total.

The nearest field of reality outside of the immediately physical one is the area of dreams. This field has been given very little study. It represents in many ways a meeting ground between psychic and physical existence. You realize here that the terms psychic and physical are merely designations used for the sake of convenience.

I have mentioned before that in its own way the dream universe is as permanent as the physical universe. Basically its structure is somewhat the same, in that it is composed of atoms and molecules. These particles however simply exist within a different perspective. The inner logic is much more consistent within the dream universe, and action is permitted greater freedom in several important respects.

The interrelationship between the waking state and the sleeping state has never been clearly understood. One of the main differences between the waking and sleeping states is merely the almost complete change of focus that is involved. When you are using intellectual methods alone you will necessarily fall short in any study of the dream reality. Man is indeed his intellect, but he is much else besides.

The intuitions must go hand in hand with the intellect. The intellect is useful in interpreting your data in terms that the ego can understand. The intuitions come close to mankind's source, and it is through the intuitions that information pertaining to the dream reality will come.

The experience involved in learning to change your own focus of awareness will be most beneficial. It will even add to the beneficial nature of your own dreams. You do not have to sleep to <u>dream</u>. Every individual has had his daydreams, and here you can see more clearly this change of focus. I meant to mention this earlier. Ruburt can request levitation dreams, and he will have them.

(*Jane already has; two nights ago.*)

Now. If the basic personality is fairly well balanced, then his existence in the dream reality will reinforce his physical existence. The opposite will also hold true. You are involved in a juggling of realities. The dream reality is simply the <u>nearest</u> reality with which you are concerned outside of your physical preoccupation. It is necessary to see the personality as it operates within both realities, if you are interested in viewing the personality as a whole. And even then unless you delve deeply you will fall short.

Studies of space and distance as they are experienced in dreams will be helpful, and our material will indeed deal with such discussions. For investigation into the nature of space and time as they are experienced within the dream framework, will tell you more about the real nature of space and time then you can ever learn through studying their distorted appearances within physical reality. This will be most important to us.

I suggest your first break.

(*Break at 9:24. Jane was dissociated as usual for a first delivery. She resumed in the same quiet and slow manner, with her eyes closed, at 9:32.*)

In normal memory you recall, obviously, but a slight percentage of your dreams, and usually these are from more surface levels.

I would suggest that you tell yourselves that you will henceforth be able to remember dreams from the deeper levels of your personality, and you should find that you will be able to do so.

(*Jane is in her second year of keeping records of her dreams, and has written down several hundred. Since September of 1965, a period of 11 months, I have recorded 185 dreams. Jane recorded 103 dreams for 1964, and so for 1965 has recorded 303 dreams, for a total of 406 dreams to date.*)

You can also tell yourselves when you wish that you will give special attention to the nature of time and space, as these appear within your dreams. You will discover then upon awakening that many perceptions concerning time and space within the dream state will remain with you.

As I mentioned, your psychological time experiences will also help you to investigate the nature of time and space to some degree.

In this sort of an investigation instructions then can be given before sleeping, and a portion of the self will indeed continue to work for you in this manner. You can indeed learn much concerning events; but what we are mainly concerned with here is the stuff of dreams, and the framework within which they have their existence.

For the framework is the same framework in which you have your physical existence. We will make you investigators even in your sleep; and you can see now how your very investigations are bound to change the nature of your dreams themselves. Only in this case nothing will be lost, and much gained. It is unfortunate that medical men who deal with the mind as a specialty have not thought of some of these connections more thoroughly.

Many problems could be worked out in the dream state. Dependency feelings that are overwhelming could be given freer and safer expression, if the patient had the suggestion given to him that he would dream of himself in dependent positions. He could then behave in the physical environment with greater confidence. He could to some extent have his cake and eat it too.

For once more, to the basic personality an experience is important according to its vividness or significance on an intimate basis. The personality does not differentiate between a waking or a sleeping experience in any real manner. This also is not clearly understood. Dream therapy could offer great advantages, but here again it could be dangerous in the hands of unscrupulous or rigid personalities.

The rigidity of a personality is its downfall. We will have some sessions dealing with dream therapy. Through such therapy actions would be allowed greater spontaneity, and channels would not be clogged by impeding actions to any great degree. Dream therapy would actually involve no more than lending a helping hand to a phenomena that already occurs.

Both psychological and physical illnesses could be largely avoided in such a manner. Rather harmlessly, aggressive tendencies could also be given freedom. The individual involved would experience the aggressiveness, and yet he would hurt no one. Suggestions could even be given so that he learned to understand his own aggressiveness through watching himself in the dream state.

This is not as farfetched as it might seem. Much seemingly erratic antisocial behavior could be avoided through such dream therapy. I will even say that crimes of the grossest sort could be prevented. The desired but feared actions would not then gather up toward an explosion. The habitual, overly-aggressive or overly-dependent tendencies would not result in habitual aggressive or dependent behavior, for each individual action would be harmlessly expressed.

If I may indulge in a fantasy, theoretically you could indeed imagine a massive experiment in dream therapy, where wars were fought by the sleeping and not by the waking nations. We will discuss this whole question very thoroughly, as I have been leading up to it for a while.

I am not suggesting that you substitute dream reality for your so-called waking reality. I am mainly suggesting that the two can reinforce each other to a larger degree than you recognize. Also it is difficult for you to accept the idea that experience within dreams is as vivid and valid a part of the personality as its waking experience.

The inner ego is quite capable of dealing with both types of experience, and it is of course to this inner ego that your own suggestions will make sense, and be acted upon.

I suggest your break.

(Break at 10:02. Jane was dissociated as usual. Her delivery had been somewhat faster this time, though still quiet. Her eyes had remained closed. She resumed in the same fashion at 10:08.)

There are however many considerations here that must be understood.

We can only begin to discuss them this evening. They are vital and must not be overlooked. When or if, for example, aggressiveness is the problem, then the preliminary suggestion should include a statement that in the dream the aggression will be <u>harmlessly</u> acted out (underline harmlessly), and <u>not</u> directed against a particular individual.

The subconscious is quite capable of handling the situation in such a manner. This may seem like a double censure, but it is in all cases the intangible element, the aggressiveness itself, that is important, and not the person or persons toward whom the individual may decide to vent the aggressiveness.

When the aggressiveness is released, then there will be no need for a victim. We do not want, in other words, to direct an individual to dream about a situation in which he is attacking a particular individual. There are many reasons for this, both telepathic realities which you do not as yet understand, and guilt patterns which would be unavoidable. This again is vital, and we shall discuss such matters to some degree.

Again, we are not attempting to substitute dream action <u>for</u> physical action, generally speaking. We are talking about specific problems that may arise that need treatment. As far as general practice is concerned, we will deal with our dreams in a much more <u>positive</u> and constructive manner, along the lines of expectation.

Problem solving will also come under this classification, where solutions are being sought. In our discussion of dependency and aggression I was speaking of potentially dangerous situations, in which an individual shows signs of being unable to cope with these psychological actions through ordinary methods of adaption. No one can deny that a war fought by dreaming men, at specified times, would be less harmful than a physical war, to return to my flight of fancy.

There would still be repercussions, however, though less disastrous, that would be unavoidable. For again, basically the personality does not differentiate between a waking and a sleeping experience. The importance of any experience is judged by the personality according to its personal vividness and significance. It is only the ego who makes other distinctions.

(Jane now took a long pause.)

This evening's session will serve as a basis for many to come.

You will hear from your Dr. Instream shortly.

(Another long pause.)

I will now bid you a fond good evening, and pleasant dreams to you both.

("Good night, Seth.")

(End at 10:25. Jane was a little more dissociated for the last delivery, she said. Her eyes had remained closed, her voice quiet. She remembered some of the material.)

SESSION 175
AUGUST 4, 1965 9 PM WEDNESDAY AS SCHEDULED

(Once again the session was held in our quiet back room. Both of us felt somewhat tired, but attributed it to the weather, which has been cloudy and oppressive for the past few days. Jane and I try to ignore such factors consciously, but have no doubt we feel the psychic effects of weather as much as anybody else.

(Jane spoke while sitting down and with her eyes closed. As in the last session her voice was very quiet and clear, and she used many pauses. We hoped to obtain more material on dream therapy. She began speaking at 9:01 actually.)

Good evening.

("Good evening, Seth.")

I see that we will have another quiet session.

We will take advantage of it by furthering several of our discussions.

I have spoken often concerning the importance of changing focus, altering the direction of consciousness. This does not involve a <u>change</u> in consciousness itself, merely a change in the direction in which consciousness is focused. This ability is obviously not only inherent within the human race, but it is used constantly in your ordinary life to some degree. Usually however this involves a rather surface change of focus, as your attentions are directed first upon specific physical areas, and then switched to other specific physical areas.

This does not involve however a change of focus in <u>depth</u>. A change to a different level entirely occurs when the individual switches focus from physical reality to other realities. In the dream state obviously we have an example of such change. One of the main reasons why this is possible within the dream state, rather than in the waking state, is that survival necessities have usually been satisfied.

(Jane now took what I term a long pause, lasting about a minute. Her pace had been slow; the above paragraph had been broken by many shorter pauses.)

Such a change of focus demands a concentration in one area to the exclusion, as a rule, of other areas. In the waking state you are usually not aware of your dreaming existence. In your dreaming existence your physical environment is replaced by your dream environment. You react to both environments whenever you are concentrated within them. Our study of the dream state will take us into many other discussions, for you will learn much about the nature of uncamouflaged reality.

There are several ways that will allow you to change the focus of your own awareness when you choose. I am speaking now of a change regarding depth and levels.

(Jane took another pause. This one lasted a minute and a half by the clock. She sat quietly, eyes closed, her hands folded in her lap. It is probably as long a pause as she has taken during the sessions. Finally she resumed speaking, her voice quiet as before.)

We will have an extremely brief session, as I can see, for various reasons, no important ones, we are falling short for this session. Or you may take a break and we will try again. We simply have a poor connection. The reasons have nothing particularly to do with any of the three of us, and occur very seldom. The conditions indeed are rather interesting in themselves, and will be discussed now or later.

("We'll take a break and see what Jane says.")

As you wish.

(Break at 9:18. Jane reported that she was dissociated as usual for a first break. She was as surprised as I was that Seth had announced a poor connection. We had no conscious ideas as to why this should be, and indeed this was the first time this problem had come up during the sessions.

(We thought our feeling tired nothing unusual, nor had we been concerned at any effect the weather might have upon us. Jane said that the extra long pause listed above was a most unusual one, however, in that it reminded her of being connected with a "dead" telephone. During most pauses, when she is aware of them, she feels that even though she may not be speaking she is still connected with a live source.

(Jane elected to try to continue the session, since she felt all right. She resumed in the same quiet voice, though with a faster pace, and with her eyes again closed, at 9:25.)

The conditions do not originate with <u>you</u> personally, though they are at your end rather than at my end, and they have to do with electromagnetic disturbances that are, to some degree, cyclic, and to which you react.

They form a sort of insulation which makes communication difficult. You can see that they occur infrequently, since this is the first time that they have annoyed us. They occur to some degree <u>fairly</u> frequently, but this period is one in which they are strong enough to exert some force.

Their action is inhibiting at your end. The weather has also a connection here, and your moods are affected by both. The period should be over by three o'clock, approximately, tomorrow afternoon, when the conditions dissipate, or begin to dissipate.

("Can this condition produce distortions in the material?")

(Naturally I wondered about this, and whether it was worth continuing the session under distortive conditions.)

Theoretically, if they affected Ruburt's ability to translate the material. There are no distortions in this evening's session, such as it is. You have felt the effects of these conditions, and they have been felt by others. They are like pockets, and are not uniformly distributed.

Your green plants are affected when the conditions prevail.

(Jane's delivery had again slowed up somewhat, so that she began to use pauses.

("The baby downstairs has been crying a lot lately, in the middle of the night. Do these conditions have anything to do with that?")

The child is also affected. I will not give you information dealing with the child this evening.

(Jane took another pause. The following material began to come through at 9:35 by our clock. Jane took many pauses while delivering it, and until just before break she sat quite still. Her eyes remained closed. Her manner was quiet and deliberate.)

I would prefer that you not ask me questions about what I am going to say.

There are four men at a table, and we are under discussion. Dr. Instream being one, I believe. If not, then the man meets his physical description closely. One other man is along in years. One is much younger. I do not know the last man's age.

A large coffee urn is nearby. Papers, no tablecloth. Someone may be taking notes. Some indecision, and a clash of dates. Straight-backed chairs. I do not hear other voices. One man may be bald in the center of his head, and one may have a mustache, or if not he is not cleanly shaven.

Flowers somewhere, in a vase or outside a window, I don't know. *(Jane shook her head.)* There seems to be something about a radio. I do not know to what this refers. A letter to you. Some cautiousness in it because of indecision, though the cautiousness may or may not be apparent.

One point should be made here. It is sometimes difficult to give specific time limits, since basically I do not perceive time as you do.

I suggest your break.

(Break at 9:45. Jane was dissociated as usual. She did not realize she was using so many pauses in giving the above data. She said she had a very "hazy" impression, as Seth talked, of a group of figures at a table. She saw nothing plainly, and so feels she is taking Seth's word for the above material.

(Jane said the above is the kind of material she would have blocked in earlier sessions as soon as she felt it coming up, although occasionally she has allowed it to come through. One instance of such data checking out concerned the Provincetown and Bill Macdonnel material of the 68th, 75th, 82nd, 83rd, and 84th sessions.

(Jane now emphasized that where she would have "stiffened up" earlier, she now feels it foolish to let the fear of failure block what might be good material. Her attitude now is that if she is wrong once, perhaps she'll do better the next time.

(Jane now resumed in the same quiet manner, sitting down and with her eyes closed. This time she began speaking again while holding a hand to her eyes, at 9:55.)

I see also a box of clippings in a drawer, perhaps a desk drawer, *(Jane took a long pause)* and an unusually-shaped object, perhaps used as a paperweight.

We will now close a very brief session. My fondest regards to you both.

("Good night, Seth.")

(End at 9:57. Jane was again dissociated as usual. She said that again she had the vaguest kind of an impression, this time of an object, perhaps the paperweight, on top of a dark wooden desk. She pointed out that Seth said nothing about the desk-top being dark.)

My sensation of Friday night, August 6, 1965.

(On the above evening I again experienced a feeling of enlargement in parts of my body. This was very similar to my experience of July 9, 1965, at Oswego State University College in Oswego, NY. See page 131. Both experiences seem to be related to sound, and both took place in the small hours of the night after I had been sleeping for some time, then awakened. In each case Jane slept on beside me.

(At Oswego, I was awakened by a party of college students in a nearby residence hall. This time I was roused by the tenants downstairs, who came home at about 2:30 AM, with company, and sat in the backyard talking. It was a very hot and humid night.

(In a drowsy state, I lay on my left side with my arms loosely crossed over my chest. I began to feel the enlargement first in my hands, then across my chest. This time I was alert as to what was happening at the first signs, and tried to encourage it without making any strenuous effort of will. The results didn't surpass those of July

9; they were just a bit different.

(My chest came to feel that it was much wider, much broader and stronger and thicker—perhaps a yard wide. My upper arms gradually grew to feel that they were as thick as my thighs. My hands, as on July 9, came to feel the size of baseball gloves. I was aware of a greatly enlarged feeling in each of the fingers to some degree, as before, but this time the feeling that my fingers were somehow united into a pawlike or clublike unit was dominant.

(The sensation was very pleasant and not at all frightening. This time I had no feeling of enlargement in my face, or in my body below the diaphragm. The sensation lasted very definitely for several minutes, giving me plenty of time to explore it, then gradually dwindled away.

(For data on my other sensations and some visions, see the following sessions: 22, 24, 26, 27, 65, 145, 146, 163, 169. Nor do these include the enlarged hand sensations that Jane and I have experienced during sessions.)

SESSION 176
AUGUST 9, 1965 9 PM MONDAY AS SCHEDULED

(On the evening of August 5, Thursday, Jane and I mailed Dr. Instream a copy of the 175th session, held August 4, 1965, and asked him to check the telepathic/clairvoyant information on pages 176-77. We had not heard from Dr. Instream recently, up to the time we mailed the letter.

(Jane's clairvoyant experiences continue. Some are more complete than others and can happen at any time of the day. Some appear while she is awake and active, others when she is in a drowsy state. They have been appearing often enough recently so that she now keeps a separate record of them. See also the notes at the beginning of the 173rd session.

(See pages 131, for Friday, July 9, 1965, and 177 and above for Friday, August 6, for the two latest examples of my experience of physical enlargement. I mentioned them to Jane just before the session tonight in hopes that Seth would mention them.

(On Sunday afternoon, August 8, Jane and I attended the funeral of my Aunt Ella Buck in Wellsburg, NY, a nearby small town. Ella was my father's sister and died at 88. My mother and father and my brother Loren and his wife and son were also there. I had seen very little of Aunt Ella over the years, and Jane had met her twice, as best we can recall. I thought it might be interesting to ask Seth to comment on Ella, so I also mentioned this subject just before the session.

(The session was a quiet one and was held in our small back room. Jane spoke

while sitting down, with her eyes closed and in a rather rapid manner, throughout the session. Occasionally she used pauses. Her voice was quiet to begin with, but where indicated it began to deepen. It did not acquire much more volume. This manifestation reminded me somewhat of the deeper voice effect Jane showed in the 172nd session. In that session Seth stated that it would become natural and easy for Jane to speak in that manner.)

Good evening.

("Good evening, Seth.")

I had intended to further our discussion concerning dream reality. Nevertheless I will be glad to discuss your aunt Ella, whose entity name is Dorinella.

(Jane hesitated over the pronunciation of Dorinella, and I had to ask Seth to spell it out.)

Her previous lives were four. Her spiritual existence this time was a very happy one. The personality however was never entirely centered within physical reality, and was able to cope with it only by remaining relatively aloof.

She was connected with your father's brother in this life. His name was Jay. She was connected with him <u>two</u> lives previously as a very beloved wife.

When we have a suitable period of time it would be most beneficial for us to discuss the various members of your present family, Joseph, in connection with their past experiences.

The [retarded] son represented the result of two main conditions. The woman could simply not bring herself to form a complete construction. Her energies were not directed in a manner that would permit her to give birth to a normal child. She deeply reacted against violence, and was overly sensitive.

She felt that it was her responsibility to have a child, and so she did. At the same time, because of the child's defect, she managed to produce a child who was relatively free of those pressures against which she reacted. She produced in other words an idiot, who was in his own way supremely invulnerable to the realization of misfortune, a child who would not grow mentally into an adult, and a child who would remain secure in a relatively eternal childhood.

(Here Jane's voice began to deepen and grow a bit louder. Jane knows rather little about my family history. Seth is correct in stating that my father's older brother, my Uncle Jay, who is also dead, was connected with Ella in this life; he was very protective toward her, and after he died eight years ago his wife continued to watch over Ella.

(I have a few boyhood memories of Ella's retarded son, also named Jay. He has been institutionalized for many years, and I do not believe Ella and her husband Wilbur saw him for a number of years prior to their deaths.)

Nor did she feel guilty. Basically she considered that she had indeed produced a human being who would remain in a sort of summer garden, secure from deep hurts and vain regret.

The child was extremely gentle in his way, and in his way he is still a gentle child. We are speaking honestly here, and so I will say that she would herself have preferred to dwell in such a dreamlike state herself. She was never a part of her century or her time, and she tried to protect her offspring according to her own limits, by seeing to it that his escape would be a more definite one than her own.

(Jane spoke while smiling, her voice going a little deeper.)

You must also realize that the entity who became her son also chose the circumstances, knowing of them in advance, for his own purposes. There are many character aspects to be considered here. For if each personality is an energy gestalt, then also each <u>family group</u> is also an energy gestalt. The actions and interactions form its characteristics and nature.

Your Ella, then, reacted against the repressed violence which has always been a part of that family structure as it is composed of its various personalities. She reacted vehemently against this repressed violence. She married a man in whom there was little aggressiveness.

Their ways were different in many respects, but they were kind to each other always. They shared a love of nature. They both hoarded the things they loved. To some extent they hoarded each other. They both dug in like squirrels, and hid.

To some extent she resembled her mother. Her vanity, however, was not a characteristic woman's vanity. Her vanity was perhaps the one characteristic that she <u>shared</u> with other members of the family. She felt she was set apart, but also that she was set apart because she could not tolerate violence. Violence frightened her deeply.

She would not admit the fear, but would change the fear to pride, saying to herself that the world was evil, and she would therefore have little to do with it. And so she did not. She was not a foolish woman. She loved her husband most deeply. She and he shared a quite mystical love of nature and of animals. They would harm no one.

I will indeed have more to say here, since I have begun. Nevertheless you may take your break.

(Break at 9:24. Jane was rather well dissociated for a first break, she said. Her eyes had remained closed, her voice fairly deep but not loud to speak of.

(I can say that as far as my own memory goes, Seth has furnished a stunningly accurate picture of Aunt Ella, her temperament, etc. The descriptions here tally

very closely with my remembered childhood impressions of Aunt Ella, when I saw her most often.

(As stated before, Jane met Ella twice, both times rather briefly some years ago, and has no idea how much she remembers of the visits subconsciously. Jane met Ella's husband Wilbur once; he died a few years ago. I remember Wilbur as a small gentle man who was a tailor and who smoked strong cigars. He had a white mustache and a gravel voice. I recall that the family accused him of drinking heavily and of not taking care of Ella, although I recall no objective evidence of this. I always liked Wilbur. After his death Ella was moved to a nursing home.

(For some data on my parents and our family group, see the following sessions: 17, 18, 21, 27, 53, 93, 94, 172, among others, in Volumes 1 through 4.

(Jane resumed in the same deeper voice, at a good pace and with her eyes closed, at 9:30.)

She was gentle, and yet displayed a characteristic hauteur, in that she felt that the world was soiled, and so she would come in contact with it as little as possible.

Your father feels this way also. But he is bitter against it, and wants what it has to offer despite himself. She did not care. She was deeply attached to the other brother. She collected buttons and string and papers, even as she collected animals. To her the buttons almost seemed to have consciousness, and when she was alone she would take out her boxes of buttons and hold some in her hands, and remember the garments to which they belonged, and when she had worn them, and how the weather had been; and she lived in a present that was deeply colored by the past.

(The material on buttons surprised me a great deal. I had forgotten about Ella's penchant for collecting things, and as far as I know had not mentioned it to Jane. Jane had no conscious memory of my doing so. As soon as Seth mentioned buttons, I immediately had a picture of Aunt Ella holding an old-fashioned red tin box, in which many buttons lay. As a boy I had been fascinated by this.)

Her husband did resent this, and he would eye her when she sat thus, but he did not say a thing. She had saved the buttons from his garments also, and she would say, "Do you remember when you wore this suit, and where we were, and what we did?"

Originally, she collected the buttons to help him in his business. His family was large and scattered. He took great pains in his work, but he was also frightened; and the world confused him and he chattered, again like a squirrel. But they were very free in their own way, and your father's family never forgave them for this freedom.

Your father wanted it but would not pay the price for it. Your mother would never think of it as freedom, but as slavery, so she had no use for either of them. She never understood the desire for freedom from worldly concerns that is part of your father's nature, and of all your natures. It was because your father was not willing to pay the price that he was attracted to your mother, although other elements also entered in here.

For part of him was determined to gain worldly success, and he was always caught between wanting freedom, but he would not pay the price, or wanting worldly success for which he was not willing to pay the price. So that part of him that wanted success was attracted to your mother, who also wanted the same thing, and he spoke to her with that part of himself only. So in the beginning she did not know about this other part of him.

He did not tell her because he knew she would have had no part of him. So when she discovered this other part of him she felt betrayed. To some extent she was, since she had been honest with him. Then when she discovered that he was not willing or able to go either way, or pay either price, she was enraged and embittered, and did not think of him as a man. So she hated this sister of his and thought: was this, this squalor, what he wanted? And she looked at Jay and was envious, and hated him for being the sort of man she wanted and did not get.

For your father was a great pretender in those early days; a dude and even a braggart, and he hid the part of himself that was aloof and sensitive, and wanted freedom. So he could be successful in no direction, for he did not know who he was.

The sister knew all this in her way. And when your parents visited her, your mother and father played the part in the beginning of the grand lady and condescending gentleman, for your father considered tailoring beneath a man.

Your mother still remembers the early days of her marriage, when she thought that she and your father would ultimately, beyond doubt, gain riches and success. She saw herself as the beautiful grand lady. She saw your father as her squire, and none of it happened. The man that she married had not told her the truth about his inner self, this itch he had for freedom from worldly concerns.

She did not have that sort of sensitivity, but she was more honest than he. I suggest your break.

(Break at 9:54. Jane was dissociated as usual. Her pace had been rather fast, her eyes had remained closed. She had no offhand conscious memory of hearing about Aunt Ella's penchant for collecting buttons, although she could have heard it easily enough from my mother, for instance.

(Jane had ended the delivery in a lighter voice. She resumed in this same voice, again while sitting down and with her eyes closed, at 10:02.)

We will go into the other questions that you had for me upon another occasion.

I do not like to deal with isolated facts. For various reasons it is easier for me to deal with blocks of related material. Much shuffling is required to give isolated facts. While I am engrossed in this particular subject I will therefore continue with it. You end up with better and more detailed information in this way, since certain associations invoke related data.

(I have long been aware that questions usually slow up the flow of the material, and have refrained from very many questions since the early sessions.

(The shuffling Seth refers to above may have to do with the material on time and the electrical field. See the following sessions among others: 122, 123, 125, 126, 128, 131, 135. According to them, Seth would have to sort through blocks of electrical intensities in order to lift out individual bits of information.)

This desire for freedom from worldly concerns is a characteristic in your family on your father's side. It has not been given any <u>creative</u> fulfillment except in your own case, for they have been thinking in terms of <u>freedom from</u> rather than <u>freedom for</u>. They did not have anything that they wanted to do with the freedom, but only escape. So your one brother with his [model] trains, and the other brother with his golf. The outlets are extremely necessary to them.

One small point here. I meant to mention a relative, Alice, who is a strong <u>masculine</u> personality; well-integrated, however, because of a unifying drive. In other circumstances, if she had children for example, there would have been great misfortune.

(Alice is a cousin to my family although we barely know her. Ella was greatly attached to her, I believe, and the two women spent some time together in the same rest home. Alice was a missionary in Korea for many years. She left the home where Ella was staying a year before Ella's death. At the funeral Sunday we heard that Alice, at 80-odd years, was still alive, traveling about the country at the moment in connection with the sale of some property.)

Another point I wanted to mention. Your father told himself that your mother, as a young woman, was sensitive and intelligent because she was beautiful. You can reread the earlier material given on your family's past lives, and you will see further involvements.

(See page 181 for a list of these sessions.)

You Aunt Ella was much less frightened of death than anyone might suppose. She loved life, if not the world, but she did not believe that death was really an end. She <u>felt</u> her <u>will</u> nearby. For several years she had begun to retreat from this existence, and as she did so she became happier.

Your parents did not understand her when she spoke to them because they were both afraid to understand. There was nothing wrong with her mind. She simply did not bother focusing her energies upon practical matters, particularly during the last years, but she was quick spiritually.

She picked up hints and signs. She responded to warmth in people, and was somewhat childlike in this manner, but she would not pay any attention to a sharp tongue. She would turn her directions elsewhere. As people can turn their backs, she would turn her inner self away.

You have been doing much better in relating yourself with your parents. You are learning that you need not go to extremes, for extremes of behavior will only serve to confuse them further, and also rob <u>you</u> of consistency and peace.

Another small note here, but a rather important one: Ruburt has nothing to fear from his mother, <u>now</u>, or after her death.

To some extent he projects his understandable but regrettable bitterness upon her, and then imagines that she aims it at Ruburt. The mother indeed has no great love for the daughter. There is a deep rage inside the mother. To some extent it is directed toward Ruburt, but Ruburt does have protection, the protection of his own love of <u>all</u> living things.

He would do his mother no harm, and for this reason she can do him no harm. The desire and the intent to do violence almost inevitably brings forth violence.

We are involved here somewhat in a basic problem, hardly Ruburt's alone, that will some day take up many sessions. For like does indeed attract like. If you hate, you will be hated. You will <u>attract</u> hate.

There are definite reasons for this. The reasons have been known and forgotten, but the very practical facts remain. If Ruburt would indeed do his mother harm if the opportunity presented itself, then he would indeed be in danger of harm. He is not capable of hurting anyone deliberately, even someone he dislikes bitterly.

His own <u>fear</u> is somewhat a danger. It is much less than it was, and <u>your</u> relationship has done much to better that situation. I will at some time say more. Ruburt's love for you, his <u>ability</u> to love in general, is his protection. So he has nothing to fear.

Loves is <u>always</u> a protection, in a quite literal manner; in a biological and electromagnetic and chemical and psychic manner.

I will now close this evening's session, and we will return to our previous discussions at our next meeting. I wish you both the heartiest good evening. And <u>I</u> look out for you two. I would help Ruburt if the need arose.

("*Good night, Seth.*"

(*End at 10:30. Jane was dissociated as usual. Her pace had been somewhat slower; her eyes had remained closed and she had remained seated.*

(We were discussing a short list of mixed questions I had drawn up to ask Seth when the opportunity presented itself, when Seth came through again. He came through, I believe, because I expressed disappointment that he hadn't mentioned my two recent sensations of physical enlargement. See the notes on pages 177-78.

(When Jane began to speak again she was lying down; she had stretched out to relax for a moment after the regular session. Now she removed her glasses, propped her head up with one hand, and began to speak from this prone position. She had briefly used a prone position once before, in the unscheduled 129th session, witnessed by Judy and Lee Wright. Now, her voice was quiet, her eyes closed. Resume at 10:33.)

We will not go deeply into the sensations this evening, mainly because I am thinking of you, and do not wish to take up more than my share of your time.

When situations arise it is sometimes necessary that additional time be spent; but when it is not necessary then it is best that you have leisure and hours to devote to your own work.

The sensations are a physical demonstration of an inner sense reaction on a psychic basis, or level, which you have not yet achieved, and cannot be expected to. The self would expand. In your relationship with your parents for example, such a psychic expansion of self would allow you to absorb your own awareness of their sometimes painful existence, and you would feel no wound yourself.

(Jane had been facing me as she spoke from her prone position, and I had noticed that her eyes had appeared to be slitted, as though preparing to open. They now did open, slowly, as she continued speaking. They were very dark and without highlights. She stared at me as she spoke for the most part, although occasionally she drew upon a cigarette that she had left burning in an ashtray beside her. Her voice remained quiet.)

You could therefore help them without being concerned with self-preservation. You must <u>now</u> be so concerned, and you are doing very well.

But with such a psychic expansion you would know that you had nothing to fear. Until you know that you have nothing to fear, then the fear is a reality and must be treated as such. This development is not an easy one, nor can it be rushed, nor can you expect it of yourself.

(Jane now sat up on the bed as she spoke.)

When such developments occur, <u>then</u> you have the awareness of the whole self, and the ego does not need to fear for its survival. The self can then act to help others, and can in no way be threatened.

The physical manifestations come first. This cannot be willed. We will say more if you wish at another occasion. If you prefer I will continue.

("Later is all right, then.")
We will then close the session.
("Good night, Seth.")

(End at 10:45. Jane blinked several times, squeezing her lids shut, then was out of her trance. Her eyes had stayed open until the end. She had been dissociated as usual. While speaking she had been aware that her eyes were open.

(For some information on Jane's mother, including reincarnational data, see the 4th and the 59th sessions, among others in Volumes 1 and 2.)

SESSION 177
AUGUST 11, 1965 9 PM WEDNESDAY AS SCHEDULED

(Bill and Peggy Gallagher were again witnesses. To date they have witnessed the following sessions: 158, 161, 162, 168 and 170.

(The session was held in our large front room. It was a warm night. The windows were of necessity open and traffic noise was quite audible, but we heard Jane without difficulty. She began speaking while sitting down and with her eyes closed. Her manner was quite active and she smiled often. Almost immediately her voice acquired a somewhat hard edge that cut through the traffic noise, and she maintained this through most of the session. The "brogue" that sometimes crops up was also quite in evidence.)

Good evening.

("Good evening, Seth.")

And welcome to our friends. I am always glad to see our Jesuit, and we shall certainly discuss the God concept for him, tonight or during another session.

I am particularly concerned however with carrying our discussion further concerning dream realities.

Our Ruburt did indeed <u>steal</u> from me a few paragraphs in his book, that were not rightfully his in one manner of speaking. In a brief communication one afternoon I explained to him the similarity between multiple personalities and the various aspects of the personality as it appeared in the dreaming and trance states.

I did not have occasion to bring this up in our sessions, and he very nicely whipped in and picked it from my palm. He did a very good job of explaining my idea, for which I am grateful.

(This occurred last Monday afternoon, August 9. Jane happened to need this bit of information for a chapter in her book, and so used it when Seth made it known. She said Seth might have mentioned it during Monday's session had he not

devoted the session to the material on my Aunt Ella.)

Nevertheless it is known that cases of legitimate multiple personality exist. Here we have several personalities, all operating within one self, each unaware of the other, and each going his own separate way.

The primary ego is equally unaware of the other personalities, who very often are actually struggling for dominancy. Now. With this in mind, consider once more the various aspects of the self in the waking and the dream states. The conscious "I" is unaware of the "I" who dreams. Indeed, the dreaming "I" seems more familiar with the waking self upon many occasions. Here you have excellent examples that correspond to your dual or multiple personality thesis.

It should be obvious that there is nothing strange in the fact that the dreaming self and the waking self appear so unfamiliar to each other. The study of hypnotism will greatly enlarge man's understanding of human personality in general. These separate states of consciousness, these multiple levels of awareness, these seemingly unrelated personality aspects, are not unnatural artificial productions, brought about through hypnosis. Hypnotism is merely a method that allows you to study the personality directly.

Its nature becomes known, for the personality, again, is not an object, nor is it an unchanging <u>unit</u>. You have been studying it in the past in a very superficial manner. It should be remembered however that hypnotism is also an action, and as such hypnotism will change the personality to some extent, as all action changes and affects other actions.

Now. These effects, these various <u>seemingly</u> separate selves that can be demonstrated through hypnosis, operate continually and quite normally in both the waking and the dream states. There is however a cooperation that exists between these seemingly separate aspects of the self. It goes without saying that some overall direction must be, and is, maintained.

I am grateful to your psychologists' ideas concerning multiple personalities, since they present excellent analogies—

(There was a knock on our door at 9:16. Jane stopped speaking but as in the 172nd session, when she was also interrupted, she gave no signs of shock or even discomfort. In a few seconds she was out of her trance.

(Our visitors were a young couple from next door, stopping briefly before continuing on other errands. They do not know about the sessions. After their departure, we agreed that our friends probably sensed that something unusual was going on. We did not ask them to stay. And as Bill Gallagher pointed out, they probably heard the deep Seth voice while in the hall outside our door; upon admittance they saw no one with which to identify such a voice. Also, although the room was well lighted the shades were closed, a practice Jane and I do not indulge in otherwise.

(*Jane said she heard the knock itself and was aware of what it meant. As long as an interruption had occurred she decided to take our first break. Her eyes had remained closed during the delivery, and she had remained seated. She had been dissociated as usual.*

(*Jane resumed in the same deep voice, which now was quite amused, and at a faster pace at 9:35.*)

I am always tempted to, when I meet your friends and acquaintances, to delve somewhat into their backgrounds. However I shall in this instance restrain myself, so that we may continue with our previous discussion.

I cannot stress too strongly the fact that any investigation into the nature of the human personality must indeed follow the lines which have been here given. The nature of reality, uncamouflaged, can be glimpsed to some degree as you study the personality in the dream state, where awareness does not operate in an ego-directed manner.

Again, the nature of space and time is glimpsed more clearly as it appears to the sleeping self, for in the dream state reality is to a large measure uncamouflaged, and the personality appears in a freer state. It should also be borne in mind that *all* aspects of the personality are part of the whole self. As such there is an overall communication between the various aspects of the self, although the separate aspects of the self may not be aware of the communications.

We have seen therefore that suggestions may be given by the waking personality to the sleeping personality, and these directions will be followed. They will be followed however by the sleeping self in its own fashion, and according to its own understanding. The solutions asked for may not appear to the conscious self in the fashion that it expects. The conscious self may not even recognize that it has been given a particular solution, and yet it may act upon the solution.

(*Jane's voice hit a louder and stronger note briefly. Again she was much amused. She sat opposite Bill Gallagher. Now, her eyes still closed, she hiked her chair closer, then pointed at him.*)

Our Jesuit with the ulcer—shall I say our ulcerated Jesuit—may derive some benefit by reading a few of our immediately previous sessions, in which we spoke of dream therapy.

In such a case it is not necessary that the conscious self recall the dreams which it requests. In many cases, in fact, it is to the ego's advantage that it remain unaware of the actual dreams involved; for the ego is indeed touchy, rigid and querulous as an old arthritic gentleman, and cranky.

Dream therapy will be discussed in many of our sessions, and definite directions will be given, whereby the waking self can to a large extent insure the help of the physical organism. The various aspects of the self communicate with each other, when they do, in a very sly fashion, for no such communication is direct. They are like relatives who do not speak to each other, yet each one knows what goes on in the other's household.

The inner ego directs all activities which are deeply subjective. The outer ego as you know deals with the manipulation of the self in the physical environment. You must remember that the whole self is more than the sum of its parts; and also, since it is action, it is never the same. It is therefore impossible at any moment to pinpoint the personality. Therefore the whole self is not only the sum of the personality as you know it in your time, it is also the sum of what it has been and what it shall be. For as I have explained action is simultaneous, and time as you think of it is caused by your own physical perception.

Therefore, in the dream state communication is possible between all portions of the self. The personality appears in its truest state if it seems, in dreams, that you are free of space and time. It is indeed because the basic self is free of space and time. If you appear to hear voices out of the past, if you seem to see into the future, it is because the dream state is a more or less faithful approximation of a basic reality in which your time and space simply do not exist.

We will be dealing rather extensively with a study of space and distance and time as they appear within the dream state, and with the freedoms that are possible for the personality within it. All of this information can be used most beneficially. It will enable the ego itself to expand its consciousness and its knowledge.

I will give you directions which will allow you to study the appearance of space and time _within_ your dreams. You will be one self dreaming, while another spying self takes notes. I will now give you both a break from taking _your_ notes, and we will then continue.

(*Break at 9:58. Jane was dissociated as usual. Her voice had been on the deeper side, with the brogue apparent at times. Her eyes had remained closed. She had remained seated.*

(*We discussed with the Gallaghers the material given on dream therapy in sessions 172-74. Bill Gallagher also wondered about using suggestion even in working out problems connected with a hobby. His hobby is rope work, and at times the designs he uses are quite complicated.*

(*Jane resumed in the same manner, her voice rather strong, at 10:10. Again, Seth was quite amused.*)

There are some very _simple_ suggestions that I can give to our confused Jesuit that may be of some help.

These are tricks known to both Joseph and Ruburt, but quite beneficial for all of that. You may give directions _to_ your subconscious when you are in your normal waking state, and it will follow them. You may for example suggest before sleeping that the next day, while you are involved in your working situation, the subconscious will be involved in working out designs for you for your own projects.

This will give you the satisfaction of making the time twice as valuable. You can indeed suggest <u>to</u> the subconscious that it carry on in such a manner regardless of your conscious concern. As a result the ego can apply itself to the job at hand while the subconscious works <u>for</u> you and your inner purposes. This is very practical, and works without much difficulty.

You may give <u>any</u> such suggestions and they will be followed. Do not however <u>strain</u> yourself trying to figure out whether or not the suggestions are being followed. Give them, then turn your attention to other matters. You may obviously also direct your subconscious to react only to constructive suggestions from any source. This is in fact an excellent habit to cultivate.

There are many ways in which you can use these tricks to your advantage. I do not exaggerate when I tell you that one simple psychic manipulation can save you much difficulty. It sounds more difficult however than it is.

(*Grinning, Jane pointed to Bill Gallagher. Her eyes were still closed, her voice a bit deep, her pace fast.*)

You can learn, even a Jesuit can learn, to change the focus of your attention within seconds. Practice is all that is required, but the practice itself will show results. When you fear any difficulty with your particular physical problem, you can immediately turn your awareness away. This is no Pollyanna gibberish.

As soon as your focus of awareness is switched the physical symptoms will vanish. It requires a knack, but it is simpler than it sounds, and you can master it. This only requires that you give suggestions to your subconscious. Tell it that it knows how to perform this manipulation, and suggest that it do so the next time you are in difficulty.

I here will suggest a brief break, and I will continue for a short time.

(*Now I saw that Jane's eyes had opened. She looked around at us all as she spoke, smiling. Her eyes were quite dark, without highlights, almost as though glazed.*)

I am very glad that we are here together, and if I cannot be merry, it is only because when I am merry I speak too loudly, and I embarrass my hosts.

(*Break at 10:23. Jane was dissociated as usual. She knew when her eyes opened, she said. As she looked around at us she felt that she saw us once removed, or as through a sheet of glass. To come out of the trance she blinked or squeezed her eyes shut several times. Her voice had maintained its deeper than usual note.*

Jane resumed with her eyes closed, and in the same deeper voice, at 10:31.)

We will indeed begin a program of sorts.

We will initiate a thorough study of the God concept, which will be begun the next time these friends are present, and will be continued when they visit us at other sessions. That is, whenever they attend a session for a while we will concern ourselves with the God concept and all of its implications.

There is some material that has already been given, and our friends should read it as a preliminary to our own study. We will therefore be concerned with the pyramid gestalts of which I have spoken, and it will be to our advantage to have this as a unit.

(Seth has actually dealt with the God concept fairly often. This would involve such related matters as the soul, energy transformation, cycles on our plane, spirituality, the "source of the source," the Crucifixion, beginnings and endings, prayer and the will to be, etc. Among others see the following sessions: 3, 24, 27, 31, 51, 62, 66, 81, 95, 96, 97, 115, 135, 146, 147, 149, 145, 151.)

I may suggest therefore Joseph that for convenience's sake the next such session simply be labeled "A" along with your usual designation, the next "B" and so forth. For your records this will allow you to refer to those sessions in a simplified manner.

It is natural then that such a study will involve us in many allied matters. I may say that Buddhism does indeed come closer in essence to reality than other religions. However, the Buddhists either have not gone far enough, or have gone too far, according to your viewpoint.

If they have gone too far, then they have been so concerned with inner reality that they have become <u>too</u> tolerant of physical disease and disasters. If they have not gone far enough, then they have not followed through sufficiently so that these physical disasters could truly be suffered without pain.

They have the knowledge to a very large degree, but they have fallen short. It is one thing to realize that all physical matter is camouflage, and they know this. But this camouflage can be most disastrous if it is not manipulated correctly. You are in no position to ignore it. You <u>are</u> in a position to understand it and to use it.

It is all very well for monks to utilize astral projection. It is all very well for them to skitter through space as if they were on pogo sticks; their knowledge is fundamental and good. The fact remains that millions of human beings who follow and practice Buddhism are told, as many religions tell their followers, "Better worlds are to come, so ignore this agony, and this hunger, and this pain, and the murder in the streets. Be in ecstasy while your belly bloats." This is not human, and it is <u>far less</u> than godly.

There is a unity and there is a joy and there is an exaltation in <u>all</u> aspects of life and consciousness. It is not to any religion's benefit that people starve.

There is nothing wrong with using spiritual knowledge in practical manners.

Fulfillment, value fulfillment, implies fulfillment of <u>all</u> abilities and <u>all</u> potentials, including quite physical potentials. The pyramid gestalts of which I have spoken have experiences far beyond those of any human being. Yet they are concerned with the least, with the existence of the least among you.

The fullest potentialities cannot be developed unless the physical aspects are also developed. Your job is to manipulate as well as you can within the physical universe, and to develop within it religious leaders of any denomination. <u>Any</u> leaders who restrict development along one level for the sake of development along other levels, betray their followers.

I could indeed continue this discussion, and <u>wear</u> you all out. However, I will now let you take a break, or Joseph if he prefers may end our session.

(*"We'll end it then. Good night, Seth."*

(*End at 10:50. Jane was dissociated as usual. Her eyes had remained closed, her voice had been good, her pace fast.*

(*Jane, the Gallaghers and I were discussing the session and related subjects when Seth came through again at 11:00. All of us were in very good humor, including Seth; the session as it continued reflected this, and a rapid-fire exchange resulted in which Jane was in and out of trance at the wink of an eye, so to speak. She manifested this same ability during the 169th session, held in Dr. Instream's office in Oswego, NY, but I would say that her switching back and forth this evening was more rapid. She said later that it was no effort at all.*

(*Jane began speaking again with her eyes closed, but they opened at times during the exchange, as they had in the last session, the 176th. Jane has resumed often lately after formally ending a session, as in the 169th, 170th, and 176th.*

(*Seth began by stating that he liked to sit in with us only as an interested participant, without bothering about notes, etc. Jane, he said, could use the practice of switching focus; and we did have the effect of a conversation among five people instead of four. There follow a few quotes from Seth as I noted them down, with some hints from Bill, Peggy and myself.*)

—Ruburt can use this practice. You see now we are using a very speedy change of focus. This ability can serve us in the future to our advantage.

(*11:01—Jane was out of her trance. She grinned and waved at us. The conversation revolved around our use of slang, and our speculations as to the source of Seth's knowledge.*)

—Ruburt has always been a doubting Thomas. And now I meet a doubting Jesuit... I have known several doubting Jesuits, but it would take me several hours to tell you about them. I have the time however....

(*11:02—Jane was out of trance again, then went back in at 11:03.*)

—No one has to watch their conversation with me. I am capable of dealing with all aspects of reality, even cloudy ones on my plane....

(*Seth continued after we all sat silently for a moment.*)

—I come and everyone is silent. I had hoped for a quiet chat... instead I meet with restraint and deadly silence.

(*Bill Gallagher had something to say, by way of analogy, about Socrates and the city street cleaners.*)

—I am convinced, young man, that you plan these remarks, they are so good. I know they are not planned, however. You are very flattering. I must therefore consider the reasons... but I have always been this way, more or less—

([Bill]: *"You have the knowledge, and I'm trying to get the knowledge."*)

I am older.

([Bill:] *"Sometimes I think I'm the older one, the way I feel."*)

You have been around... but there Joseph sits. He too has been around. I could tell you much about Joseph and Denmark, but I would not divulge the circumstances in which he was so unfortunately involved.

(*Seth had more to say about my life in Denmark in the 1600's, although nothing factual or involving dates, etc. The sum total of it was far from flattering to me. Jane was out of her trance again at 11:05. She remembered some of the material.*)

(*Seth resumed again at 11:10, again in a jocular fashion, after we had been discussing his definition of action, among other things.*)

I enjoy the emotional rapport among us here... our discussions are indeed action. Action changes me, and everyone in this room. I am no exception, even though I am here in a less conventional form. Actions change us all. We must change. I enjoy the actions... I also enjoy the buildup of your ideas. I am sincerely interested in all of your ideas—so that I can correct them. But this does not mean we cannot have an informal atmosphere.

(*Jane, smiling, was out of her trance again at 11:11. She went back into it within a couple of minutes to wind up the session.*)

—I will now, since I too know your conception of the time, leave. As always, since you are my friends, I regret leaving. There is much you do not understand about relationships, which will explain these informal gatherings... I am not completed, or finished, or fulfilled anymore than you are.

We shall on some occasion have an entirely informal evening... I shall be gentle about any connections I may make.

(*End at 11:14. Jane's eyes had been closed and she ended upon a note of humor. Her manner had been pleasant and animated throughout. Her eyes had been open at times, and very dark. At times she had switched in and out of the trance state very rapidly—more rapidly than indicated here. It had been no trouble for her.*)

(This experience reminded me that Jane might try a little experiment of her own the next time such an occasion arose for informal exchange. It was simply that it should be possible for Jane herself to ask Seth questions, then go into trance to answer them. She agreed that it should work, especially if she was capable, as Seth, of carrying on a conversation with three other people, almost simultaneously.

(During this informal exchange, Jane had been dissociated as usual. She now has participated in three such informal exchanges: during the 169th, the 170th, and the 177th.

(During tonight's exchange her voice had not been as deep as during the regular session preceding it. She had however spoken quite rapidly.)

SESSION 178
AUGUST 16, 1965 9 PM MONDAY AS SCHEDULED

(On Thursday, August 12 we received a letter from Dr. Instream that was somewhat puzzling to us; in the letter he did not mention receiving the copy of the 175th session, which we mailed on August 5. The session contained some clairvoyant-telepathic material, presumably referring to Dr. Instream or people he knows, that we were interested in checking out.

(Jane has been practicing psychological time regularly. She reports that she attains her usual good "state," with little else happening. The only suggestions she gives herself now are to the effect that she is completely relaxed, and free of space and time. She used to use many more suggestions.

(It will be remembered that in the 140th session Seth suggested Jane avoid psychological time for a while, after she had unwittingly gone too far, too fast. A week later Jane resumed psy-time on a reduced time basis. Now, even though she is back up to her regular half-hour, she has had no experiences to speak of since then. She has however had some rather startling clairvoyant experiences outside of psy-time.

(It was a very hot and humid evening and we held the session in our large front room, where we have a cooler. Because our windows were open traffic noise was rather bothersome to me. Jane spoke while sitting down and with her eyes closed. Her voice was quiet—too quiet as it developed. I had trouble hearing her, and shortly after she began speaking she hiked her chair closer to my table, and her voice acquired a little more volume. She used many pauses.)

Good evening.

("Good evening, Seth.")

We see that Ruburt is trying too hard outside of our sessions.

He is doing very well in our sessions. However in his psychological time experiments he is trying too hard. This leads to a constriction. We want an expansion.

(Jane moved her chair closer again, after I had asked her to repeat a few words.)

He is not to worry concerning any investigations of our sessions. Affairs will be handled very naturally.

We are concerned with our material. Witnesses however are beneficial for the development of his own confidence, and the development of his own confidence facilitates the development of his abilities.

There will be a period of relaxation following the completion of his book, and during this time there will be a release of psychic energy that he will use most beneficially. He forgets to open up when he becomes overly concerned about his abilities. However, in the dream state he has been teaching himself to achieve greater freedom, and the results will show.

(Since Seth began discoursing on dream suggestion and health in the 172nd session, both Jane and I have been experimenting with these ideas. Jane has had quite a few interesting dreams since then, as a result of her suggestions.)

He must avoid a do-or-die attitude. He does best when he allows his mind to wander, and not when he hems it in. In his psychological time experiments lately, he has concentrated with his will, though he did not realize he was doing so. Again, this leads to a constriction.

His book will be successful in many ways, and there will be other such books. On a subconscious basis Ruburt actually suggested his recent levitation dreams, with most effective results. He was not confident enough of his own abilities, and the dream success was most beneficial from this viewpoint.

In many ways his nature is extremely spontaneous in a natural fashion, and it is this attribute that is important to us. We will indeed try our own tests on various occasions. Our results will depend to a large degree upon the development of Ruburt's abilities, and upon his own confidence. This is quite natural. He tries too hard with his own tests. When he forgets to try he does very well.

(The above passage refers to tests Jane uses on herself. Sometimes these involve Dr. Rhine's Zener cards, sometimes objects sealed in envelopes, etc. Jane has not really extended herself in such tests, mostly due to a lack of time. She is interested in learning what other abilities she may have, however, outside of these sessions.)

There are many details here that we shall discuss most thoroughly. He must remember however in his psychological time experiments that to focus outward, within and through the universe, is to expand and focus inward simultaneously. He must seek the expansion before he seeks the results or effects of the expansion.

It would help if he let himself go in the same way that he does when he works on his poetry. It will indeed be beneficial for you both to suggest to your subconscious that it enable you to develop your psychic abilities, and then consciously <u>forget</u> the matter.

Ruburt does allow himself this freedom, until he begins to brood about it. We will begin slowly to further develop his abilities in our sessions. We may even ourselves initiate such a program.

I am not primarily concerned with effects, as you know. They can be beneficial however from several viewpoints, and they can also give Ruburt confidence. Any such effects however will happen within the framework of our sessions, and we must always work in an atmosphere of mutual integrity.

I suggest your break, and we will then turn to other matters.

(*Break at 9:22. Jane was dissociated as usual for a first break. Her eyes had remained closed; her voice had been loud enough to rise above the traffic noise. The noise had bothered me, but Jane said that as she was speaking she was aware of no distractions.*

(*She had used many pauses, some of them close to a minute long. Her "brogue" had also been apparent at times. She resumed at a somewhat faster rate, again with her eyes closed, at 9:30.*)

Now. The connections between the dreaming self and the waking self, and between the dream universe and the physical universe, exist on chemical, electromagnetic and psychic levels.

They are completely interwoven. Effects in one are reflected in the other[s]. As you have already supposed Joseph, suggestions received during the sleeping state are often carried out by the waking personality.

(*It might be interesting to digress a moment to discuss the point raised by Seth in the last paragraph. I believe he is referring here to an experience of mine. As far as I can recall, this was the first time I became consciously aware that a dream could influence waking action.*

(*On Tuesday night, June 22, I had five dreams which I wrote in my dream notebook the next morning. Dream number five was a very short one, in color. In it I found myself approaching a certain traffic light in my car. I was on a side street, two blocks from the printing plant where I work. In the dream I sat waiting for some little time for the light to turn green, giving me access to the main highway, Lake Street. I seldom take this route in actuality, since this particular light is set to favor the heavy flow of traffic on Lake Street. Anyone approaching it as I did in my dream can wait for up to a couple of minutes for it to change.*

(*As usual, after writing down the dream upon arising I promptly forgot it. I left the house for work. Sometimes I drive to work by different routes, for variety. On this particular morning, June 23, I did so. I then found myself traveling down this particular side street, approaching the light in question, but without remembering the dream to this moment.*

(When I was a few car lengths from the light, the dream suddenly popped into my mind. Just as in the dream, I found myself stopping for a red light. The effect was so startling that I at once began to wonder whether it was possible to act out dream suggestions in waking life. My self-questioning was particularly intriguing because I could have chosen from a half-dozen routes to work; yet I had picked a course that enabled me to act out the dream of the night before, while not being consciously aware of the dream.)

Suggestions made by the waking personality are also carried out by the sleeping self. The characteristics of the sleeping personality therefore partially determine the physical existence of the waking self. Solutions to problems are sought and received and worked for in the dream state. The physical environment is directly affected then by the activities of the dreaming self.

Abilities unused by the waking personality are utilized in the dream state. A study of dream activities will often allow the waking personality to recognize abilities of which it is not aware, to discover talents that are not being used. Such a study can be most beneficial in allowing the personality to utilize all of its capabilities. There is no doubt that the whole self is a composite formed by the various aspects of the personality as it is seen in the waking and dream states, and at other levels of operation.

There are levels of which we have not yet spoken. The repository of potentiality however is contained within those layers that are not conscious. As a rule the ego <u>chooses</u> those elements from this repository which it feels will be most beneficial in dealing with physical reality.

In many instances however, because of environment and other influences, the ego accepts few of the abilities available, and therefore hampers the full development of personality. Of necessity the ego discards more than it accepts, and this is why Ruburt runs into difficulties when he becomes too egotistically concerned.

In actuality the ego itself definitely benefits by allowing greater flexibility. It does become more active, and to some degree more permissive under such conditions, but the flexibility involved adds to its strength in beneficial ways.

Ego concern is a very jealous concern, and it is directly connected to the personality's concept of survival necessities within the physical universe. The ego that is overly fearful for survival will allow little potential to show itself unless that potential is directly connected with <u>physical</u> survival. Actually what happens here is that the ego sells the personality short, out of fear, and denies those very abilities that are needed, <u>and in practical terms</u>.

I will suggest your break, and we will continue along these lines.

(Break at 9:48. Jane was dissociated as usual. Her eyes had remained closed, her voice had been a bit stronger, her pace had picked up quite a bit during the delivery. Her brogue had again been apparent at times.

(She resumed in the same manner at 9:57.)

The ego that ignores too many of the possibilities of the inner self is soon in dire difficulty, and is forced to realize that it has been considering survival in a very limited light.

For the personality in such circumstances will shrivel up, and ultimately the physical self will die ahead of its time, and despite all emergency efforts made by the ego, unless it makes the necessary effort. Survival within the physical universe, as within all others, is determined by the full development of potential.

The greatest possible development allows the greatest possible security, for such development shows itself physically and in all other manners. The entire gestalt simply works better and more efficiently and more joyfully, from the smallest cell to the most organized aspects of personality.

You may find it helpful, and certainly fascinating, to study your own dreams, looking at them for the purpose of searching in their framework for abilities of which the ego is not aware.

(Jane now took a long pause, then smiled.)

Your own talents have worked for the survival of your personality, Joseph. They have given you a strength that you would not possess if your ego had not allowed them to emerge. You may not think of your artistic abilities as serving any practical purpose, insofar as survival is concerned, and yet they have been your main security, and in very practical ways.

Without a sense of joy and inner accomplishment and development of potential, the personality will not only fail to flourish, but the inner self will refuse to maintain the physical structure adequately. This is extremely important. Superficial measures will not fool the inner self.

We will discuss for some sessions the nature of dreams, practically speaking, from many viewpoints. Other suggestions will be given for general benefit. I hope in the future to make these points clear enough so that you will be able to discover definite connections where you have not before, that will tie in waking and dreaming situations with rather surprising results.

By far the most immediately helpful suggestions have to do with dream therapy, with problem solving, and the search for abilities as shown within the dream state.

The energy used in constructing dreams is every bit as <u>intense</u> as the energy used in the waking state, but there is no depletion because the sleeping self uses energy more naturally, realizing that it is available, and being more free in its operation.

The energy is used in a more diffused manner however, than in the waking state. It does not have to be focused in one main direction only. It is as intense, but it has a wider radius. There is no strain involved.

This is one of the reasons why health suggestions given immediately before sleep are so effective. Incidentally, they are excellent practice. Expectation can also aid you. In this case suggestions should be given leading to dreams in which a desired situation is accomplished. The dream will then increase and activate your own expectations. And as you know, the expectations themselves have much to do with whether or not any given situation will occur. Further detailed discussions will be held on all of these points, before these matters are covered.

I will now close our session. And <u>Ruburt</u> should reread particularly the first portion of the session several times.

My heartiest wishes to you both.

("Good night, Seth."

(End at 10:20. Jane was dissociated as usual. Her eyes had remained closed. Her pace had been good, her voice average and with an occasional touch of brogue. The hot and humid evening had not bothered her during deliveries.)

SESSION 179
AUGUST 18, 1965 9 PM WEDNESDAY AS SCHEDULED

(In the last session Seth had commented favorably on trying some tests with Jane and me. An hour or so before this evening's session, without telling Jane beforehand, I made a black ink drawing of the symbol below on a small sheet of paper. [This was to be our first "envelope test".]

(I folded it once, put it in an envelope, then sealed this envelope in another so there was no chance of seeing through paper. My idea was to hand the envelope to Jane just before she went into trance for the session. I wanted to see how much, if any, of the contents Jane or Seth could describe.

(Interestingly enough, Jane came back to my studio as I was writing down the above paragraph in longhand. I usually write these preliminary notes before the session to

save time. I tried to divert her attention now but she read the words "without telling Jane beforehand." She left the studio when I asked her to, but I now thought she had been alerted to something unusual, and might be anticipating a test of some sort. I had not wanted to make her nervous.

(I picked the symbol above because Seth had dealt with a version of this in the 68th, 75th, 83rd and 84th sessions, in connection with Bill Macdonnel's trip to Provincetown, MA, last summer. Seth insisted that Bill had seen a symbol similar to this on a rowboat at Provincetown, although Bill did not recall it. Other data Seth gave us about Bill's trip was verified. Note that I added my own initials to the symbol above. My idea was that using such a design as a test would summon up a little more emotional involvement, since Bill was included along with Seth, Jane and me.

(I was not sure whether the test would be telepathic or clairvoyant, or a combination. I felt it would now be different since Jane was probably alerted. She confirmed this just before the session when she asked me about it, so I gave her the envelope at 8:57. She agreed to some nervousness, though not a great deal. She also said she thought Seth might address the session to Dr. Instream, and that if he did she would prefer not to be distracted. Thus she might not deal with the envelope.

(Because it was another very hot and humid night we held the session in our large front room, where air circulation is better. Traffic noise was a problem once more; our windows of course had to be open, although the blinds were drawn. The quality of the air seemed to aggravate the noise, and quite often during the session Jane appeared to pause until the noise abated temporarily. I felt that the noise, being such a problem, was influencing the quality of the session.

(Strangely enough, Jane did not speak in an overly loud voice. In the beginning she spoke while sitting down and with her eyes closed. She leaned forward in her rocker, holding the envelope in her clasped hands. She used many pauses, some of them quite long.)

Good evening.

("Good evening, Seth.")

I would like to make a few points here in connection with the letter which you recently received from Dr. Instream.

First of all, I have no information of setting up any unreasonable nor impossible conditions. An atmosphere of trust, mutual trust, would however seem to be indispensable. Spontaneity must be allowed for.

These two factors are extremely important. I do not set them as conditions. It is simply a fact that little will be achieved without them.

(Cars and trucks rumbled and boomed by outside, and Jane sat quietly until the noise subsided somewhat. Seth refers above to Dr. Instream's letter of August 10.)

Another meeting between Dr. Instream and myself would be advantageous, so that we could speak plainly. Perhaps such a meeting would facilitate mutual understanding, without which such a venture has little hope of success.

Our main problem is simply Ruburt's own confidence, or lack of it. This, in time, will not bother us. I spoke plainly in our recorded session, nor do I regret so doing. I am not only objective, I am also, perhaps unfortunately, given to bluntness.

(Another long pause, until the traffic noise subsided. The recorded session that Seth addressed to Dr. Instream is the 170th.)

I did say quite plainly that I would cooperate in any such endeavor that is conducted with integrity, and so I shall. When I spoke of terms, saying that my terms should be met, I was not, again, speaking of any impossible conditions; merely that spontaneity, trust and integrity be necessary factors in our endeavor.

It is quite true however that proof is not necessary from my standpoint. It is quite necessary perhaps from your standpoint. This is quite understandable, and since I realize this I do not see how it becomes an issue. Particularly since I have more than once stressed that I <u>would</u> cooperate.

My emotional response however was quite legitimate. I would prefer that <u>some</u> informal meeting be held if possible between us, as a preliminary to our venture. I do not necessarily stand on ceremony, but I do feel that <u>some</u> friendly discussion would be seeming under the circumstances.

For one thing, I would like to know specifically what Dr. Instream has in mind, and prefer that we work it from that angle. This could be discussed between us.

I now suggest your break.

(Break at 9:18. Jane said she was dissociated as usual for a first delivery. Her eyes remained closed. She used many pauses other than those indicated, and said she was aware of the traffic noise at times. She held the test envelope for the entire delivery.

(Her voice had been rather quiet, and remained so. Again with her eyes closed, and holding the envelope, she resumed at 9:26.)

Such a meeting would help to set Ruburt at ease.

It is important however that he does not feel under pressure. The idea of tests somewhat upsets him, but this can be overcome without too much difficulty in time.

I would consider it a gesture of courtesy if Dr. Instream acquainted himself with some of our material.

Now, for ourselves: Ruburt must work some things through on his own, as he knows. There is no doubt that the whole affair still seems strange to him, and he is acclimating himself to new conditions as they arise.

It is understandable that he becomes uneasy at times under such circumstances. It is an excellent idea that he has taken up his painting again, for this turns his awareness to other matters. We shall endeavor to handle our relationships with the outside world in such a way that your private situations are not bothered any more than absolutely necessary.

(*Another long pause. Jane sat learning forward, her head down, holding the test envelope.*)

Ruburt has been lately in a period in which he has been seeking knowledge as to his own abilities. This has been reflected in his dream activities, as well as in his waking situation. The concentration upon psychic phenomena in general, including his concentration in his book, has somewhat made him weary. This is very temporary, and already he is beginning to find new reserves of energy. I am <u>easy</u> on him now, however, for the above mentioned reasons.

We will try to see what we can do with your envelope. It contains paper with writing on it, printed or perhaps typewritten, and also I believe handwritten. It may be in the nature of a license, but it is of some legal nature rather than a personal note, blue or green and white, the handwritten material on printed lines. I believe it belongs to you, Joseph, and while it is yours that it has a legal connotation.

(*Jane took a pause of average length. She sat with her eyes closed, still holding the envelope though not actively fingering it. She had delivered the above information quietly and steadily.*)

It seems that another person is also somehow involved with it, a male.

(*Another pause, longer this time.*)

Ruburt has been somewhat uneasy at the thought of a test. To some degree this may affect our results. However, the <u>very fact</u> that he permitted the test to be conducted shows that his attitude is improving.

I will now suggest a short break.

(*Break at 9:43. Jane was dissociated as usual. Traffic had become noisy again, and she said she thought Seth took the break now because of this. Jane had realized she was discussing the envelope. When she opened it she was quite disappointed with the results. I was pleased.*

(*We had no idea of how to interpret such an experiment, or even whether there is a one best way. Would "errors" of omission be counted? Seth did not mention a symbol at all, yet used the words handwritten and printed. To me printed means mechanically produced; to Jane printed means hand lettering, as were my initials beneath the symbol.*

(*Seth did not mention two envelopes, although Jane said she knew there were two involved. It is also obvious that touch alone could give information as to whether the envelope contained paper, some kind of cardboard or other heavier material, or perhaps metal.*

(I was puzzled as to why Seth, or Jane, was so definite about the envelope containing a license or some sort of similar document, when Jane revealed that at last break she had thought the envelopes did contain a license. We thought it most interesting that the data based on Jane's conscious thoughts proved to be that in error. It will be remembered that Seth/Jane paused before delivering the last line of information concerning the envelopes. This information I consider a direct hit. Another person, Bill Macdonnel, is involved with the symbol. See my notes on pages 199-200.

(I can say that when Seth/Jane paused before delivering this last line, I had the feeling that some kind of inner shift in control had taken place; that Seth rather than Jane was responsible for the last line of material. There was no objective evidence on which I could base this feeling, yet I sensed it. And of course I knew as Jane delivered it that the material about a license was not correct.

(Jane said that Seth himself was definite about another male being involved with the contents of the envelope. Her own thought, as she spoke, was that a female was involved; but Seth, she said, would not allow her to say a female was involved. Thus it seems that in giving the material on the envelope, Jane was drawing upon a couple of levels of awareness at once.

(Traffic noise was still audible. Jane resumed in a bit louder voice, with her eyes closed, at 9:57.)

We will not have a long session.

The combination of the traffic and the test, of which Ruburt was aware, served, though only slightly, to dismay him. However there are some points I would like to make.

We are dealing here with something rather unusual, in that we are attempting to permit two personalities to exist side by side, so to speak. Ruburt is not in a deep trance state. I do not supersede his own personality. He <u>allows</u> me, in our sessions, to coexist with himself.

A deeper trance state would allow us to get less distorted results on such a test as this, initially, but our results will improve. And such experiments will be helpful in that the various layers of the two personalities, Ruburt's and my own, will be seen in their operating procedures.

Ruburt will learn very quickly through such practice. It must be remembered that this is new to him, and upon occasion he must distinguish between my communications and his own thoughts. This sort of practice will be most beneficial, and though he may not think so consciously it will build his confidence.

("Were you aware that he was distorting the information while he was speaking?"

(Jane paused and frowned.)

On one level, yes. However, this is a rather permissive relationship in many respects, and one of my primary concerns has been to allow both of you to recognize and develop your own abilities.

The distortions that appeared are most helpful, in that they allow Ruburt to differentiate between my communications and his own thoughts. At times he has had difficulty in this respect, as is perfectly natural. This does not occur when he does not know in advance that a test is planned, when I speak spontaneously; as for example when on one occasion I gave definite details concerning your Mark's vacation.

(Mark is Bill Macdonnel's entity name. Again, see the 68th, 75th, 83rd and 84th sessions, and pages 199-200. Bill verified just about all of the details Seth gave us concerning Bill's trip to Provincetown last summer.)

The features which hung in front of his face did not bother him, since he did not know what I had planned to do. For the record incidentally, let us add that this occurred in full light.

(See the 68th session. During this session, in which Bill Macdonnel saw an apparition for upwards of an hour, Bill and I saw an independent set of features that appeared to hang just in front of Jane's features.)

The repetition of such tests will be beneficial, and his abilities to let material through undistorted will grow. You can benefit however in the meantime even from failures. We are attempting to develop Ruburt's abilities. They are not fully developed by any means.

(Jane had spoken for much of the evening with her head down at a slight angle. Very recently she had lifted it somewhat, and I saw that her eyes appeared to be slitted. Now they opened, at 10:15. She looked at me casually. Her eyes were very dark, without highlights.

(Jane's cigarettes lay on the table beside her. She lit one as she continued speaking, in a quiet voice. Traffic noise had quieted. She did not stare at me continually.)

My interest is in the development of the abilities. Proofs will be a natural result. I communicate with you through Ruburt. I am to some extent therefore dependent upon him. It is up to me to train him, and tests such as this will help us in this endeavor.

My only concern is that he is not frightened off. I believe however that our foundation is strong enough so that we can safely proceed in this direction.

Your idea Joseph was a good one basically, for practice. It was hardly scientific enough, even if the results were 100 percent accurate, which they were not, for Dr. Instream. But it is a beginning.

Using such a procedure in each session will do much to eliminate Ruburt's uneasiness and to build his confidence. The emotional impetus however is lacking. In some manner perhaps in the future we can do something to build in an emotional impetus of some sort, as it will be conducive to success.

(Jane's eyes now closed at times as she spoke. Her voice was quiet and she was still smoking.)

Some similar experiments might be conducted with our friendly Jesuit, and she who dislikes the feline family.

(Here Seth refers to Bill and Peggy Gallagher, who have witnessed several sessions. Last week they agreed to participate in some tests. In the beginning the experiments would involve such simple procedures as having the Gallaghers, while at their home, focus upon objects Jane and I have not seen, at appointed hours during sessions held in our own home.)

Such experiments could be done on your own, and also in connection with our sessions.

("We'd like to try them in connection with the sessions.")

I am perfectly willing. You may have some difficulties with Ruburt, but I presume you can get around this.

I suggest a brief break.

(Break at 10:24. Jane was dissociated as usual. Her eyes were open as break came; she blinked several times and was out of her trance. While speaking she had been aware that her eyes were open. Her voice had been quiet.

(We had anticipated a regular break, but hardly had we relaxed when Seth came through again. This time Jane spoke with her eyes closed for the most part, in a quiet voice, and with pauses. Resume at 10:25.)

On second thought I will make a few comments and end our session.

A meeting with Dr. Instream will build up Ruburt's confidence, in that he will feel that he knows with whom he is dealing. I know, but Ruburt needs to feel a friendly reinforcement on the doctor's part.

This is not strictly necessary, but it would be advantageous. He reacts to the emotional atmosphere, and his abilities will operate best if he feels that he is investigating these matters along with interested parties, than if he feels that he is being skeptically observed.

(Jane's eyes now opened again, and she lit a cigarette while speaking.)

There must be a friendly cooperation. Even scientific investigations can flourish in such an atmosphere. We will now end the session. My heartiest wishes to you both, and my regards to Dr. Instream.

("Good night, Seth.")

(End at 10:30. Jane was dissociated as usual. She ended the session with her eyes closed. Her voice was quiet.

(Again, we had barely begun to discuss the session when Seth came through briefly. Jane spoke with her eyes closed. Her voice was quiet and she continued to smoke. Resume at 10:31.)

All in all, we did not do badly, considering that Ruburt was forewarned that a test would in fact take place.

You will get better results either if Ruburt does not know in advance that a test of any kind will be given, or if such tests become so commonplace that they no longer concern him.

An emotional rapport of some sort, established between Ruburt and Dr. Instream, would definitely help us.

(Jane took a long pause.)

Such an informal meeting as I have suggested, perhaps on Ruburt's home ground, again, would reinforce such rapport. And a frank as well as objective attitude on the part of Dr. Instream in his letters would also help.

Ruburt feels to some extent that there is a lack here.

("Good night, Seth.")

(End at 10:33. Jane was dissociated as usual. Her eyes remained closed. She said she would prefer that tests be given often, so that she can become used to them; as she has become used to speaking while sitting down, and with her eyes open occasionally.)

SESSION 180
AUGUST 23, 1965 9 PM MONDAY AS SCHEDULED

(Jane has finished her ESP book for all practical purposes, and has been looking through the Seth material for a suitable quote to end the final chapter. I suggested she ask Seth for a few appropriate words this evening.

(Jane has been improving in her psychological time experiments since Seth advised her that she was trying too hard in the 178th session. Today she attained an excellent state.

(As I had for the 179th session, I prepared a test envelope in case we had a chance to use it during the session. This time the double envelopes contained a black and white photo I took of Jane at York Beach, ME, a little over a year ago this month. I thought this would have an extra emotional content, as did the symbol I used in the first test. [This is to be our second such test.]

(It will be remembered that it was at York Beach, in August 1963, that Jane and I saw the fragments we had ourselves created, according to Seth, in the dancing establishment called the Driftwood Lounge. This was some months before the sessions

began. *The snapshot was taken on the beach perhaps 200 yards from the Driftwood. For York Beach material see sessiosms 9, 15, 17, 69, and 80 in Volumes 1 and 2.*

(*I took care that Jane did not see me preparing the envelopes this evening, although she was well aware a test might take place. We had discussed the matter earlier in the day but she had not given me an unequivocal yes or no answer, as to whether we should make such tests an everyday procedure during sessions. See Seth's comments on this in the last session.*

(*Tonight's session was held in our back room. My writing table is beside a bookcase, and before the session I slipped the test envelope between a couple of books without Jane being present. Thus I could easily reach it during the session.*

(*Jane spoke while sitting down and with her eyes closed for the entire session. Her voice was quiet, and although she used pauses her delivery was for the most part quite rapid. She began speaking at 8:59.*)

Good evening.

("Good evening, Seth.")

Our Ruburt is indeed relaxing, having just finished his book, and he has my congratulations.

There may be a pleasant languor for a few days. He should think of other matters at least briefly, and concern himself with innocent pleasures so that he may be renewed.

His painting will serve him well in this respect, and his psychic energies will indeed be refreshed and renewed.

The book will definitely be a success, and a financial one, that will represent his initiation into a field to which he will contribute in no small manner. The book will represent the beginning also of financial success. The reasons are fairly simple, for this field is one in which Ruburt's innermost energies and interests are already rooted.

It was far from inevitable that he <u>turn</u> to this field but the innermost portions of his personality were drawn to it, and within this field he can develop his abilities, mature, and contribute. Because of this intense focus, there <u>will be</u> financial success.

Within, I believe, three months after the book is accepted, another book will be assured; and then at that time, or very shortly after, it will be contracted for.

Your own abilities, Joseph, have been at a plateau level, from which they will begin to rise, at which time another plateau will be reached, and the process continued. Such plateau levels are beneficial to the whole personality, since they allow time for adoptions.

I would like to add a few notes here. Ruburt was simply not confident enough in the Father Trainor episode last evening to adequately perform the inner manipulations necessary, without your presence. The first occasion was completely spontaneous, and his ego was not aroused.

(*Sunday, August 22nd, Jane discovered the tape recording of the first two Father Trainor episodes was deteriorating, for unknown reasons. Last evening she tried a rereading of the two poems involved, but stopped before getting through G. K. Chesterton's* Lepanto. *She began the reading all right but soon felt a sense of strain. She turned off the recorder.*

(*Bill Macdonnel was present but I was working in my studio. Jane said my absence annoyed her somewhat. Perhaps too cautiously, I had advised her against the attempt earlier in the day, since she had expressed general fatigue. She was also not quite sure of how sympathetic Bill was to the attempt. See the 131st and 158th sessions for details on the Father Trainor experiments in Volumes 3 and 4.*

(*Now Jane smiled, speaking quietly along.*)

I see you have no tests for me this evening. Soon perhaps I shall have some for you.

(*This was a perfect opportunity for me to slip the test envelope out of its hiding place on the bookshelf, reach across my small writing table and drop the envelope into Jane's lap. It was 9:10. Her eyes remained closed and she did not touch the envelope.*

("*There's one for you.*")

I shall still have some for you. They will involve dreams, and we will work for awhile in an effort to train you so that clairvoyant dreams can be received at your suggestion. This may involve somewhat more than you suppose, but nevertheless you should learn to handle the sleep state well enough so that some success is achieved.

We will be involved when we are alone with variations of the dream condition, and with dream therapy, and the nature and classification of dreams. You should find the material highly interesting.

The stuff or fabric or makeup of dreams has not been covered here, nor have we discussed the actual ways in which the personality uses energy to construct his dreams and project them. All of these matters will be thoroughly covered.

(*Jane now smiled again. She picked up the test envelope and held it in both hands, lightly fingering it briefly without heavily bending it, twisting it, etc. It was 9:14. Her eyes remained closed. She paused rather briefly, then delivered the following material in a quiet voice, with gentle emphasis at times, and with average pauses.*)

We will see now what we can do with your own little test, and with our friend Ruburt.

Inside the envelope, heavy paper or light cardboard. I sense color, perhaps orange, yellow; but I get the impression of something sunny, as an orange-yellow color would be. I also have the impression of black, and two people.

The numbers 4, 6, perhaps of an age or date, and a border. I <u>think</u> now of a border of flowers, and of the two people, a man and a woman, and J. B. I think also of hills.

You may now take your break.

(*Break at 9:18. Jane was dissociated as usual for a first delivery. She was greatly pleased at the results of the test, and so was I. Neither of us regard these tests as scientific but we do consider them a beginning toward scientific tests.*

(*Jane said she felt it when I dropped the test envelope into her lap. This did not make her nervous however; she was "already Seth," she said. In the first test she had the envelope in her possession before the session began, and could not but help know that a test was in the offing.*

(*Jane said that when Seth began speaking she tried to keep herself out of it as much as possible. She had the feeling that Seth was in the foreground, she was in the background. She did not feel nervous while giving the data.*

(*Also, while she was giving the data Jane experienced a concept. She had the mental picture of a border, of something square, as the photograph is, with a border around it. She had no indication of size; the photograph is 4" x 4". And also again, at this time Jane had a "distant" thought or impression of the error she made in the first test regarding a license, but felt content that she was keeping herself in the background.*

(*The orange-yellow-sunny interpretation of this photograph is particularly intriguing to us because it was taken on an extremely bright day; we remember it well because some other pictures I took on this roll, of rocks and the sea, were overexposed because of brightness and reflections. It is of course a black-and-white photo. The two people involved, a man and woman, could be Jane, and me who took the picture. I am 46 <u>now</u>, but was 45 when I took the picture.*

(*Jane does not know what association led her to mention a border of flowers. Most striking of all perhaps, she said that when she heard herself speak the initials J. B., she knew that Seth meant Jane Butts, the subject of the photograph. She recalls wondering at the time why she did not say her own name aloud. The reference to hills is clearly seen in the photo: Jane sits on a group of craggy high rocks on the Maine seacoast. With the figure painted out of the photo the rocks would easily resemble any number of aerial shots of denuded mountain ranges, or hills, depending on scale.*

(*And again we consider the ways of various levels of the mind. With all of the above data Seth, or Jane, did not use the word photograph.*

(*For some other material on concepts see the following sessions: 149, 151, 153, 164.*

(*The session resumed with Jane again sitting down and speaking with her eyes closed. Her voice was quiet and rather fast. She smiled in recollection of her ebullient feelings. Resume at 9:35.)*

I am pleased that Ruburt is so pleased.

If I can satisfy him, then indeed we will be able to satisfy anyone, for he is so stubborn.

He has learned much however since our last session, and you can see that it was much better that we allowed the distortions to come through in our first test, since it allowed him to learn more about the simultaneous existence of our consciousnesses during a session.

I may therefore myself congratulate him. There are few limitations upon what we can do, and most of these limitations are human limitations, existing on Ruburt's part rather than on my own. He is quick to learn however, once he makes up his mind and is willing to learn.

These informal tests are an excellent method of building up his self-confidence. And his self-confidence is absolutely necessary to us.

It is best that we work in this manner to begin with, in his home territory. Later it will make no difference if he progresses, as I believe that he will. For the <u>immediate</u> present, and for the immediate present only, such tests should be conducted here. He is concerned too much about the object which your friends are using for the other test, and for now I am afraid that he will <u>unwittingly</u> distort this material in this respect.

("Do you know what the object is?")

I <u>know</u> what the object is.

(Seth/Jane spoke quietly but firmly in answer to my question. The object in question is one that Jane's friend, Peggy Gallagher, is carrying about with her in her handbag. I do not know what it is.

(Peggy has had the object here in our apartment on a couple of visits not connected with the Seth sessions, and of course told Jane about it. Peggy began to carry it about with her a week or so ago after Jane and I had asked if Peggy and Bill, her husband, would cooperate with us in some future tests.

(Perhaps also Peggy began carrying the object because recently Jane has had several clairvoyant experiences involving the Gallaghers, and other mutual friends, that have been verified.)

In a very short time, as his confidence is built up, we will not have the difficulty. I <u>believe</u> however that he will be able to take part in such tests when your friends are present and the object is concealed. But he should not be forewarned.

It is important that these affairs be spontaneous, at least for a while. When he feels under test conditions he will not do well until his confidence is strengthened; and we shall see that it is.

We will learn much through these endeavors, for they will provide lessons

SESSION 180

in themselves, and will be excellent examples of the precise manner in which extrasensory perceptions, as you prefer to call them, are received and interpreted. The role of association will be found to play an important part.

I suggest a short break.

(Break at 9:48. Jane was dissociated as usual. Her eyes had remained closed. Her voice had been quiet and rather fast, although she had used pauses too.

(Jane said she felt that Seth was trying to come through with material on the Gallagher object, and that she was trying not to block it. She had the feeling Seth wanted to say it was rock; the other day Jane had the conscious impression that it was tin or galvanized metal, of the sort Bill Gallagher uses in fashioning some of his modern sculpture.

(I would like to note here that the Gallaghers have not pressed Jane to name the object, in trance or otherwise, nor have I. Jane has certainly been aware of it, since she has mentioned it to me at odd times during the last few days. Therefore I was somewhat surprised that either Jane or Seth might be considering an attempt to name it now.

(Jane resumed in the same quiet and fast pace, with her eyes closed, at 9:55.)

We have our beginning.

I am interested in these matters because they will show the ways in which the personality handles such data. They will be demonstrations to point up our own text, because I will handle them in that way.

They will <u>end up</u> providing proofs that your scientists require, but they will serve a purpose closer to <u>my</u> heart, in that they will display the operating procedure of the human personality as it manipulates inner perceptions.

We will build up Ruburt's confidence until he will be sure enough of <u>himself</u> in relationship to me, so that he will be able to let undistorted material come through where tests are concerned.

There has never been any real problem in this respect with the material, because it did not egotistically alarm him. For a beginning he is doing very well. In a light trance state, some quite complicated manipulations are necessary in this sort of situation.

He will actually be building up confidence in <u>me</u>, and therefore he will allow me to come through when it is required that I do so in any investigations. For regardless of my own <u>occasional</u> irascibility with the behavior of your scientific communities, such men seek after truth, and there are few enough involved in that search.

We will try to arrange <u>my</u> tests for you as far as clairvoyant dreams and suggestion are concerned, so that these tests also add definite objective knowledge to the nature of clairvoyance in general.

The human personality has no limitations except those which it accepts. There are no limits to its development or growth, if it will accept no limits. There are no boundaries to the self except those boundaries which the self arbitrarily creates and perpetuates. There is no <u>veil</u> through which human perception cannot see, except the veil of ignorance which is pulled down by the materialistic ego.

That which appears empty, such as your space, is empty only for those who will not perceive, who are blind because they <u>fear</u> to perceive that which the ego cannot understand. The ego however is also capable of greater knowledge and potentiality and scope.

It dwells in the physical universe, but it can indeed also perceive and appreciate other realities. The ego is part of the personality, and as such it can partake of <u>sturdier, heartier</u>, more <u>vivid</u> realities. The personality can dwell, and does dwell, in many worlds at once.

The inquiring intuitions and the searching self, like summer winds, can travel in small and large spaces, can know of actualities that are more minute than pinheads and more massive than galaxies.

The power and ability of the human personality, in a most practical manner, can be seen as unlimited.

Ruburt can use this to close his book if he so desires.

(*See my notes at the start of session 180, page 206.*)

You may now take a break and I will continue, or you may end the session as you prefer. As always I await your pleasure.

(*"We'll take a short break."*)

(*Break at 10:14. Jane was dissociated as usual. She ended the delivery with a smile. She felt very good. Her eyes remained closed, her voice quiet. She thought she might very well use Seth's material above to end her book.*)

(*She resumed in the same quiet fashion, at a somewhat slower pace and still with her eyes closed, at 10:20.*)

I am not going to keep you much longer.

It is most helpful however that at least now Ruburt can definitely differentiate between our two consciousnesses; or at least he is learning to do so.

This will be helpful in other respects also. The practice will soon show excellent results. He will simply know which channels are which, and therefore can change his frequency, so to speak, with a surer hand. This has been a most enlightening session for you, and we have achieved results that do not show here yet. Do you have any questions, Joseph?

(*"Was there any element of telepathy involved between you and me, in the test this evening?"*)

In tonight's test?

("Yes.")

Tonight's test dealt with clairvoyance. Although I happened to pick up my information in that way, and it could have just as easily been obtained through telepathic communication. In the future I imagine that tests will be worked out in whatever manner is needed.

("How about in the first test?")

(See the 179th session.)

The first test was the same.

I myself operate well in that way. In many instances however data can be received in either manner, and telepathy may well be involved in other tests. I, for my own reasons and peculiarities, usually obtain such information clairvoyantly; and we will have much to say concerning the ways in which such information is received and interpreted, as this is very important.

If you have any questions I will do my best to answer them. Or if not we will end the session.

("I have no more for now.")

My congratulations then. Your part in these sessions is extremely important, as I expect that you know.

("Yes. Good night, Seth.")

(End at 10:28. Jane was dissociated as usual. Her eyes had remained closed. Her voice had been quiet and rapid for the most part.)

SESSION 181
AUGUST 25, 1965 9 PM WEDNESDAY AS SCHEDULED

(Jane has decided to use the passages on unlimited human potentialities, given by Seth in the last session, to close out her ESP book.

(Jane began speaking while sitting down and with her eyes closed, at 8:59. Her voice was quiet, her pace rather rapid even though she used pauses.)

Good evening.

("Good evening, Seth.")

The ego skims the topmost surface of reality and experience.

This is not the result of any inherent egotistical quality. It is true that the ego's responsibility is with the relationship between the self and the physical environment. It must of necessity be focused within the confines of physical reality.

Nevertheless it is fully capable of perceiving far more than Western man allows it to perceive. Fear and ignorance and superstition quite obviously limit the potentialities of the ego, and therefore to some degree limit even its effectiveness within the physical universe.

The ego itself in many instances cannot experience <u>directly</u> certain intuitions and psychological experiences, but it can experience them insofar as it can be aware of them on an intellectual basis. When training forces the ego to become too rigid, and to limit its perception of other realities, then the intuitions will not be accepted by the ego because intuitional experience will not fit into the framework of reality as the ego sees it.

The ego, because of its responsibility, will therefore fight against what it then considers an unknown threat to survival. Struggles are therefore initiated which are entirely unnecessary. We want to bring intuitional comprehension to a point where the ego will accept it.

In our dream experiments therefore, this is one of the purposes that we hope to achieve. The ego is not equipped of itself to delve <u>directly</u> into nonphysical realities. If the ego is trained to be flexible however, it will accept such knowledge from the subconscious, and other wider horizons of the self.

Our ego must have its feet upon the solid earth, it is out of its element, naked and in an unfamiliar environment, outside of the normal characteristics of physical existence. Its basic distrust of dream experience is necessary for the overall balance of the personality. Physical reality is a rock to which the ego must cling, and from which it achieves its power, energy, position, and reason for existence.

This provides necessary balance and necessary control, and results in the sturdy anchorage of the personality in the environment in which it must survive. You have here one of the main reasons why you must request the subconscious to enable you to recall your dreams. The ego would see no reason for such a memory, and on general principles attempts to repress them.

Again however, through this excellent balance and these fine controls, the ego will accept knowledge derived from the dream state, as a man might accept a message from a distant land in which he does not care to dwell, and whose environment would both mystify and frighten him.

In our dream experiments then, we will allow you to bring such messages to the ego. We will attempt to map this exotic country in such a way that the ego can understand what is there in terms of resources, that can be used for its own benefit. We shall map this dream state from various perspectives, until you know it very well.

I suggest your break.

(*Break at 9:16. Jane was dissociated as usual for a first delivery. Her eyes had remained closed. She resumed with the same fast and quiet delivery, again with her eyes closed, at 9:20.)*

For several reasons we will have a fairly brief session this evening.

I want to give you some more material to further fill out our outline for future sessions dealing with dream reality. I have intended to give you both an evening off entirely, out of the goodness of my heart, and because we will be concerned very soon now with relatively significant discussions, and a break will do you good.

Instead of missing a session however, I decided to give you this small preliminary material this evening, and then dismiss school early.

(Jane smiled. She had been speaking with quiet amusement.)

We will be involved with a study of the characteristics of the dream world <u>in general</u>, and attempt to isolate it as a separate reality simply for the purposes of examination. Then we shall consider it rather carefully in its relation to physical reality, using comparisons and dissimilarities.

This will <u>then</u> allow us to proceed into the relationship between the waking and sleeping personality, and discover the many ways in which the personality's aims and goals are not only reflected but sometimes achieved in and through the dream condition.

Usually the dream state is considered from a negative standpoint, and compared unfavorably with waking reality. Emphasis is laid upon those conditions present in the waking condition, and absent in the dream state.

We shall however consider those aspects of consciousness which are present within the dream environment, and absent in the physical environment. No study of human personality can pretend to be thorough that does not take into consideration the importance of the dream reality.

In our final discussions we will, in a practical manner, discuss the ways in which conscious goals can be achieved with the help of the sleeping personality. All of this material will be reinforced with experiments that I hope you will conduct yourselves.

(Again Jane smiled. I had noticed that her eyes had become slitted again as she spoke. They now opened. They were very dark, without highlights. She lit a cigarette as she continued speaking.)

It is amazing how man regrets the hours spent in sleep, for he does not realize how hard he works when his ego is unaware.

We hope to make it clear. We hope to let you catch yourselves in the act. This phase of our endeavors will be fascinating to you in its scope. You will not, again, regret the hours spent in sleep, for you will see how productive they can be, and you will realize how they are woven into the tapestry that makes up your entire experience.

We will deal also, as I mentioned previously, with the nature of space, time and distance as they appear in the dream environment. And some of our experiments in this line will be very illuminating.

Here the ego cannot go, but it can benefit from the information that is given to it, and perhaps in time even a shadow of the ego may pass through that strange land, and feel in some small way at home.

I believe that I will now end our session, unless there is anything that you prefer to discuss.

("No, I guess not.")

My best wishes then to you both; and I quite enjoyed the quiet and relaxed atmosphere.

("Good night, Seth.")

(End at 9:39. Jane was dissociated as usual. Her eyes closed, then opened and she was out of the trance. She had looked at me only casually while delivering the material. Her voice had remained quiet and rather fast.

(Oddly enough, looking back, Jane could not say whether or not she realized her eyes were open. But she was sure she was aware of this while she was speaking.)

SESSION 182
AUGUST 28, 1965 10:30 PM SATURDAY UNSCHEDULED

(No session was expected for tonight. Bill and Peggy Gallagher visited us unexpectedly at about 8:30 PM. The four of us decided to try a sitting like we had on Friday evening, August 20, 1965. That didn't develop into a session; Seth didn't speak. I have separate notes on it, showing how Jane expressed voice contact with an entity professing to be a female Gallagher. The details given by the entity were however not overtly familiar to Bill or Peggy. After the sitting we concluded that although something had taken place, the information was probably garbled.

(To begin tonight, the four of us sat at our small coffee table, holding hands. The room was lit by a candle within three feet of us on another table, and by reflected light from the kitchen on one side of the living room, and from the bedroom on the other side. Jane began speaking, asking if anyone was present. I had hesitated to speak, because on a previous occasion while trying this procedure I had inadvertently brought in Seth. See the 129th session, witnessed by Judy and Lee Wright.

(This time however Jane brought Seth in herself. We had clustered around the coffee table for perhaps five or six minutes when Seth came through. We broke our handclasps and relaxed for an informal exchange that lasted until 1:23 AM, with rather frequent breaks.

SESSION 182

(Jane's eyes opened perhaps ten minutes after she began to speak, and remained open for most of the session thereafter. She smoked, looked about at us, etc. Her eyes were very dark, without highlights. None of us saw any indication of feature change, nor did Seth tell us to be alert for such. Seth's manner was quite energetic, the voice on the strong side but not really loud. Twice in a frisky mood, the voice climbed very briefly in volume; both times this happened near the end of the session.

(I made no attempt to take notes, nor did Peggy. What follows is my reconstruction from memory, made immediately after the session ended. I kept my notebook beside our bed also, and whenever I thought of something to add I did so, up until noon of the next day. Jane then read the notes and suggested any corrections she happened to remember. Peggy and Bill did most of the talking during the session. They are reading the early sessions now, and so what developed was a rather condensed review of some of the main tenets of the material, for their benefit.

(Seth periodically asked if any of us had questions. For myself I avoided questions that might lead to answers I would wish to have on paper. The Gallaghers' questions were of a more general nature usually; and many of them had to do with Bill's family history. Seth usually addressed Bill as the "friendly or inquiring Jesuit," and Peggy as the "cat lover."

(Much of the session was a kind of review, as the 162nd session was, which the Gallaghers also witnessed, with Lorraine Shafer. The material on the construction of matter was gone over. Seth talked a good deal on the cooperation of all living things in maintaining our universe, and of how it's so very wrong for civilized human beings to kill. He dwelt upon this at some length. I believe a remark Bill made before the session began, about animals, led to this.

(There were a few new bits and pieces of information throughout the session. One is to the effect that although Seth's contact with Jane and me is his first venture into education on our plane, [which he had told us many sessions ago], he is also in contact with other groups on other planes. These other groups are not physical in our terms. Seth said that these other groups also have their wrongs, as we have ours. Killing is not one of them however, nor are wars.

(A new physical effect concerned the candle, standing on the table against the wall perhaps three feet from our group. All the windows in the apartment were closed with the exception of one kitchen window, because the night was extremely windy; this wind aggravated my hay fever. The candle burned with a low flame, one perhaps a quarter-inch high. Seth, talking about physical effects, said that he could probably have levitated the small coffee table we sat around tonight, with Ruburt's help. But Ruburt still needs to develop his abilities further, Seth said. Abruptly the candle flame shot up to a noticeable degree, at least twice its previous height. The increase in

brightness was plainly noticeable, causing all of us to look at the candle. Seth then said he had caused the flame to grow. It stayed brighter for several minutes as he continued talking, then died down. Bill confirmed my own thought at the time, that a stray burst of wind had affected the flame. We had no way of knowing if wind was responsible or not; the kitchen window was perhaps fifteen feet away, and around a corner. Seth went on to say that the candle flame would not grow higher again, because Ruburt was alerted to the effect now, and was watching it.

(Seth said my special sensitivity to windy days during hay fever season, [and one I was well aware of], stemmed from an incident that took place while I was traveling to California with my parents when I was about three years old. [This would be about 1922.] On a windy day on the prairie, somewhere west of the Mississippi, but short of the West Coast, I stood by a hill with my parents. My mother and father were arguing loudly. Father threatened to leave my mother and my brother and me. My father also had hay fever. I had had attacks before, but after this incident I had hay fever each year. [I have always had it since I can consciously remember.] When I remarked that my father had got rid of _his_ hay fever, Seth said _he gave it to me_. Seth said this is a common occurrence in illnesses being passed about among a family group. I identified with my father out of fear, Seth went on, because he threatened to leave me and thus must be all powerful; and since my father had hay fever, I acquired hay fever as a mistaken sign of strength.

(Seth dwelt upon the Tibetan monks who use astral projection, and follow their strict religion, while the peasantry live miserable practical daily lives, without hope for the most part. This is not right. He said the monks use psychic energy, which all of us have available; but they don't use it for any great ends, and thus are shallow.

(Peggy asked Seth about a recent dream in which she saw numbers in various corners. Seth named the numbers as 4 and 2; the month of April was represented by 4, with 2 being that day of the month. He did not say what this meant however.

(Bill's mother, who was also an arthritic cripple like Jane's mother, was a very aggressive personality, a masculine one, who developed arthritis in order to lose her mobility and thus avoid harming Bill's father and the children. She felt a growing rage and aggressiveness she could not control. Seth said association worked here, in that Jane could perceive this data because her own mother has arthritis. Bill's mother was very fond of flowers.

(Bill's mother was fascinated by the relationships of numbers, Seth said, and the color blue. After the session Bill revealed that his mother had been a bookkeeper, which Jane and I did not know previously. Peggy recalled that Bill's mother had been buried in a blue dress, which upset Bill's father very much; and that Bill's mother had many blue dresses in her wardrobe.

(Seth told Bill he subconsciously blamed his father for his mother's condition, after Bill remarked that whenever he and his father were together for a few minutes they would end up arguing. Also, when a small child Bill had overheard a sexual encounter between his parents, in which his mother cried out. Bill took it to mean his father had hurt his mother. Later when his mother fell ill, Bill made the subconscious connection with her illness and this earlier incident, and blamed his father for his mother's illness.

(Bill's mother tried to project her illness to other members of the family, as often happens also. This involved guilt feelings on her part.

(Seth slipped in some personal material on Walter Zeh before "Ruburt catches me in the act." He prefaced this by saying that we were all friends here tonight, presumably I suppose if the information was considered to be personal. Just before this he had mentioned again the similarity between Jane's mother and Bill's mother. Now he said that Walter Zeh had also been an invalid in a previous life, and a female. For reasons he didn't go into now, Jane owed Walter Zeh a debt, which she has paid in full. Jane had been attracted to him also in an attempt to make up to him, because she hadn't been able to make up to her invalid mother. In his previous life Walter Zeh had been crippled because of an accident.

(Also it was necessary that this episode in Jane's life take place before I came along, and be gotten out of the way and done with. It had to be done first.

(Seth made one short remark I would have liked to question him further on, to the effect that we would have plenty of go-arounds with "your parapsychologists." He did not elaborate.

(Seth told Bill that a summer Sunday in 1946 is very important to him subconsciously. It involved Bill's father William [Jane hadn't known the name of Bill's father], and an older man with brown hair whom Bill looked upon as being in a position of authority. There was some kind of disagreement as to Bill's choice of a career [Bill had left the Navy not long before], an argument with Bill's father; ever after that Bill didn't get along with his father. Bill did not follow his father's suggestions, I believe.

(Walter Zeh is a fragment personality, and a disturbed one. Because he had been an invalid in a past life, he tried to slow down Jane's development in this life to a crawl. Yet Walter has learned much and is doing very well.

(Seth told Bill that his mother had been very close to another female in the family, though not a daughter. They had talked about childbirth, etc. Bill thinks the other woman was possibly the wife of his father's brother.

(Seth said he had unfortunately been involved with some other groups on our plane, in seance gatherings. He spoke very harshly of such "idiotic" gatherings and personalities. At the same time Seth stated he was not a spirit, although if he materialized in the middle of the floor we would pay more attention and not take him for granted.

(*During his discussion on the creation of matter, Seth used the coffee table and a wineglass in making his points about how each of us creates his own world, with its own atoms and molecules. This led also into a discussion of the consciousness of each atom and molecule, etc., and our agreement telepathically on such things as the placement of objects in space. See sessions 66 and 68 in Volume 1.*

(*A Freudian slip that Jane made in reference to her own mother in the past tense, "was," whereas Seth wanted Jane to say "is," was duly noted. Jane, he said, would be perfectly happy never to see her mother again.*

(*Right after the session began, Seth showed how Jane's personal subconscious memories had, during the sitting with the Gallaghers, on August 20, distorted the material we received. What actually happened was that Jane's maternal grandmother tried to get through, but Jane wanted to get Bill's mother, and so named the entity speaking as a Gallagher. Seth mentioned that Jane's own memories of the shredded-wheat incident should have told her what had happened. Also, Jane confused the corner grocery in her neighborhood with the grocery in Bill's neighborhood, which was located in the middle of a block. Much, Seth said, Jane had picked up telepathically from Bill. Bill had looked up to the man running the grocery store in his neighborhood.*

(*Toward the end of the session Seth said he thought the object Peggy has been carrying in her handbag has "something to do with rock," and that a man had somehow been connected with it, or its origin. The problem here is getting the information through Ruburt, without distortion. See the 180th session. The Gallaghers said nothing about the object at this point, nor did I. Later at break I forgot to ask them about it.*

(*Bill's mother exerted a "pull" on his father which the father subconsciously resented. Her illness was not the result of events in this life only, but of past lives also.*

(*I told Seth I hadn't felt like going out dancing tonight because of the windy weather, and that I thought Jane would be disappointed. I had wished some company would drop in. This was just before darkness fell. As soon as the Gallaghers entered, they told us they had thought about us while eating dinner in Ithaca, NY, some 30-odd miles away, and had decided to stop by just in case we were home, even though it was Saturday evening. Seth said there had been telepathic communication between us, and as near as we could calculate we had been thinking about each other at roughly the same time.*

(*The number 5 is connected with Bill's 1946 date and incident, but Seth could not say in what way, or how.*

(*Bill and Peggy agreed that Seth's material on his parents seems to fit them psychologically, although some of the information given concerning Bill's subconscious feelings toward his father was a surprise to Bill. At one point Seth asked Bill to not say so much when he answered a question, because this led Ruburt to start to actively and consciously consider the material and to make his own interpretations, which could be distorted. Seth also asked Bill not to tell us any more about his family relationships; presumably so that more material Seth came through with in future sessions could be checked with Bill's knowledge, as in the blue dress and the bookkeeping incidents.*

(Possibly Peggy and Bill could dream about events of interest to them, that were discussed this evening, if they used suggestion. They could also use the pendulum, though they might need more subconscious practice. Seth repeated often that Peggy and Bill should read more of the material.

(Speaking of the fact that civilized man should not kill, Seth said the whole idea of killing is fallacious to begin with: an enemy who is "dead" is far more harmful than one who is still alive. Here he was dealing with the basic unity of all consciousness again. Killing is not thought of as an end in itself on other planes, he repeated. But it is wrong to kill on our plane when we do consider it an end.

(Seth told me that tests similar to our envelope tests, or perhaps involving objects, could probably be held here in the apartment when others such as the Gallaghers are present. Ruburt's confidence is the big factor. This restriction to home grounds is a very temporary one, and later Ruburt can deal with objects at a greater distance.

(Bill's mother had lived a previous life in China. Bill's family was involved in very complicated psychic relationships. Bill told Seth he thought that on the whole his ulcer is a little better since he and Peggy had first attended a session, the 158th, of May 30, 1965. Seth told Bill the ulcer is a parasite, and that he no longer needs it.

(The session had been going for perhaps half an hour when Bill suggested to Peggy that they leave because the hour was growing late. He felt tired. Seth then said he would wake Bill up, or get him interested, and he proceeded to do this by launching into the discussion on Bill's mother.

(Ruburt has abilities of his own that sometimes get mixed up with Seth's. There was much telepathy going on tonight. Regarding the individual constructions of the world of matter, each with its own set of atoms and molecules, Seth said that these individual worlds are not as much alike as one might think, even though there is telepathic agreement on such things as the placement of objects in space, etc. We focus on the similarities and ignore the differences to a large extent.

(So far man's behavior has him headed for destruction rather than survival. Seth repeated several times that for civilized man to kill is wrong. An animal in the jungle killing for food is one thing. To kill for the sake of killing is another. When a wild animal kills, the killed is replaced in the natural scheme of things. No gap is left, and the balance of nature is maintained. When man kills he rips out a part of himself that he has created. Man will stop killing when he realizes this, and that

death is not an ending but a change of form.

(Just before the Gallaghers left, Seth/Jane's voice began to grow very loud just for a sentence or two. We all clapped our hands over our ears, and Seth had mercy on us. The voice was somewhat unusual, Seth told us; he himself was not interested greatly in physical effects or proofs, but realized they might be necessary to us, or scientists. He was interested, he said, in effects like the voice, or Jane's facial changes. There was much that he and Ruburt could do; there was also much they could not do. It depended upon Jane's confidence to a great extent.

(Seth told Bill and Peggy, in connection with the subconscious construction of their individual worlds, that they really lived in many worlds at once. At the end of the session Seth told the Gallaghers he had deliberately given the information about Bill's mother being a bookkeeper and liking the color blue, in order to show them that valid information had been produced, no matter what its source.

(As Bill opened the hall door, Jane, standing beside him, came through as Seth, very loud, for a few words. But it was enough to make him shut the door quickly. When Seth then departed, usual good nights were said, the Gallaghers left and the session was over.

(End at 1:23 AM. Jane felt fine in spite of the length of the session. Indeed, it was she who initiated it during our casual conversation, after the Gallaghers had been here for a while. Her eyes had remained open for the most part until the end, and she had been dissociated as usual.

(Addition: Also, Seth said, when a person gets sick, they <u>want</u> the illness—a reference to my hay fever, taken from my father.

(The Gallaghers later confirmed that Bill's mother was very fond of flowers.

(Seth told the Gallaghers they should record their dreams, and study the symbolisms therein. Dreams are very cunningly constructed by the whole self so that one symbol can have meaning to many layers of the self.

(Seth said the material on individual constructions of the world of matter can be verified mathematically.

(Jane's maternal grandmother is on a midplane—at least one, and perhaps more, lives to come yet. [Or Bill's mother, I can't recall]. Later: we believe Bill's mother is the one on the midplane.)

SESSION 183
AUGUST 30, 1965 9 PM MONDAY AS SCHEDULED

(This afternoon while painting I had a vision. With my inner eye I saw the face of an older man, facing to the left in full color. I made two pencil drawings of

SESSION 183   223

the image. It was quite clear, especially about the eyes, nose and mouth; and later I realized that I had been "seeing" it for at least a few moments, almost absent-mindedly, before I understood what was happening.

(For what it is worth, earlier in the afternoon I had been wishing I had a model handy, for I felt like doing some quick sketches as a relief from the constant oil painting. It is difficult for me to get models when I have the time to use them. For some other material on my visions, see the 22nd and 47th sessions, in Vols. 1 and 2.

(I had prepared a test envelope to give to Jane during the 181st session, of August 25, but did not do so because of the short session. When the envelope was not used I did not mention it to her, but saved it for tonight's session. It contained part of a calendar page for April 1965. I came across the calendar beneath a stack of books and on the spur of the moment decided to use it for the test, wondering whether this type of cut and dried subject matter would have as much emotional pull for Seth/Jane as the subject matter of the first two tests. See the 179th and 180th sessions. Jane was out of the house when I prepared the usual double envelope.

(As will be seen, there were some very interesting developments because I chose this particular subject for a test.

(The session was held in our small back room. Jane began speaking while sitting down and with her eyes closed. Her voice was quiet and she used pauses, although her pace picked up considerably as first break approached.)

Good evening.

("Good evening, Seth.")

I had told you that I had considered giving you a night off. Instead, we had an extra session.

The experience was a good one for Ruburt, since it served to give him additional and much-needed confidence. I attempted to give several definite characteristics that would serve to identify your Jesuit's mother, and I believe that we succeeded.

(Bill and Peggy Gallagher witnessed the unscheduled session, the 182nd, on Saturday August 28. The Jesuit tag has come to be a standard one for Bill, and quite a humorous one in Seth's view.

(During the session Seth gave an accurate psychological account of Bill Gallagher's mother, according to Bill. She is now dead, and Jane and I never met her. Bill has told us very little about her, other than that she was an arthritic cripple like Jane's mother is. Three points in particular were quite authentic, according to Bill. Seth stated that his mother "was fascinated by numbers," loved the color blue, and was inordinately fond of flowers. After the session Bill Gallagher told us his mother had been a bookkeeper, was buried wearing a blue dress—blue was her favorite color—and that she was indeed very fond of flowers.)

Now, before we plunge into the nature and characteristics of dream reality, let us briefly consider the relationship between emotions, space, and distance as they occur within the waking conditions.

An emotion obviously does not take up physical space, yet it takes up varying amounts of psychic space according to its intensity. It seems to recede in time and to shrink in psychic space as the intensity of it begins to diminish. An intensive emotion will represent the present in time, a particular instant of <u>now</u>.

Whenever circumstances tend to revitalize such a charged emotion, that particular now will be re-created. The emotion will once again rush into the psychic space which is formed by elements in the personality's psychological environment. The immediate emotion of any moment, therefore, forms the framework of your present time within the waking state. As the emotion diminishes it takes up <u>less</u> of your psychic space, fills up less of your inner environment, and you seem to yourself to recede from it.

As far as distance, physical distance, is concerned, this whole idea is subconsciously taken into consideration. That which appears ahead of you in distance, and has not yet been experienced, under usual circumstances has not yet entered the psychic space of inner environment. When you reach this imaginary physical experience, and if you are emotionally involved in it, then it becomes the PRESENT, in capital letters.

The moment is remembered because the emotions experienced at the time almost completely fill the psychic space, forcing all other experiences out. The stronger the emotion the more vivid the moment becomes, the more totally it is recalled. And even in future years such past instances can be experienced as vividly as any present experience. In other words, to some large extent such a strong emotion unites experience and knocks down the artificial barrier of past, present and future.

I will let you take your break.

(*Break at 9:17. Jane was dissociated as usual for a first delivery. Her eyes had remained closed, her voice quiet but fast. She had used some pauses however. She resumed in the same manner, with some longer pauses, at 9:26.*)

As we have often stated, inner experience is the only <u>true</u> dimension of existence.

Because of the physical structure, experiences within your system have a slow-motion distortion which creates the appearance of time. Time as you know it, waking time, is intimately connected with the emotions and with emotional intensities. Now. There is also a connection here that can be explored most clearly by using color designations.

Red is the most <u>present</u> or immediate of colors. The cool colors are more contemplative, or more indicative of contemplation. They do not however have the same type of intensity. They leave room within psychic space for other emotional experiences also.

There are electrical connotations here also that are important, electrical components that compose the emotional experience, and that tend to show themselves in certain auras of color. Within the dreaming state however inner experience is not limited as it is in the waking condition, so that the time barrier can be largely dispensed with. There is an additional psychic space to be filled.

(For some related material concerning time, intensities and moment points, see the following sessions: 149, 150, 151, 152.)

Experiences are more directly felt, although the same sort of differences occur here as far as intensities are involved. In the dream state as in the waking state, experiences vary in their intensity. There is however a more mobile element and an easier movement <u>through</u> experiences. Transitions are more rare in the dream state, since physical time lapses are not necessary.

Spontaneity is more the rule. Images appear and disappear, for there is no necessity to construct them as continuous physical constructions. There is therefore greater opportunity for new creations. These dream experiences take up psychic space, as do waking experiences. Their intensity is immediately felt however without any reliance upon physical time.

They are felt according to their intensity only. You might say, returning to our analogy, that there is more color-mixing within the dream state, and the materials are immediately at hand. Distance is then seen in its true light, not in relation to physical space but in its basic relationship to emotional intensity. As you seem in the waking condition to travel out of an experience, or as you seem to separate yourself from it, then physical time enters into your awareness.

When you directly experience an emotional event, when you are at its heart, so to speak, then you do not seem to experience physical time. Only as you move to the outskirts of the experience does such time realization enter in. The dream experience however is always free of the realization of physical time, practically, for you experience dream events directly from the center of awareness.

You move from the outskirts of one dream into the core of another without a change of intensity, and therefore without the sense of physical time passing. It goes without saying that a sense of time may or may not be interwoven in any given dream sequence, but you as the dreamer are not conscious of the physical hours that pass as you sleep.

You may take a break.

(Break at 9:49. Jane was dissociated as usual. Her eyes had remained closed, her pace had been rather fast.

(Our bed is in the small back room we usually use for sessions. During break Jane sat on it while she smoked a cigarette. The break was rather long, and Jane had started on her second cigarette. She was still on the bed when Seth came through again. Jane has yet to speak from the prone position for any amount of time. She came close to it this evening, leaning back upon an elbow quite often.

(Her eyes opened soon after she began speaking, and she continued smoking. She was quite restless. Most of the time she spoke from a sitting position. Her eyes closed at times for a sentence or two. They were very dark, and her voice was quiet and fast. Resume at 10:00.)

In the dream reality you have the opportunity to work out solutions to problems within a larger framework in a psychic environment, where there is no immediate necessity for physical construction.

This function is extremely important, and represents one of the main ways in which problem-solving is dealt with by the personality. This is also the reason why the plays of Shakespeare have endured the centuries. The dramas are not true to life in physical terms, but are true to life in psychic terms.

The creative abilities have full reign within the dream state, and it is here that the personality first tests its creative intensities and methods. The personality's physical environment therefore is greatly colored and formed by his dream existence. There is some leakage from waking-life experience to dream experience, but this leakage usually represents the material needed, or the problem to be solved. Mental events and dream events are primary. The individual first manipulates situations within the dream reality, and then transposes his characteristic method of handling them upon the physical reality.

It is true, as Ruburt has discovered, that these dream elements are interwound. Events are indeed clairvoyantly perceived in the dream state. On the other hand in many instances the sleeping personality solves a problem, and therefore causes the physical event because it is the result of the dream work involved.

In many cases he perceives in a dream a future physical event, and then within the dream situation acts out various possible solutions, until he hits upon the most agreeable one. In the dream state the personality actually has at its command a stupendous amount of subconscious information of which the ego is not aware. It is actually more practical therefore to seek the solution in the dreaming state, or in periods of dissociation if you prefer. The amount of data available to the subconscious is simply superior in quality and larger in quantity to that available to the ego, and this information can be used effectively through suggestion.

The subconscious in sleep has great freedom, and has at its command information gained through past experience in this life and in other lives. In the intense focus of awareness that occurs within the dream state, the inner self is able to direct all of its energies for the purpose of solving a given problem.

It is able to use all of its vast information, gained through previous experience, and all of its knowledge, to solve the problem at hand. Literally, the whole inner personality is able to focus upon any given problem, completely free of distractions, using the subconscious language of symbols. This language is crisper in its fashion, and more concise and more inclusive than any written language. For as we have explained, each symbol has various meanings to all layers of the self.

(*Among many others, see the 92nd, 93rd and 94th sessions in Volume 3.*)

Computerlike, the data is instantly made available exactly when and where it is needed. The ego is indeed equipped to handle physical reality. Its purpose is the manipulation of the personality within the physical universe. Its most effective method of procedure however is to form the problem concisely, and then to feed it to the subconscious before the personality enters the dreaming state.

This requires on the ego's part an excellent ability to perceive correctly the elements of the physical situation, to express it in terms that the subconscious can understand, and to deliver the message properly. The subconscious will then break the physical data given to it down into its psychic components, translate it into symbols; and the inner self, at the request of the subconscious, will then focus all of the energies at its command to deliver the most acceptable solution, taking the entire needs of the whole self into consideration.

The solution therefore may not necessarily be accepted completely as the best solution by the ego. The ego is aware of the physical situation only in its relationship to itself. It is not aware of the internal situation. The solution however must be made in relation to the total conditions. It is extremely important then that the ego correctly interprets the physical situation, for this is the information that it will give to the computer, so to speak.

You may take a break or you may end the session.

(*"We'll take a short break then."*

Break at 10:26. Jane was well dissociated. It was one of those instances, she said, where she was "totally involved" with the material she was delivering. She felt as though she was inside the material. Her eyes had been open most of the time, and she had been quite restless. Her pace had been fast.

During break Jane mentioned that Seth had not yet discussed my vision, noted on page 223. Nor had I given her the test envelope. I had discovered that I was reluctant to break into the material when it was going so well, and when Jane gave such an indication of involvement with it. I thought it might introduce an alien note, and also that it might interfere with the results of the test itself.

(I did not mention the envelope, and in view of the late hour decided to forget about it for this evening. Jane began speaking while sitting cross-legged on the bed. Her eyes opened again shortly after she began. She was smoking, and her voice was quiet and fast. Resume at 10:33.)

I have several points to make here.

We cannot cover everything I had in mind for this evening, or this session would run well over its ordinary allotted time.

To follow the above material, let us emphasize the importance here of a <u>clear</u>, honest, perceptive intellect, for it is largely upon the intellect that the ego depends. The intellect collects from the physical environment those situations and conditions which affect, or will affect, the ego.

The intellect chooses from the total physical situation those elements with which the personality will ultimately have to deal. The intellect is discriminating and selective. An ego that is overly rigid will inhibit the intellect from perceiving various portions of physical reality, and therefore distort the appearance of reality, limiting the intellect's abilities.

Necessary and vital information is therefore not collected. The problem is not seen in any total light, but in a distorted manner. This distorted picture is then delivered to the subconscious, which is able to make <u>some</u> corrections. It still cannot view the physical situation as clearly as can the ego under best conditions.

When the ego is of such a rigid nature that it distorts physical reality out of all context, then however the personality had better rely upon the subconscious even in this respect, for the subconscious will at least perceive those elements of physical reality that immediately threaten the whole self.

This material this evening will be extremely useful and practical to you both. We will discuss it more thoroughly in another session.

(Jane closed her eyes and smiled.)

A very brief word here concerning your Mark. Putting up with him will not seem a chore if you realize that psychic energy is not only being used when you do so, but <u>within reason</u>, when you do so unresentfully, you are gaining psychic energies through interactions.

(Mark is Bill Macdonnel's entity name.)

The very act of dealing with him kindly utilizes your own abilities in many ways, stretches the limitations of your sympathy and understanding, and of your patience, yes; but in so doing you become stronger and better able to deal with your fellow human beings in general, with benefits to all.

I am not speaking of overdoing this, as you understand. There is an analogy here, perhaps not flattering to Mark, but I do not mean it unkindly.

Are your hands tired?

(Jane looked at me. The pace had been rather fast.

("No.")

You recall that I told you animals relied upon the psychic energy of their owners. So do weaker personalities to some extent rely upon stronger ones. Now this could result in a draining of available energies, but when this occurs it is only because you are not as strong as usual. When energy is withdrawn for this reason, the individual who is used to relying upon it will feel bewildered and resentful, and abandoned without knowing the reason.

The use of energy in such a way does <u>not</u> however, and should not, ordinarily drain you. To the contrary, again within reason, it should invigorate you, allow you to draw upon additional energy, and give you practical experience in doing so.

I say to you within reason, but if your abilities were fully developed I would not have to use that phrase, for you would be so renewed in <u>any</u> encounter that no such question would arise.

The you does not necessarily apply to you, Joseph.

I will give you a few sentences concerning your vision. Or you may take a break, or I will save it for the beginning of our next session.

("You can continue.")

(See my notes on page 223.)

The man was an acquaintance of yours in a life many centuries ago. He no longer experiences earthly or physical existence. I know of him. I do not know him. He was a teacher, and is one now. He was a relative when Ruburt was Seth. He knows of our relationship, and was curious.

(The very first sessions dealt a good deal with reincarnation. Jane and me did not ask for this kind of data; it just came that way through the Ouija board and we accepted it at face value. Frank Watts, it will be remembered, was our communicator; the present Seth entity did not announce his presence until the 4th session, when he superseded Frank Watts.

(In the 3rd session, December 6, 1963, Frank Watts told Jane and me that we had lived lives in Mesopotamia, our first, in the 4th century BC. Frank Watts and I were females, Jane was a male, our brother, and his name was Seth.

(In the 54th session Seth went into considerable detail in explaining the construction of entities. He could not give us this information earlier, he said, because we would have leaped to the conclusion that he was Ruburt's [Jane's] subconscious mind; this is not so. As everything else does, entities constantly change. To quote Seth: "Ruburt is <u>not</u> myself <u>now</u>, in his present life; he is nevertheless an extension and

materialization of the <u>Seth</u> that <u>I was at one time</u>... He grew, evolved and expanded in terms of a particular, personal set of value fulfillments... He is now an actual gestalt, a personality that was one of the <u>probable</u> personalities into which Seth could grow. I represent another, I am another."

(Seth then continued to explain how I am also an offshoot of that early Seth entity. Thus Jane, myself, and our present communicator, Seth, are related psychically; it is this that makes our sessions possible, according to Seth.)

I will now end an excellent, rather lengthy session. I do suggest that you study this material carefully this evening.

Do you have no tests for me?

(Jane, still sitting cross-legged on the bed, smiled and leaned forward. Her request caught me by surprise, and it took me a few moments to fish the test envelope out of its hiding place and lay it on the bed before her. It was 10:58; I thought it much too late for a test.)

You must give me a moment.

("Yes.")

(She picked up the envelope, fingered it lightly without bending it, and waved it at me briefly. Her eyes were still closed.)

I have the following impressions, that are somehow connected with what we have here.

The number five, and several buildings. Much space. Something to do with two people, and a yard. Wind, and blue, perhaps a dress.

I would here like to make a suggestion, that tests be given to Ruburt fairly close to the middle of a session, rather than at the beginning or end.

I also get the impression of a string, of what I do not know. Did I mention the number five?

("Yes.")

Perhaps 1965, and a road. I will now end the session.

(Jane laid the envelope down. Her eyes were still closed.

("Good night, Seth."

(End at 11:02. Jane was dissociated as usual. She said that as I fumbled around trying to find the test envelope, she was forced to wait. During this period she spoke to Seth: "Okay, I'm staying in the background, so you can come through loud and clear," or words to this effect.

(When she opened the test envelope to see a clipping of a section of a calendar page, containing numbers and a few spots of red and yellow, Jane was quite disappointed. Her reaction was similar to my own as I listened to her recitation of the test data. A very interesting fact now dawned on both of us when we looked at the <u>back</u> of the clipping; for here we found most of the data Seth had given was quite correct.

(In making up the test, I had unwittingly focused my conscious attention on the calendar side of the paper. This was the first time I had used a test object containing material on <u>both sides</u> of the paper. The makeup of this particular calendar consisted of the days of the month on one side, and a drawing in color on the other.

(The test paper was folded once. The number five was on the calendar side, in the upper center. Directly back of the number, on the other side of the paper, were two buildings, one an erected house, with just above it a floor plan of another. There was a yard, and trees, and a blue simulation of blueprint paper in back of the floor plan.

(Returning to the outside, calendar side of the test paper, there were several strings of numbers. The calendar month was April 1965, although the year date doesn't show. Returning to the other side of the paper, we see that a road leads up to the garage attached to the drawing of the erected house.

(Thus it seems that Seth traveled through the thickness of the paper, picking up impressions as he went along, and did this at least twice. He also mentioned "two people...perhaps a dress." There were no people on either side of the test paper. Checking the whole calendar however, we noted there was a drawing of a man and a woman on the upper section of this particular page, but that I had left them behind in clipping out the test section. They would be about four inches removed from the clipping, and stood before another drawing of a house. We do not know if this is a legitimate interpretation of something "somehow connected with what we have here."

(Wind is an intangible, and is not overtly indicated in the drawing. These are a draftsman's drawings, quite precise in detail. The background material is rather freely and loosely brushed in, so that a breezy and modern effect is indicated. We do not know if this effect prompted Seth's mention of wind. The effect of the drawing was one of "much space."

(Jane said she had not expected any test, and so did not feel nervous about anything forthcoming.

(Also, the calendar is from a building-supply company: "Lumber. Hardware. Paint. Masonry. Supplies. Roofing.")

SESSION 184
SEPTEMBER 3, 1965   10:30 PM   FRIDAY   UNSCHEDULED

PART ONE
(Tonight's unscheduled session is arbitrarily divided into two parts in order to present the envelope test data first. I have verbatim notes on this; I asked Seth to speak slowly enough for notes on the test and he agreed. The rest of the session material is

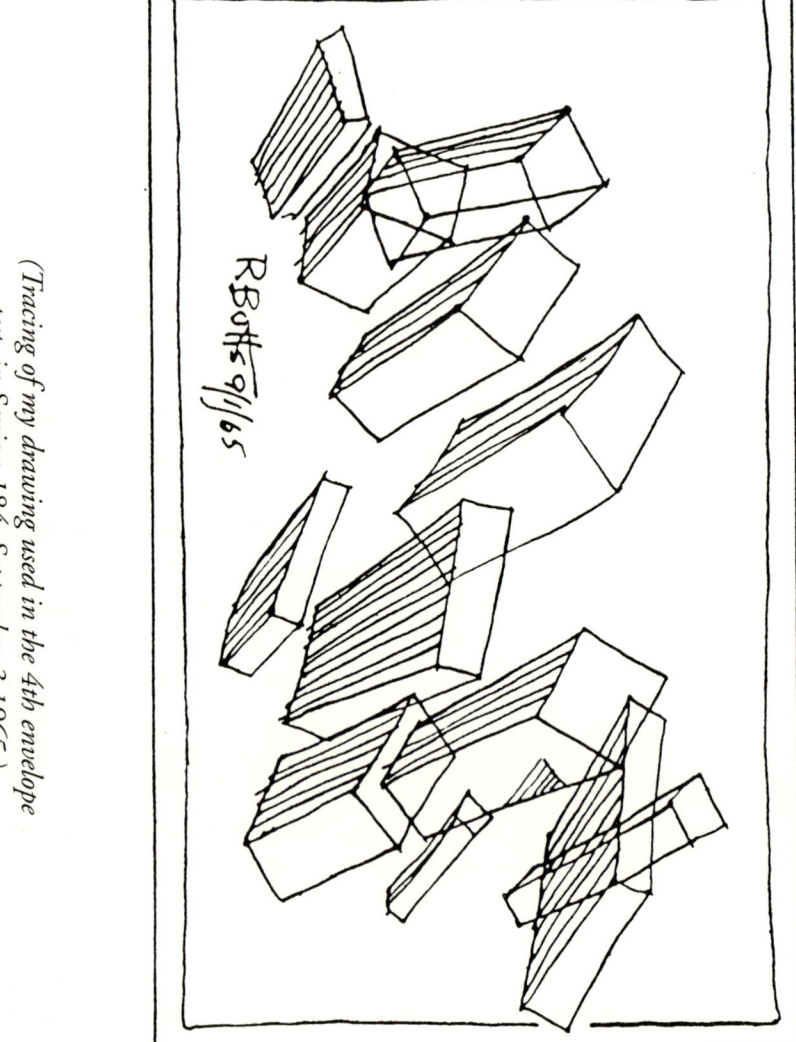

(Tracing of my drawing used in the 4th envelope test, in Session 184, September 3, 1965.)

presented in summary form in Part Two.

(Jane, her ESP book finished and mailed, has some free time for a change. She has copied the 179th, 180th and 183rd sessions to send to Dr. Instream. She also plans to write him a letter. As it developed, she will be copying Part One of this session to send to Dr. Instream also, for even though the session was unscheduled an envelope test developed. Once again parts of the test results were unexpected. The whole test was very interesting; and all the more so because it was Jane's first before witnesses.

(Our regularly scheduled session for last Wednesday, September 1, was not held because Jane and I had unexpected visitors. A few details here are of interest because the visitors became entangled with the test results mentioned above.

(Actually the young couple calling on us live in a downstairs apartment. They have been married about a month. Both of them work at my place of employment, Artistic Card Co., in Elmira. I secured the apartment for them when a vacancy developed just before their marriage. The young lady works with me in the art department. Her husband is a salesman who travels at irregular intervals, but quite often.

(Our friends in question do not know about the sessions. They visited us at 8:30 PM Wednesday, and before Jane and I realized it session time had come. We like our new neighbors a good deal and did not resent their calling, but we did dislike missing the session. They left us at about 10:30. Jane and I did not consider having a session then; I also thought Jane could use the break in routine.

(I had prepared the usual test envelope that Wednesday afternoon while Jane was napping, as she usually does on session days. When the session did not materialize I saved the envelope for the next session, which I thought would be on Monday, September 6.

(The double envelope contained a simple line drawing I executed in black ink on ordinary white paper. It was folded once. I chose this subject matter in an effort to see how Seth would handle more abstract subjects. The drawing is reproduced on page 232; it is a pen tracing made from the original on a light table.

(Bill and Peggy Gallagher, who have witnessed several sessions, visited us this evening, Friday, September 3. Our conversation touched upon many subjects. They read the 183rd session, dealing with Jane's third envelope test. No session had been planned for this evening but as the four of us sat around our coffee table Seth came through at about 10:30 PM.

(Seth told us that he merely wanted to join in the general conversation, as he had during the unscheduled 182nd session last weekend, which the Gallaghers also witnessed. Seth requested that we continue our exchange without notes on my part and without weighty questions. Jane's eyes were closed in the beginning, her voice

average in volume. She was nevertheless quite active in her chair. After perhaps half an hour her eyes opened. They were very dark. She smoked as she talked with us, and at times got to her feet as Seth. This last is something she has not done for many sessions.

(Much was said before the envelope test developed, and this is summarized in Part Two. At about 11:50 PM Seth surprised me by asking if I had a test prepared. I replied that I had and went back to my studio to get the envelope I had readied for last Wednesday's session, and my pen and notebook. Jane, as Seth, sat quietly talking with the Gallaghers while I was gone; I wondered if the enforced delay would give her time to become nervous.

(Normal lights were on in the living room where we had gathered. Jane took the double envelope. She held it without making any obvious attempts to guess at its contents by feeling. She sat with her eyes closed now and her head down somewhat as she faced the three of us. She did not appear to be nervous, and her voice remained average. Pauses will be indicated. The first paragraph that follows consists of the excerpts I noted down. Begin at approximately 11:51 PM.)

We will go slowly with this, Joseph... The first test in the presence of witnesses... We are not bothered by light... We will be silent for a moment however.

(Jane paused. The following material is verbatim until otherwise noted.)

These are impressions of what it is I hold.

I have the impression of the number 3 or 7, or perhaps 3 and 7, *(pause)* and of a road, and something spectacular.

I am aware of course of the double envelope. *(Pause.)* Something 10 times, and a familiar location. A spread of sorts, as perhaps of a spread of grass.

An unpleasant circumstance occurred before or after, in which a woman was involved. The color gray, and a multiplicity of design. *(Pause.)*

Perhaps crisscross shapes, and a sign.

I will now suggest a break.

(Break at midnight. Jane's eyes now opened. She had been dissociated as usual. She asked me to open the test envelope. She said she had no idea whether the information given was correct.

(In the first test, given in the 179th session, I had found myself mystified over part of the data. Now, the four of us found ourselves puzzling over the first part of tonight's test data. As will be seen however most of it is connected with the test object. We are learning that our confusion stems from the unexpected and sometimes far-reaching turns that such connections can take.

(Jane herself made the possible connection that the "...unpleasant circumstance... in which a woman was involved," could be entangled with the day I made the drawing; this being last Wednesday, when we missed our regular session because of visitors. See my notes on page 233. Seth's information following this statement

connected itself with the drawing easily enough, even to the "color gray," which arises from the shadow effect I achieved in the drawing by using closely-spaced parallel lines.

(Bill Gallagher pointed out that my name and date on the drawing, besides being a "sign," also contained a combination of 10 letters and numbers, as "something 10 times." We do not know what to make of such interpretations.

(Seth came through again at 12:10 AM, as we were discussing possible distortions of the test data. Once more Jane spoke while sitting down and with her eyes closed. Her voice was quiet but faster than before, so the following short account consists of the excerpts I noted down. Resume at 12:10 AM.)

Once again there was some confusion of channels... as there was in our first test when we were alone... But tonight we succeeded in getting Ruburt painlessly across that first-test-before-witnesses barrier... And it was a barrier to him. Such tests are very good training for him... He needs it... It is a beginning.

We held many sessions before we tried such tests... while we waited for Ruburt's confidence and abilities to develop... They are still growing. They need even more developing, and they shall be.

(End at 12:12. Jane was dissociated as usual.

(Bill and Peggy Gallagher now left. I thought the session had ended, but as Jane and I sat talking Seth came through once more. The following material still concerns tonight's test, and is verbatim because once again I asked Seth to speak slowly. Jane's eyes were closed in the beginning, her voice quiet. Resume at 12:20.)

We were not selective enough. We will have to learn to be more selective.

The road referred to your neighbor, the male, who is a salesman, and who travels on the road often. It was he and his wife who were referred to here in the unpleasant episode. This was associated with the test because the session for which you prepared the test was not held because of their visit.

(Jane paused, then opened her eyes. She lit a cigarette.)

I did not realize that this would not help you, that this information would not help you here. This was not Ruburt's distortion, but my own misunderstanding.

The 3 and 7 referred to a visual image, not too clear, of 7 designs, separated somewhat from 3 other designs. The road was a distortion, but only superficially, for it was meant as a symbol to describe the man involved, and I could not get Ruburt to say <u>salesman</u>. It was a misunderstanding actually, rather than a distortion.

I could not get the meaning <u>clearer</u> to Ruburt, but he did not <u>distort</u> the meaning. He came as close as he could under the circumstances.

("Thank you, Seth.")

(End at 12:25. Jane was dissociated as usual. She had no visual images that *she was aware of, she said, while giving the original test data. As far as she knew she had let Seth through without thinking about anything herself. Again, see my notes on page 233. It appears that many impressions can attach themselves to such a simple thing as a small pen drawing.*

(Referring to the drawing, it can be seen that there is an interlocking group of 7 designs or blocks on the right, and a like group of 3 on the left. My literal mind also notes a single block beneath each of the larger groups, but Seth did not refer to these. We suppose the "familiar location" can refer to our own apartment wherein I made the drawing; or perhaps to the apartment house itself, in which our visitors also live. And surely the drawing contains a "multiplicitude of designs" and "crisscross shapes".

(The drawing can be "a spread of sorts," but we see no particular connection with grass, nor with "something spectacular." I did not think to query Seth about these points as we sat talking near the end of the session.

(The session ended at 1:10 AM. Through it all Jane had been dissociated as usual. There had been rather frequent breaks. Jane now went to bed, and I began to make notes to supplement what I had already written down. I would like to add here one more piece of information given by Seth, concerning an earlier test, before concluding Part One. This was given after the Gallaghers had left.

(It will be remembered that in connection with the test photograph used in the 180th session, Seth/Jane stated: "...and a border. I think *now of a border of flowers..." The test photograph has a white border. Seth now informed me that in the 180th session Jane distorted the information about the border of the photo into a border of flowers because of her personal childhood associations. He said Jane has an early memory of a border of flowers around a garden.*

(After tonight's session Jane said she vaguely remembers a small plot of grass and vegetables, bordered by flowers, maintained by her grandfather in the backyard of her home in Saratoga Springs, NY. This would be quite an early memory for her. She had not made any conscious connection with this memory and the border data given in connection with the second test, however, until Seth mentioned it tonight.)

PART TWO

(The following material is a summary of other topics covered in the unscheduled 184th session, witnessed by Bill and Peggy Gallagher. Some of the material was of course obtained while the Gallaghers were present, and was in actuality intermingled with the test data discussed in Part One. Part Two depends on my memory and on Jane's to some extent. I am fairly certain of it. Material I recall but vaguely is omitted.

(Almost at the beginning of the session Jane, as Seth, pointed at me and said my head would be clear for the rest of the evening. Hay fever had been bothering me a great deal during the day. Seth said the reason I am bothered more at home than

at work, where I feel remarkably good, is that the house dust in the apartment reminds me of house dust at home, and of my mother, when I was a child.

(As Seth suggested, it developed that my head was good for the next few hours, and I was more than willing to comply with the suggestion. Seth said I could have information concerning my parents and my hay fever at any time during a regular session, so I could get it all in writing. He said he prefers to deal with blocks of material in this fashion.

(Seth told me I have improved in my relations with my parents, even though this is hard to see for me, at times. I am doing all I am capable of for them at the moment. In the future I will expand enough to be able to include them in my awareness without fear of personal threat, which impedes me at the moment. My parents need love as a child needs love, unquestionably, and this I cannot give at the moment. I should not feel guilty at this. My parents visited my brother Loren for four days during the week of August 29 to September 3. Seth said this was more than an ordinary visit as far as the folks are concerned, in that they were looking for the type of love described above from Loren and his wife also. Loren is 45; I'm 46; Jane 37.

(It would be a great help if I could learn to talk with my parents in a conversational way, about inconsequential things.

(In this summary I give all the information I can recall on a particular subject at the same time, for convenience's sake, although it may have been scattered throughout the session. Thus some of the above material was given to me after the Gallaghers had left.

(Seth deplored our ideas on war and peace, which must improve if we are to survive. This led into a discussion about computers, and Bill Gallagher's personal idea of studying up on them for future use in business. Seth said computers would transform human life. He said Bill's personal ideas were good ones; the inherent danger with them had to do with the type of salesman's personality, the feeling of superiority and of having power over others, that might color the use of computers. He told Bill that it would require strict discipline on his part if he worked with computers in such a fashion.

(After the Gallaghers had left Seth told me Bill Gallagher had "great bursts" of energy. Bill and Peggy, he said, were very good for us and the sessions, in that they contributed. I do not recall more on this particular point. Seth told Bill that if he follows the material given on the construction of matter and suggestion, and applies it, he can be rid of his ulcer within a year. It will require discipline. Bill should read the material because the intellectual integrity behind it will appeal to him. Then he will understand how he creates his own ulcer.

(Seth told Bill he didn't seem to have enough time in the day because he had the common habit of chopping time up into segments of minutes. A conception of *time close to psychological time would give Bill enough time to do all he wants to do.*

(*In the beginning of the session Seth asked us to continue as we had been; he wanted the convivial party air. When we fell silent, or adopted the usual more formal session air, he demanded to know what had happened to all the jokes. On one occasion his voice began to climb in strength and volume, half jokingly. Bill and I implored him to keep the voice under control. For the most part however the conversation moved along quite easily.*

(*At this time Jane, as Seth, stood up and picked up our cat Willy. Her eyes were open. Her voice was loud also, and Willy immediately squirmed out of her arms and darted away, his ears back. "See," Seth/Jane said, "Your pussy doesn't know who his mistress is right now...." Actually, Seth said, Willy knows him well, having grown used to his appearances. Many many sessions ago Willy had occasionally reacted to Seth's appearance, usually just before a session began, or at the very beginning itself.*

(*At one point I remarked to Bill Gallagher that I used to have two favorite questions for Seth: "What do you do between sessions?" and "How's my old friend Frank Watts?" Seth's answer to my first question was "What do you do?" He now gave essentially that answer when Peggy asked my old question tonight. Commenting on Frank Watts, the personality Jane and I first contacted on the Ouija board to begin these sessions, Seth told me that there were records in town pertaining to Frank Watts, if we would stir ourselves to look for them.*

(*When Peggy asked him if the records pertained to Frank Watts being a teacher, Seth gave an answer I do not recall, except that I am sure it was not a direct yes or no. Frank Watts, Seth did tell us, is doing very well. Seth also said in a quietly humorous way that Frank Watts was still a fathead, as he had told us many sessions ago. In Volume 1, see the 11th session, held on January 1, 1964.*

(*Seth told me that if possible I should go out dancing as usual with Jane tomorrow night, Saturday, if I felt good enough. As it developed we did not go.*

(*A few days ago Peggy Gallagher had brought Jane a copy of the latest Cosmopolitan magazine, and suggested that Jane query them about running some excerpts from her ESP book. In view of Cosmo's drastically revised format, Jane agreed to try. Naturally we wondered how the ESP subject would be received by a popular magazine, and this gave us a chance to try an experiment that we had discussed before.*

(*This was simply to determine if Jane herself, as Jane, could ask Seth a question, then go into trance and deliver the answer as Seth. Since Jane had been switching focus often tonight, I suggested that now was as good a time to try the technique as any. With a little urging Jane, a little self-consciously, asked Seth about what kind of a reception such a query would get from the editors at Cosmo, whether they would buy such an article, etc.*

(She then closed her eyes, went into trance, and delivered the answer. It was entirely in the affirmative.

(Seth stated that the editors at Cosmo would be interested, and that in answer to Jane's query, which would consist of a chapter from her ESP book plus a letter outlining her ideas on adapting it for the magazine, they would send a letter of interest. Such an article, Seth said, would not be immediately bought by Cosmopolitan, but would eventually. The editors would ask for some changes. In the beginning they would be merely interested. Seth mentioned no time limit concerning the sale.

(This past week Jane learned the editor of Topper magazine that they had bought a short story of hers, The Mission. She was of course greatly pleased by this news. Seth now told us that Jane would sell more stories out of that batch she had written up before starting the ESP book. It will be remembered that Seth had something to say about Jane's sales of short stories and books in the 104th session. The predictions given in that session 10 months ago are still working out. See Volume 3.

(Seth said the oil sketch I have begun of my vision, described in the notes for the 183rd session, is very good. It is promising to be one of my best pieces of work.

(Yoga exercises are excellent because they teach concentration. Jane, Peggy and I had been trying some earlier in the evening.

(Jane, Seth said, needs a rest after finishing her ESP book. Even a day or two of rest will help, in terms of subconscious value fulfillment. The individual must have such rest periodically, in one form or another. Sometimes such value fulfillment cannot be really attained for years, Seth told us. At other times it is achieved in a moment or two.

(Jane is at loose ends now, and quite restless. She will be calmer when she starts her next project. In the meantime she worries, Seth said, about my opinion of her because the money is slow in coming. She also worries about a delay before her next project is accepted, remembering the long delay between her first novel, The Rebellers, *and the acceptance of the ESP book—at least a year. I reassured Seth that I am not worried about Jane or her contributions in any way. Seth told me that Jane is pulling her weight psychically in our household, and that money will follow.*

(At one time our cat Willy became sick on the rug, and Seth broke from the discussion to enable Jane to take care of Willy.

(Seth briefly discussed the candle-flame effect mentioned in the 182nd Session, saying the phenomenon was so successful because Jane had no forewarning of it.

(Seth said in answer to a remark by Bill Gallagher about tattoos, that he himself had never been tattooed. Our friend Mark had, however, in his Denmark existence when he was a sailor. Mark is the entity name for Bill Macdonnel. According to Seth, Jane and I knew Mark in Denmark in the 1600's. Mark, Seth told us, had a large angel tattooed on his chest as a good luck charm, and believed it to be a

protection against storms at sea.

(Seth had some very interesting comments to make when the conversation turned to flying saucers, and the recent rash of reports on such craft in the newspapers. The craft do exist, Seth said, and the action of governments in relation to them leaves much to be desired. I believe he used the word pitiable in this connection. Also, government people cannot bear to admit something they cannot explain.

(Seth said that nevertheless the government had a point when they tried to prevent public panic by denying the existence of such craft. A great danger at this particular time would be that an admission of the saucer's existence would, strangely enough, serve to unite the far-left and far-right extremist groups in this country. These groups would unite in declaring the craft to be Russian, that they were much advanced over anything we have; this whole furor would create panic, Seth said. In six months such reasoning would not apply, because of impending developments in this country. This would presumably be because of the impending elections, though Seth didn't say this in so many words. In answer to my question he said Barry Goldwater would not be one of the far-rightists to cause trouble. Nothing was said about the source of the saucers, their inhabitants, etc.

(Bill Gallagher has something of a cold, and Seth gave him instructions for using suggestion upon retiring tonight. If he executed the suggestions properly, Seth told Bill he would wake up tomorrow to find his cold vastly improved. He would not be rid of it overnight, but would be well on the way to disposing of it.

(One disquieting subject arose after the Gallaghers had left, and Jane, Seth and I were talking quietly. Seth surprised me by mentioning our neighbor across the hall, Leonard Yaudes. We have known him for several years but he does not know of the sessions. Seth began by saying that the following information was on the edge of Ruburt's awareness and that he was not very well focused upon it. It had to do with the possibility of an accident or an unpleasantness for Leonard sometime within the next three months. Seth then mentioned the period from September 15 to October 15, after saying that possibly he could focus a little more intently upon the problem.

(Seth said one other person would be involved, but he would not say whether it would be a male or female.

(At first I had thought Seth meant that Jane and I would be involved in the trouble seen for Leonard, but Seth reassured me by saying we would not. It did not involve a disaster for Leonard, he said, nor a crippling accident; he used the word unpleasant often, and did not commit himself beyond this.

(Any trouble that developed would be the result of present trends involving Leonard, and at this time these trends were so general it was impossible to pinpoint future events with any certainty. If the present trends were changed, the personality of the future trouble would change also. Jane and I know Leonard fairly well, but

actually know little of his inner feelings, his friends, etc. We have no idea of what Seth means by trends. I had become concerned about attempting to warn Leonard in some fashion, but Seth said this could not be done.

(In case of a specific predicted event such a warning could be given, and if heeded could head off trouble. Seth told us that in this case there was nothing we could do. The present trend would have to continue before trouble really was a possibility. Nevertheless Jane and I will be alert on Leonard's behalf, especially between September 15 and October 15.

(The session ended at 1:10 AM. Jane had been dissociated as usual while speaking as Seth. Much of the time her eyes had been open. She had smoked many cigarettes. Her voice had usually been quiet, her pace a conversational one, which means that usually it is a little too fast for me to take notes. Jane felt no unusual fatigue at the end of the session.

242   THE EARLY SESSIONS

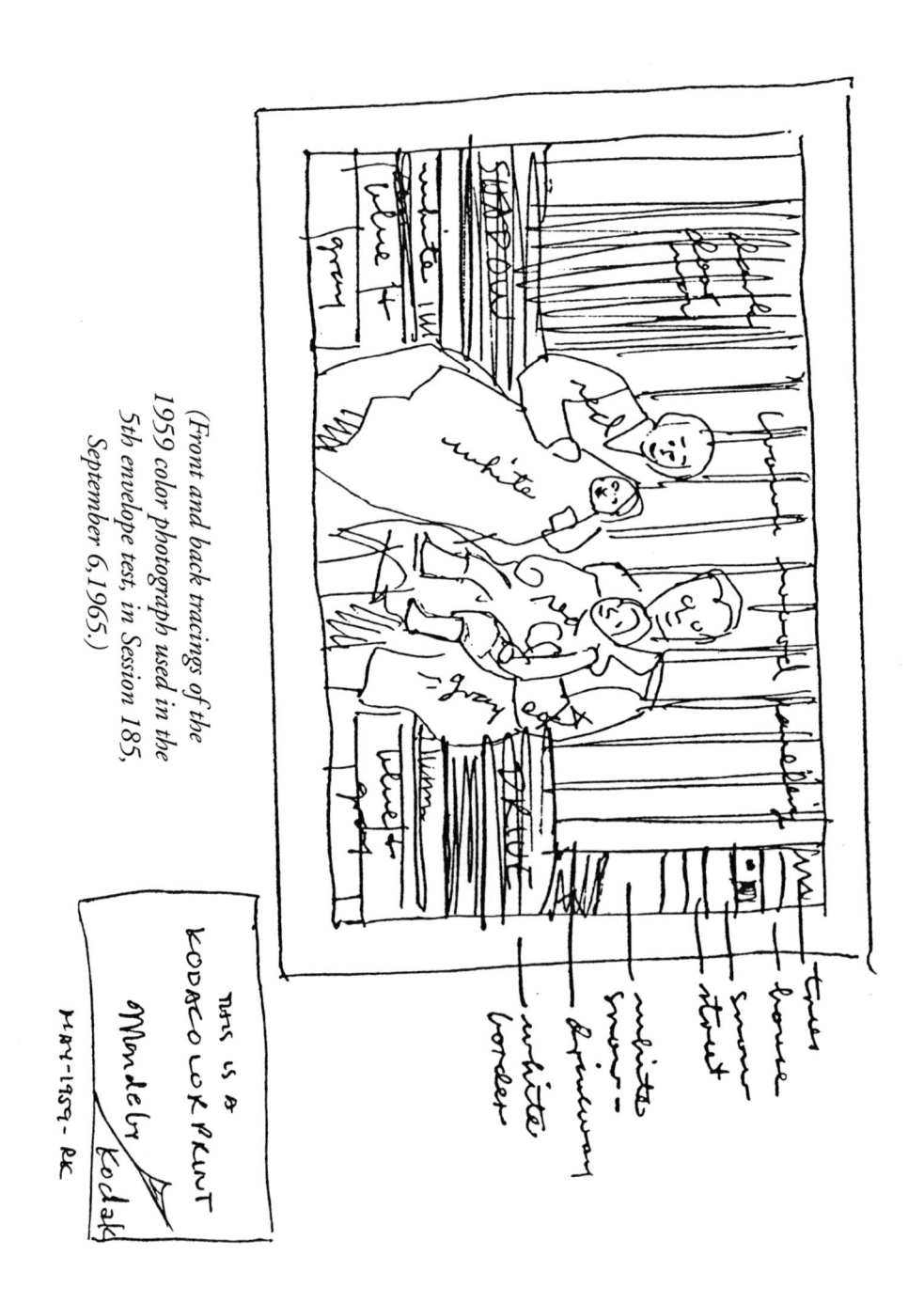

(Front and back tracings of the 1959 color photograph used in the 5th envelope test, in Session 185, September 6, 1965.)

SESSION 185
SEPTEMBER 6, 1965 9 PM MONDAY AS SCHEDULED

(Since today was a holiday, Jane and I had some extra time. We used part of it to copy the 179th, 180th and 183rd sessions, plus Part One of the 184th, to send to Dr. Instream. We also agreed on a letter to him. Jane will mail the material tomorrow.

(Once again I planned an envelope test for the session, should the opportunity arise. I prepared the usual double envelope while Jane was working at the front of the apartment. For the test I used a color photograph of my brother Bill, his wife and two young children, taken in Webster, NY, in 1959. I found the photo accidentally in my files earlier in the day while looking for something else. I knew Jane hadn't seen it for some time, perhaps years. Bill is 37 years old.

(The photo is of a winter scene, with brilliant contrasts of light and shadow. I have indicated the colors crudely in my tracing on page 242. The group of four sit on the edge of a concrete patio at the back of Bill's house. I did not mention a test to Jane, but she is well aware that they are in the offing now; earlier in the day she casually mentioned tests, without asking specifically whether I had one planned for tonight.

(The session was held in our small back room. The window was closed, for my hay fever bothered me most of the day. In spite of this however, I believe I have been helping myself to some extent through suggestion. Jane began speaking while sitting down as usual, with her eyes closed. Her voice was quiet. She began rather slowly, but soon picked up her pace considerably.)

Good evening.

("Good evening, Seth.")

For this session we will leave our material concerning dreams, to discuss another matter. We will however return to the dream data at our next session.

A while earlier this evening Ruburt read something that made him wonder whether or not he had, or could develop, healing ability. I decided to speak about the general subject this evening.

It is an extremely interesting one, though somewhat complicated. This ability is a natural one, operating to some degree or another within every personality. It is a natural protective mechanism of inner origin, directly affecting matter. It is a self-correcting mechanism. The individual's health is determined by his ability to take advantage of, or to use, this mechanism.

The term mechanism may be a poor one, but I use it now to emphasize the physical aspects of its nature. When the ego is resilient this mechanism works automatically and well. It is the ego in many cases who clogs the works, so to speak.

Ruburt has for years done fairly well in this matter, automatically regulating large areas of his health, with as you know some small failures, such as the sinus condition mainly, and the faulty eyesight.

(*My hay fever bothered me enough so that I made some noise using a tissue. Jane sat quietly waiting, her eyes closed.*)

Are you ready?

("*Yes.*")

Generally he has done very well in regulating the physical organs, however, and in maintaining a level of effectiveness that is most unusual, considering his early unhealthy psychic environment.

We will now tell you, Joseph, that your head will be clear for the rest of this evening.

("*Okay.*"

(*I was glad to hear this, and had been wondering whether Seth would give me this suggestion without my asking. He had done likewise in the unscheduled 184th session last Friday, and the suggestion had worked well for me. Whatever its source I had certainly responded.*)

There are ways in which this natural ability can be strengthened, and it may be of benefit that we discuss them. These ways will not only be helpful in facilitating these automatic health correction tendencies, but will also be generally beneficial as far as <u>all</u> inner abilities are concerned.

They will allow you to increase your clairvoyant and telepathic abilities. They will aid in astral projection training. They will increase your powers of concentration, and will also show themselves in your own work.

It goes without saying that you must bring to all your experiences more than a mere wish to be different, more than a mere curiosity. In order for you to operate effectively in any area there must be in your makeup a strong, positive and definite desire to benefit the race of man. Intellectual knowledge is important, but the desire to benefit your fellow human beings must be emotional as well as intellectual.

These suggestions which I am about to give you will aid immeasurably if they are followed.

They demand a certain discipline it is true, and according to your desire you will find the discipline easy or difficult. I could have given you <u>all</u> of these suggestions at an earlier date, but you would not have been ready for them. In giving them to you, I take into consideration your own backgrounds, and I have made concessions accordingly.

(*Jane's eyes opened briefly. She looked at me then closed them again.*)

Your meals could be somewhat simpler. I would here suggest very few fried foods. You have too many of these. I would suggest less heavy foods. Fresh fruits and vegetables are excellent. Meat, but not fatty meats, and not an overabundance of meats. You will enjoy your meals more and you will savor the individual tastes with more discrimination.

I will give you the suggestions, and then I will give you the <u>reasons</u> behind them. I will have some little more to say concerning diet. You do well as it is, avoiding thick sauces and gravies. There is no fear here of short-circuiting necessary vitamin needs. I am mainly suggesting a change in the way food is prepared, and whenever possible a reliance upon fresh vegetables and fruits. Frozen are preferable to canned.

It is important obviously not to overeat. In general small fairly frequent meals are preferable to three <u>heavy</u> meals.

I suggest your break.

(*Break at 9:27. Jane had been dissociated as usual. Her delivery had been rather fast. Her eyes had remained closed after the one look she gave me.*

(*Seth's comments on our meals rather surprised us, since we are quite careful about our diet as it is. We do eat fried foods, of course, but decided we could cut down on these.*

(*I thought my head was a little better, following Seth's suggestion; but the difference was slight and I hoped for more improvement. It was a relief not to be sneezing however. During break I mentioned that each new tack the material takes usually leaves some other subject dangling. I expressed concern because Jane was interested in receiving all the material on dreams that she could get. She thought her next book might deal with dreams.*

(*Jane's eyes opened again after a few sentences following break. She looked at me but casually as she spoke, and at times let her eyes close. I would say her eyes were open about half of the time until next break. Her voice remained quiet. Resume at 9:35.*)

Now my dear Joseph, this material concerning health will indeed tie in very well with our dream material, which is one of the reasons why it is being inserted here.

We shall have our sessions for many years. There is no fear that any of the material will be left dangling in midair. The material will change now and then in the balance of its components, for it too must change and grow. The identity of the material must change and grow if it will endure.

Theoretically, it would be better indeed if you were vegetarians. However at this time I do not suggest it. There is no doubt, for various reasons, however, that many benefits are connected with this particular dietary habit. I repeat: I do not suggest it for you, for various reasons. Moderation will do us as well.

You would do better with fruits for dessert more often.

Now aside from these dietary suggestions, I also believe other patterns of behavior could be adopted. The isometric exercises, for now, are excellent and should be followed by both of you. The two Eastern exercises, done occasionally by Ruburt, should be adopted by you both as a matter of routine daily.

Later other such Eastern exercises should be added. The walks should indeed be systematically continued. Deep breathing should always be adopted during such walks. When the walk entails an errand the <u>walking itself</u> should be the important matter. You should attempt to feel yourselves a part of the environment through which you pass, and attempt to enter into it rather than feel yourselves as observers.

Ruburt should drink no more than five cups of coffee daily at the most. If he is not giving up his cigarettes, then as you suggested moderation should be used. The present fifteen a day will do for now, but this should be reduced to ten when it is feasible.

I mentioned in the past those suggestions given by Ruburt to himself, concerning the continued health of the physical organism. You should both utilize this practice. In our dream material we will go deeply into the nature of health suggestions given in connection with the dream situation, and such suggestions may be considered a part of this evening's list. All of these—you may call them rules if you prefer—all of these rules then are for your own benefit, and are personalized, formed by me taking into consideration your own needs, strong points and weaknesses. Therefore they apply, the dietary suggestions and the exercise suggestions, to you only.

We can and will give a <u>general</u> list, but it is always better if this list be implemented by personal consultation. You have done much better in the overall in health maintenance than you did in the past; since you are both in excellent <u>organic</u> condition you can say that you have both done well. However there is a large difference between a general state that is free of disease and a state of exuberant health, in which the inner and outer selves are perfectly attuned.

Such a state is far from impossible, and we shall see that you achieve it. The rules that I have given you are an absolute necessity if that state is to be achieved. And it is only in that state that the inner self can utilize its abilities.

You may take your break. I will then have a few words to say concerning the connection between diet, personality, and health. All of which incidentally is reflected in the dream state, and in the nature of dreams themselves.

(*Break at 9:56. Jane was well dissociated. Although her voice had been rather average this evening, she said now that she felt it to be strong subjectively. Jane told me it is hard to explain, but at times she feels she is more a part of the voice than at other times.*

(Her pace had been good, her eyes closed at times. Usually she opened them and stared at me to emphasize a point.

(I was now aware of some improvement in the state of my head, and felt much better. I hoped the improvement would continue. Jane now resumed while sitting down, and with her eyes closed, at 10:02.)

Joseph, you can help yourself considerably by giving yourself suggestions, beginning tonight, as you fall off to sleep, to the effect that your head will be clear tomorrow. Suggest that while you sleep your inner self will make whatever corrections or adjustments are necessary to bring about this end.

This should be done <u>every</u> night during your season, and will <u>immeasurably</u> help you. The same suggestions should be given by Ruburt for the sinus condition. He has helped your health often, automatically. He is a health-giving personality in this respect, <u>generally</u> speaking.

The <u>nervous</u> cigarette habit does not help him however, for it diverts his energies. Obviously it is a symptom. Moderation at least will be of great benefit, if <u>he</u> follows our suggestions.

(It was 10:06. Reaching over, I dropped the test envelope in Jane's lap as she spoke. Her eyes were closed. They did not open now, nor did her delivery falter. Actually she gave no sign that she was aware of the envelope. I chose this method of introducing the envelope into Jane's awareness to see if it would halt or interfere with the material of the moment, and was pleased to see that it did not. I had taken care to see that Jane had not seen the test envelope during breaks, or before the session.)

His efficiency in this healing process can indeed grow.

A little more here concerning diet. You are indeed to a large extent what you eat. You are bound up in the cycle of earth relationships. The eating of meat without doubt focuses the physical mechanism closely to the physical system. There is nothing wrong with this. If you are trying to develop inner abilities however, and if you wish to <u>allow</u> yourself a mobility of focus, then moderation in this respect must be used. Eggs and milk and cheeses can be substituted occasionally without changing your overall eating habits.

(It was 10:11. Jane had been speaking with pauses. Now she paused again, then picked up the test envelope. Her eyes were still closed. As during her previous four tests she held the double envelope lightly in both hands. She did not appear to be nervous.)

We will now see about your envelope. Give me a moment.

(Jane's pause was very brief.)

I have an impression of a road or a <u>tree</u>; that is, of such parallel lines. I have an impression of afternoon, an impression of three people, of dirt or dirt color, and shadows or shadow shapes, perhaps of pyramid form.

Again, I have the impression of a white border, and perhaps on the other side, of writing. The shadow shapes are dark, and contrasted with light. I have the impression of chimney shapes.

Ruburt has the impression of the school fence across the street from the house in which he lived, and <u>he</u> is thinking of a particular photograph of his own that involved his house, the street, part of the fence, and perhaps some children. We are letting <u>all</u> of this come through.

I now suggest your break.

(*Break at 10:15. Jane had been dissociated as usual. Her eyes had remained closed, her voice quiet. She delivered the test data without hesitation or fumbling. She told me she had felt the envelope drop into her lap but that it had not bothered her.*

(*Once again the test data was interesting. This was the first time, also, that Seth had separated his own data from that of Ruburt's, or Jane's. Refer to my tracing of the photograph on page 242. Seth's data can be seen to apply rather directly, with the exception that the photo is of four people instead of three. This is dealt with after break, along with the matter of chimney shapes.*

(*Jane told me that in the past she would have given her own interpretation of the photograph she had in mind along with Seth's information. On one level she had a distinct impression of her own photograph. But now she allowed Seth to separate the two impressions.*

(*Jane resumed while sitting down and with her eyes closed, and in a quiet voice, at 10:21.*)

Now. We let all of this material come through purposely, so that you can learn from it.

For one thing, we are trying to teach Ruburt preciseness in word formation. I am not able yet to give him a visual image during a test. Therefore the information must be passed on verbally.

The parallel lines and the tree did refer to the wooden boards of the wall, which are obviously parallel, each board being distinct and clear.

I was able to transfer to him the pattern of the people. This is where three came through. The child, the baby image, did not come through clearly. The road is obvious.

Now, I knew this was a photograph. Ruburt however, through association, made certain deductions. He picked up from me the fact that children were involved. He picked up the road and the pyramid shapes. This led him to think of his old home, <u>for in the afternoon the shadow of its roof</u> threw a <u>pyramid</u> shadow form upon the road.

The children that <u>I</u> perceived, he projected into this picture of his, a photograph in which children were indeed involved. The photograph used in the test was taken in the afternoon. The chimney was not in the picture. I saw the chimney of the other house in the test photograph, but this does not show there.

These tests are most advantageous, and should be continued. We will endeavor to teach Ruburt so that more precise data is received.

We will now end the session, though I would continue if you prefer.

("I guess we can use the rest.")

My heartiest regards; and follow my suggestions, both of you.

("Yes. Good night, Seth."

(End at 10:31. Jane was dissociated as usual. As before, her eyes had alternated between opening and closing. Her pace had been good. She said that Seth was in a good mood and would have liked to continue the session.

(During last break we had speculated about the photograph being taken in the afternoon, because of the elongated shadows on the white snow. I will check with my brother in Webster, hoping he can remember after six years. It seems reasonable to agree with Seth; I do not believe such shadows can be found in the morning during the winter months.

(See my sketch of the photo on page 242. The baby, in white sits on the lap of my brother's wife, Ida. The pattern of his clothing and blanket forms a triangular shape, very similar to the shadow shapes on the snow; these forms can be called pyramid easily enough. The baby perhaps did not come through as well as the other three figures because of a lack of contrast.

(The photograph has a white border, and a stamp with writing on the reverse side. No chimneys show in the photo. The house across the street is very small in the photo; for Seth to make an association with that house is most intriguing to us. As in the last test, the process of association involved proved to be most interesting.

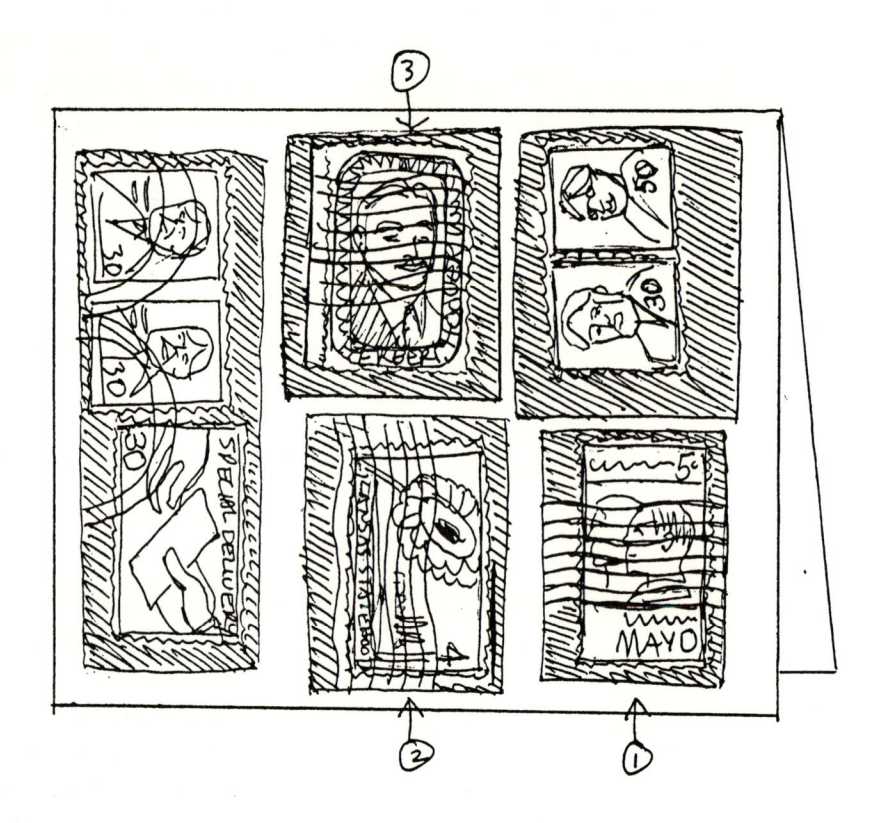

(Tracing of cancelled United States postage stamps used in the 6th envelope test, Session 186, September 8, 1965.)

SESSION 186
SEPTEMBER 8, 1965 9 PM WEDNESDAY AS SCHEDULED

(It will be recalled that in the 185th session Seth gave me some tips on how to help my hay fever through suggestion upon retiring at night. It has been a rough season and I was very uncomfortable over the Labor Day weekend. I had been using suggestion at various times through the day; trying Seth's method, I noticed an amazing improvement at once. I slept well the night of the 6th, and sneezed but five times the whole following day. The improvement has maintained itself, and soon now the season will be over. I can truthfully say the change in my condition has been magical. I am on a much-reduced dosage of my prescription antihistamine. I have learned I can do without it, but taking the drug removes the last of the lingering traces. For

some reason, the suggestions given before falling off to sleep are very potent.

(*Ever since mailing in the finished manuscript of her ESP book Jane has been very restless. She is very eager to get to work on her next project, but keeps struggling among many ideas, notes, etc. I suggested to her that she skip tonight's session if she felt so nervous, but she decided to hold it regardless.*)

(*I had prepared the usual double test envelope earlier in the day, but doubted it would be used if Jane was not in a good mood for the session. This time I cemented a collection of used U.S. postage stamps, still on original paper, to a folded piece of white paper. See my tracing on page 250. I sandwiched this paper between two pieces of bristol board to prevent identification by touch, and slipped the assemblage into the usual two envelopes.*)

(*The session was held in our small back room. Jane began speaking while sitting down and with her eyes closed. Her voice was average, her pace good. She used a few pauses.*)

Good evening.

("*Good evening, Seth.*")

We are indeed endeavoring to run through the storm clouds.

I do not know how long our session will be. We will have to discover what we can do here. I will direct some remarks personally to Ruburt.

First of all, he has not relaxed since he mailed his book, really.

Since he finished his ego has held him in a tight clamp. After the psychic excitement and effort and discipline involved in the venture of the book, there simply must be a complete relaxation, a letting go. There must be time for the organism to renew itself.

It makes no difference that physical time does not exist as you imagine, since you act as if it does. For this reason physical time is involved. Ruburt has been at himself constantly for new ideas, trying to force himself to plunge into something new. There must be a recharge of energies.

The conscious mind, the ego, must be momentarily diverted, so that the intuitive self is allowed freedom. He should know that inspiration does not come from the ego. He knows this intellectually, but upon this occasion he insists in using his ego as a whip to force speed. In the past he was more sensible in this respect.

When he is working his plunge into creativity is deep. It is not in his nature to go halfway. If he had taken more time off <u>completely</u>, he would not be in his present position.

It will not do if he resents the time he thinks is lost in relaxation or other pursuits. His intuitive nature will respond easily and enthusiastically when he stops trying to beat it into submission.

He has forgotten the daily joy that comes through simple observation of the day. I here suggest most strongly that until the following Monday at the earliest, he does not work at his writing or his records, that he does not consciously brood over them, and that he divert himself by changing the focus of his conscious awareness.

Surely this is not too bitter a pill. It may require effort but relaxation is necessary, or the period of transition will be needlessly prolonged. He can do what he likes: putter in his apartment, visit friends, paint, read, walk. It would be preferable if he did change his environment during this period, physically, by walking outdoors or visiting.

The psychological-time experiments should also be suspended. When the conscious mind is so diverted the intuitions can do their work. You did well Joseph, teaching him discipline, but as he never goes halfway, so sometimes he learns his lessons too well. One point here also: you pace yourselves differently in your work.

I suggest a break, and we will see what we can do.

(Break at 9:19. Jane was dissociated as usual.

(As in the 183rd session, Jane began to speak after break while sitting upright and cross-legged on the bed. She was still out of sorts and restless. She sat with a hand to her eyes, her head down. Her eyes were closed, her voice quiet. The pace was slower now, with more frequent pauses. Resume at 9:28.)

Now. Generally speaking, this automatic mechanism that adjusts the whole health structure works very well when the personality is in the dream state.

It is very susceptible to suggestion. Ruburt's jesting remark this evening that he would suggest refreshing dreams was actually an excellent one. The personality can indeed refresh itself in such a manner, and often does automatically.

(Jane now took a long pause. She still sat with her head down, resting in one hand.)

I did have a suggestion myself, that involved some small effort on Ruburt's part. It, if followed, would do him good however. It would be most beneficial for him to do some sketching at the riverbanks. The sketches could then be used for paintings.

(Another long pause. The pace was getting to be so slow that I expected the session to end at any moment.)

It goes without saying that suggestion before sleep will also help. It is the ego that is rigid, not the subconscious.

Do you have any tests for me this evening?

("Yes."

(It was 9:34. Jane smiled as she asked the question. Again I was surprised, not

expecting any interest in a test tonight. I fished the envelope out and handed it to her. She held it in her right hand. Her position was the same, head down, eyes closed.)

We will see what we can do. Please give me a moment.

I have the impression of something splendid. Perhaps a scene. Two or three people, and some connection with water.

(Another pause. Jane sat without moving.)

I also have the <u>impression</u> of a tavern of some sort, or place of refreshment; of tall parallel lines, and of horizontal parallel lines. Also lines on the other side, and of someone stubborn.

I have the impression of 3 6, perhaps an age or part of an address, and something that only partially appears, that is half visible. Maybe something to do with a man, woman and a child. There is something to do with a child somehow involved.

You may take a break to check our results.

(Break at 9:39. Jane was dissociated as usual. Her eyes had remained closed, her voice quiet. She had used many pauses in giving the test data, although she hadn't appeared to be nervous. During the whole passage, she sat almost without moving, holding the test envelope almost motionless in her right hand. She had no visual impressions while speaking, she said.

(Jane regarded the test results as very poor, at first glance. I didn't know what to think. Some of the information applied at first glance; other parts of it, I thought, were impressions attached to the test objects themselves, as in the 185th session.

(Still sitting upright on the bed, Jane resumed with her eyes closed, in a quiet voice and with pauses, at 9:47.)

Ruburt was not at his best this evening, so we did not get specific-enough information. I knew you had a test prepared however, and thought that we should go ahead.

("Did you pick that test information up from me telepathically?")

The fact of a test, yes.

("After the session began?")

Yes.

I would, overall, suggest that Ruburt not return to work until spontaneously he desires to do so. This will happen rather quickly if he relaxes. Wait until an idea presses him for expression.

I am going to close. However, I will see that all in all we have not lost out. Ruburt should remember that his reaction is a normal one. Our next session will indeed be a full and excellent one. My heartiest wishes to you both.

("Good night, Seth."

(End at 9:54. Jane was dissociated as usual. Her eyes remained closed until the

end of the session, her voice quiet. Seth said no more about the results of the test, and in view of Jane's state I thought it best not to query him about it tonight.

(From the sketch on page 250 it can be seen that parallel lines, both horizontal and tall, or vertical, are present; these are the customary wavy lines of cancellation. See stamps numbered 1, 2, and 3 on the sketch. On the envelope paper beneath stamp #2 is a green printed box of the type used for prepaid mail, but I do not know if this is what Seth means by "lines on the other side." This could also refer to the letters the stamps once serviced.

(Herbert Hoover, the Mayo brothers, Susan B. Anthony and Robert E. Lee appear on some of the stamps; I suppose any of these could be connected with "something splendid." Stamp #2 depicts a scene in Kansas. Seth mentioned two or three people; the stamps depict a total of nine people, plus two hands on the special delivery stamp. Are these hands "something that only partially appears?" The same thing could be said about any bust depicted.

(No water scene appears specifically on any stamp, or a child. Men and women are shown. As far as I can tell no portion of an address shows, or a tavern or place of refreshment. Nor do we know what to make of "someone stubborn," unless this was a personality trait of one of the people depicted on the stamps. I could speculate that Jane's constant nagging at herself to begin another project was stubborn, in that she refused to relax. This is hardly the kind of test data we seek however. 3 6 is Jane's age, but we discount this also.

(Perhaps a later session will clear up some of these points.)

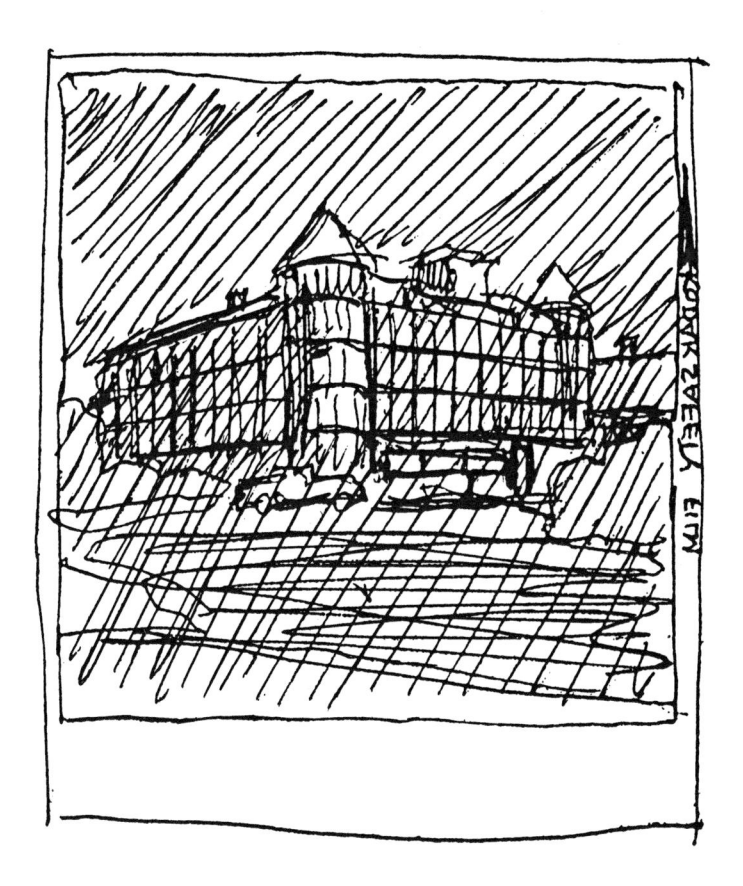

(Tracing of the photographic negative used in the 7th envelope test, in Session 187, September 13, 1965.)

SESSION 187
SEPTEMBER 13, 1965 9 PM MONDAY AS SCHEDULED

(While at work last Thursday, September 9, at 11 AM, I had a vision of the type described on page 223. This time, while bending over my desk, I saw with inner vision a rusty opened sardine can lying on a worn wooden shelf. The colors were very vivid, the detail needle sharp. I saw clearly if briefly the flecks of rust on the can and the grain of the wood. The scene was lit by strong sunlight from my left, so that long shadows were cast to the right by the humble can.

(Earlier in the day I prepared the 7th envelope test for the session tonight. This time I picked a negative I had taken during our vacation in 1964 at York Beach, ME. The subject was the Driftwood Hotel, situated but a stone's throw from the beach. This place has strong emotional attachments for Jane and me. It will be remembered that it was in the dancing room of the Driftwood that Jane and I saw the personality fragments we had ourselves created, on our vacation in York Beach in 1963. See the 9th session in Volume 1. We had this experience several months before these sessions began. See the sketch of the negative on page 255 of this Volume 4.

(Bill and Peggy Gallagher were witnesses for tonight's session, and the session was held in our large front room. Traffic noise was not a problem, the windows being closed because of the cool night. Jane began speaking while sitting in her favorite Kennedy rocking chair. Her eyes were closed, her voice good but not loud, her pace a little fast. She used few pauses, and sat much of the time learning forward with her hands clasped before her and her head tilted down slightly. She began speaking at 8:59.)

Good evening.

("Good evening, Seth.")

My heartiest welcome to our dear friends, the Jesuit and the cat lover.

I am going to speak this evening concerning our dream reality, although I promised our guests earlier that we would discuss the God concept. However we took valuable time out in order to put our Ruburt in line, and so we are somewhat behind.

I am pleased that he has been following my suggestions.

And I hope that our Jesuit will also follow those instructions I have given him. We will here consider the dream reality in an isolated manner, as if it were a thing disconnected from normal consciousness, although in reality it is not so disconnected.

Joseph, you will let me know if and when I speak too swiftly.

("Yes.")

(By now Jane's accent, which might be termed a brogue of sorts, had become quite noticeable.)

I spoke in a recent session concerning the connection between distance and emotions. The true reality of distance as you know it is dependent upon the intensity of emotion, and has nothing to do with your idea of space. The emotion which is intense is felt at its peak as present in time, and immediately here in terms of distance.

Emotions take up a certain amount of what we call psychic space within the personality's awareness. As the intensity of the emotion fades, so it seems to you that it recedes in time. But this is an illusion caused by the limitations of your outer senses. Now. In the dream state the outer senses are to a large degree restrained in their activity. Therefore the dream state more clearly represents the actual nature of time. Intense emotions within the dream state are experienced as present time, and the personality moves easily through these emotional intensities without experiencing the sense of passing time, although any given dream may contain within it its own time element.

The dreamer is not aware of the actual passing of physical hours. He is only aware of the <u>interior</u> time element as it appears within the framework of his dream. The personality will be seen to operate in some manners that would be considered quite normal, if he were in the waking state.

He acts, speaks, walks, talks, makes certain deductions. He responds to <u>interior</u> stimuli. The personality also operates within the dream state in ways that would not be considered normal in the waking state. He travels through space in moments. He speaks with those who do not exist within physical reality. He sees parents who have died in physical ways, and in his dreams he knows, on many occasions, what other characters think within the dream context.

(Jane smiled, then paused for emphasis.)

You see, then, that while the personality can act in a more or less normal manner while in the dream state, he can also act in ways that are denied him in periods of so-called normal consciousness. He has freedoms and abilities and talents in the dream state of which his waking self may be unfamiliar.

It would seem to be that the waking personality could learn much from his sleeping counterpart, and this is indeed the case. Theoretically speaking, and in theory only, anything that a personality can do or achieve in the sleeping state, he can do and achieve in the waking state. The limitations are those adopted by the ego, in many cases for good reason.

However the limitations can be diminished, and the waking personality can avail himself of many characteristics shown by the sleeping self.

I will suggest your break, and we shall continue.

(Break at 9:20. Jane was dissociated as usual for a first delivery. Her eyes had remained closed. Her pace had picked up as time passed, and by break her delivery was quite fast and businesslike.

(Bill Gallagher voiced the thought that during delivery there is always a change in Jane's face, but that he couldn't articulate it. He said he has been aware of this since the first session he and Peggy witnessed, the 158th.

(Jane resumed while sitting down and with her eyes closed once more. Again her brogue was apparent, her voice good, her pace fast. Resume at 9:33.)

The sleeping personality is as close to the inner self as you will come in this existence, for here the personality is soon <u>free</u> of the camouflage concerns with which it must be involved in the waking condition.

In the sleeping state we see the personality as it is in operation. We see its abilities and its limitations. Our friend, the Jesuit, will do well to read our dream material, for dreams are a reflection of the needs of a personality and of the abilities. The focus of attention and concentration are magnified a thousandfold in the dream state, and dreams form the basis for your physical environment.

First, problems are worked out within the dream framework. Answers and solutions are arrived at. These answers and solutions are then transformed into physical reality. No dream is meaningless. No dream lacks purpose. Each dream has meaning to all levels of the personality, and one dream object is a symbol which is translated by all layers of the self, in a mathematics which is more complicated than any dealt with by your physical computers.

As we have suggested in the past, the dream state can indeed work for your benefit in a more efficient manner, if proper suggestions are given before sleep. The dream fabric itself, the dream drama, is woven of many threads, and <u>all</u> aspects of the personality <u>contribute</u> some of the ingredients.

One dream will enable the ego to solve pressing immediate problems. The dream drama will enable the personality to act out various possibilities which are experienced as reality. The most effective drama is then reacted to in physical reality.

This same dream, however, will deal with many other actualities. It will serve as a method of communication between the various portions of the self. It will deliver information concerning past and future, and if proper suggestions are given it, then the self will use the dream drama particularly to better the overall condition of the personality.

There are chemical and electrical connections that cannot be ignored here. For a dream has a chemical reality and an electrical reality. It is built up, on one level, of chemical components that have an electrical basis, and it is through these connections that transformation within the nerve structure of the <u>physical</u> organism is made.

The pituitary gland is of great importance here, and the thyroid gland of secondary importance. Negative electrical charges are responsible mainly for the <u>durability</u> of any given dream. The mind, as you know, does not appear within physical reality, although the brain is indeed of physical origin.

Our dreams therefore occupy the same space as is occupied by the mind—no space at all. There still must be a connection with the physical organism, and here our chemical and electrical components enter in. Each dream is actually built up through a chemical synthesis that follows strong electrical pathways.

You recall that all experience has an electrical reality, deposited from birth within the physical cells of the body, so that at physical death we have an electrical counterpart of the physical being with all memory and experience intact.

Were such experience a part of the physical self, and dependent upon it, the personality could hardly survive physical death. And were dreams so connected to the physical self, then whole areas of the personality would dissolve with physical extinction.

As it is these dreams, having an electrical reality, are deposited in coded form, with all other experience, <u>within</u> but independent of the physical cells. Dream experience is as real to the personality as waking experience. Only the ego makes any distinction. Therefore the personality that has survived makes no distinction on its own.

I suggest your break, and we shall continue. It is nice to have such friendly guests. I do not grow weary of speaking to Joseph but it is good to have an audience, particularly when one is a Jesuit in spirit, although I believe he does not follow certain Jesuit rules.

([Bill G:] *"You're a most interesting speaker, Seth."*)

I try.

(*Break at 9:57. Jane was quite well dissociated, she said. Her eyes had remained closed. Her pace had been fast, her voice good, with more than a touch of brogue at times.*

(Bill Gallagher said that in his opinion Jane, when speaking as Jane, doesn't move her facial muscles the same as Seth does. Seth forms his words more carefully and distinctly, Bill said, and this effort shows.

(Jane resumed in the same manner, again with her eyes closed, at 10:11.)

We have said this often. However, suggestions should always be given before sleep, that the subconscious will maintain the organic integrity of the physical organism. This is basic.

Suggestions should also be given so that a harmonious relationship be maintained among all levels of the personality structure. Suggestions should be given that constructive tendencies are given free reign. Perhaps more important, suggestions should be given that <u>only</u> constructive suggestions will be reacted to. These suggestions give you a leeway.

(*Jane now paused and smiled. Her eyes opened. She looked at Bill Gallagher.*)

I am very pleased, for I opened Ruburt's eyes earlier, and our Jesuit missed it. When I can put one over on him, then indeed I am doing well.

(*I missed it too, of course. My eyes are down most of the time as I write, although I have cultivated the habit of looking up at Jane quickly every sentence or so, as a matter of routine.*

(Jane's eyes were very dark, without highlights. She looked casually at the three of us.)

These simple suggestions will serve to guard the personality from many unfortunate circumstances, and if they are given nightly they will serve as an adequate protection against organic disease, such as ulcers.

(*Jane grinned and pointed at Bill.*)

A man who has an ulcer, Joseph, he thinks differently than a man who does not have an ulcer. Suggestions such as these will keep problems such as these in the background.

Such suggestions will serve to protect the integrity of the physical organism, for these suggestions also have an electrical reality and a chemical reality, as your fear of cats has a chemical and an electrical reality that forces you to act within that framework.

(*Jane was now speaking to Peggy.*)

You have created the framework, and you can remove the framework, as he has created the framework within which an ulcer can have reality.

(*Our cat, Willy, had been sitting at the foot of Jane's chair. As if by signal Willy now got up and walked toward Peggy, who sat but a few feet away. He brushed against her leg and she involuntarily jumped. The timing was perfect. We all laughed.*)

I am amused.

Because suggestions do have an electrical and a chemical reality, they can therefore change the framework within which you operate. Theoretically there are no limitations to what any of you can do. Practically the limitations are your own, and practically it is within your province to change them or not to change them.

Because suggestions are formed of the same stuff that forms your physical reality, suggestions can indeed change the framework within which you operate. This is no Pollyanna hogwash. Many of the ways and the means have been given. My suggestions, if followed, will be fair enough proof of the validity of our material.

Do you have a test for me this evening?

("*Yes.*"

(*It was 10:23. The material had been so interesting that I had forgotten the time. I had planned to hand Jane the test envelope at about 10:00. Her eyes had been open up to this point, but she now closed them and sat waiting quietly while I handed the envelope to Bill; he passed it to Jane. She held it lightly in both hands, her eyes still closed.*)

I ask that you give us a moment.

These will be impressions. I have the impression of four, f-o-u-r, of something. Of gray, of mood or color. (*Pause. Jane shook her head as if in doubt.*) The impression of a masterpiece of some kind in connection with what I hold.

(Pause.) And something federal. *(Pause.)*

Ruburt has the impression of something to do with a toothbrush, or toothbrush salesman.

I have the impression of a door, and of horizontal parallel lines, and a mass. *(Pause.)*

I do not bother to state the material is light. It would be obvious; or that we have sealed envelopes. I have the impression of dark, and of a voice, and of initials. I would say again, J. B.

We will now take a break or end the session.

("We'll take a very short break then.")

(Break at 10:28. Jane was dissociated as usual. She said she had no visual data during the material on the test; just the thought of the toothbrush and of herself. Her eyes remained closed until break.

(Peggy said that she watched me rather than Jane during the test, and that I did not betray by facial movement anything about whether Jane was doing well on the test, or not well.

(As usual, some of the test material obviously applied, and other statements seemingly did not. By now however we have learned that material in the latter category is not necessarily distorted; it could merely be another example of the sometimes far-reaching impressions that attach themselves to test objects. Seth has said very little about the reasons for this. So we were now curious to learn what application, if any, such statements as four, a masterpiece, a voice, etc., had to the test object. Again see my sketch of the photographic negative on page 255.

(Jane resumed in the same good voice, and with her eyes closed, at 10:40.)

The photograph was taken at four o'clock in the afternoon.

The voice referred to a singer who sang on the bandstand while you danced.

The federal represented all I could get through to Ruburt, I am sorry to say, concerning the fact that the building was a large one. He had the idea from my information of a large federal building.

The other statements are obvious. We are in a training period, and will progress. And I hope rapidly.

(I did not realize at the time that Seth did not explain the masterpiece statement; I could have asked otherwise. Jane's manner now turned more humorous. Her eyes opened again. She smiled, and looked back and forth among the three of us as she spoke with quite a bit of animation.)

Ruburt is still rather nervous in our tests; even with his good friends present, oh he is so frightened! However we are making headway in this respect, and he will learn with experience.

He is hardheaded. In many ways this is to our benefit. In the overall we will want more specific information. It must come in a more clear manner, and so it shall.

We shall do things here. It may take time.

(Jane's eyes had closed briefly. Now she looked at Peggy and smiled.)

Our cat lover is embarrassed when he looks at me.

([Peggy smiling:] "Why would you say that? You said "he" when you spoke to me.")

Because—I say he advisedly, and we shall go into that at a later occasion—because <u>he</u> is not sure who he is looking at. A natural reaction.

(This little exchange was interesting to Jane and me. It will be remembered that Jane's entity name is Ruburt, and that Seth refers to Ruburt as "he"; our interpretation of this being that Jane's entity is male-oriented in the overall sense. Many sessions ago however Seth explained that this male or female orientation had little if anything to do with sex as we conceive it.

(Peggy's entity name is Aniac, given by Seth in the 158th session. Seth has given little information on Peg's entity, but his use of "he" evidently means that Peg's entity, like Jane's, is male-oriented.

(Jane now pointed at Bill.)

<u>He</u> is so busy looking that he is hardly embarrassed.

(This was a reference to Bill's habit of closely scrutinizing Jane as she delivers the material.

([Peggy:] "I don't think embarrassed is the right word.")

You may choose a better one.

([Bill:] "You fell into the trap, Peggy.")

I watch Joseph's hand. I will be glad to give suggestions when you remind me, so that your hand will not tire, and so that I do not tire our friends.

I will indeed, with due regrets, end our session. For I do indeed hesitate as always to leave you—

(Jane's voice abruptly rose in volume until it became very loud. I winced; the strong voice subsided quickly.)

—and it is not because I am weary—

("Yes.")

—but because I have sympathy for the limitations of your endurance. I will answer any questions put to me kindly.

([Peggy:] "Why did you say that a man who has ulcers thinks differently?")

Simple questions. It is because the man thinks differently that he has the ulcer, for the ulcer is the result of his characteristic method of thought. It is the result of his characteristic manner of viewing reality. This causes him to add to his self-image, in reality, that disability. The ulcer is formed intimately from the electrical reality that composes his thoughts. Do you find that a satisfactory answer?

([Peggy:] "Yes, very definitely."

(Jane turned to Bill.)

And do you—should I say dear father—

([Bill:] "Yes, my son—")

—have any questions or remarks?

([Bill, still laughing:] "I'm afraid not. Not at this time.")

I will then close the session. My heartiest regards to you all. <u>Good evening</u>!

(Jane really blasted out the good evening.

([Bill:] "Good night, Seth, and thank you."

("Good night, Seth."

(End at 10:50. Jane was dissociated as usual. It was evident that Seth enjoyed the exchange at the end of the session. Jane's eyes remained open until the end.)

SESSION 188
SEPTEMBER 15, 1965 9 PM WEDNESDAY AS SCHEDULED

(As it developed tonight's session was a short one. Several of the young people I work with planned to gather this evening in the downstairs apartment. The young couple mentioned in the 184th session live downstairs, and I also work with them. There was talk at work this morning that the whole group might visit us this evening. I relayed the information to Jane at noon, and suggested she decide whether she wanted to hold a session with the idea that it might be interrupted.

(Jane's first thought was to skip the session, but as the party downstairs got under way in a quiet fashion, and we were not called upon as 9 PM approached, she decided to hold it as usual.

(Shortly before session time Jane told me she had the thought that dreams and astral travel, or the astral body, were somehow connected. The session was held in our small back room. Jane began speaking while sitting down and with her eyes closed. Her voice was quiet, her pace quite slow and with pauses.)

Good evening.

("Good evening, Seth.")

Ruburt <u>prepares</u> himself in certain ways for our sessions. He forms a certain psychic and psychological framework, within which we operate. When there is question as to whether or not a particular session will be held, it is more difficult for him to make these preparations.

We will now continue with our previous discussion, and carry it further.

There are indeed connections between what is called ectoplasm and the composition of dream images. They are not the same thing, but they are closely allied. What is called the astral body is also composed of some of the same components.

It goes without saying that dream images certainly have form to the dreamer, even as physical objects have form. The astral body also has a form. These forms do not take up space in the way that physical objects do. There is less density, but there is still observable form. The images that appear in dreams exist as forms in another dimension. They are free of the necessity to follow physical rules of time and growth. They are constructed more immediately and directly and spontaneously than are physical objects.

There must be a connection however with the physical organism, and the connection, the physical connection, is both electrical and chemical. The connection between what you might call materializations, and the physical organism, are also electrical and chemical. The same applies to the connection between the astral body and the physical body.

Dream images are indeed, in density, between the tangible nature of physical objects and the intangible reality that is entirely independent of physical matter. The dream reality cannot be <u>entirely</u> disconnected from the material universe because of its connections with human personality. There is a dependence here.

The dream images however are projections sent out, so to speak, by the personality, and many astral projections occur within the dream state of which the waking personality is unaware. In this case the projection is simply of a kind that allows manipulation back and forth between two realities. The dreamer who dreams he was in Paris may well have been there.

Dream images, not astral projections, operate within certain electrical limits, limits that form the boundaries of the dream universe. Dream images are nevertheless <u>almost</u> fibrous projections, almost a thinned-out composition, more plastic basically than physical matter, but composed of a number of the same properties. For again there must be this connection between the nature of dreams and the matter of physical reality.

(*During her delivery of the above paragraph Jane's eyes opened, then closed. They were very dark. She continued to open and close them until break.*)

We will use an analogy for its excellent implications. It is as if the personality in sleep projected out of himself bits of himself, of his own physical matter, thinned out, stretched into an amazing plasticity; plastic properties that can change instantly from one form to another. He goes out with these portions of himself, but because of the nature of reality projections cannot be recalled.

I suggest your break.

(Break at 9:25. Jane said she was dissociated as usual for a first break. She reported a "weird" feeling however. She was aware that the material was good, yet at the same time she felt annoyed and distracted. We thought this stemmed from the fear of interruption because of the party downstairs, though we heard nothing.

(Jane said she was even conscious of my movements, slight as they were. The night seemed rather close also, so we had to open a window. Even though the window was on the side of the house, we immediately became aware of some traffic noise.

(Jane resumed in the same quiet voice, with pauses, and with her eyes closed, at 9:36.)

Dreams are a continuous process.

You create them both waking and sleeping, although you are not aware of them in the waking state. You constantly project and constantly emit energy in meaningful patterns on as many layers of activity as possible.

These are quite legitimate realities that continue in their own fashion, even though you are no longer concerned with them. They remain <u>connected</u> to you, that is to the personality, however, and are a part of the overall reality of the self. You partake of their energy.

(Jane had been using pauses while speaking. Now however she took what turned out to be the longest pause that I have noted during these sessions. It was just two minutes long by the clock. During this time she sat quite still in her chair, her eyes closed, her head down with one hand lifted to her face.)

Oftentimes you send out dream images within a dream framework from your own nerve centers. These then work out problems for you, and the answer is given to you subconsciously.

This material will be extremely interesting, and is somewhat difficult. Because Ruburt is not at his best I am going to close our session, and give you this material at our next regular meeting.

The reality and the framework within which these sessions exist have electrical and chemical organizations also, that require a delicate focus that was upset this evening. It is simply more difficult then for Ruburt to make the necessary inner adjustments.

Distractions, or <u>fear</u> of distractions, have their own reality, and set up strongly positive electrical charges which can be detrimental, although other conditions, chemical and electrical conditions, must also be considered. We do have a good start however.

My heartiest regards to you both. If there is anything you would like to say, Joseph, by all means do so.

("I guess not."

(I didn't think it wise, considering Jane's mood.)
Then we will end our session.
("Good night, Seth.")
(End at 9:49. Jane was dissociated as usual. She was however still bothered and upset; this time the traffic noise contributed. Her eyes remained closed, her voice quiet.

(Jane said she was even conscious of the sound my pen made on the paper as I wrote. I always work on several thicknesses of paper so that writing noise is not a problem, and use a ballpoint pen to avoid scratching noises. Ordinarily Jane has excellent hearing; she must have super acuity in the trance state.

(Copy of the test page of script used for the 7th envelope test, in the 189th session, September 20, 1965. This is a random page, unnumbered. The original is double-spaced:)

(His wife was drinking a cup of coffee in the kitchen. "I saw a station wagon just like your father's," Bob Hagel said.

("Great. Just what we need. He'll be coming any day now, though. You just wait and see."

("Things pile up, don't they?" he said.

("I'm all goose-pimply thinking about everything. All kinds of decisions. I'm waiting for them to totter down on us like a pile of bricks." She grinned sheepishly. He sat down, but she stared at the table. Everything seemed threatened, curled at the edges, burnt black and in need of replacement. Her wide gray eyes were anxious, her slim almost boyish body had an impatient agility. She shook her head emphatically so that her short curly black hair bobbed up and down.

(Bob Hagel grinned at her, yet for a moment he didn't know what to say. He had a sick feeling in the pit of his stomach. While he hadn't made any conscious decision to leave the valley, he felt as if he had. He felt as if the whole thing was out of his hands. He sat there in his paint-stained khakis, a man almost forty, brave, cowardly, cocky. Before he spoke he tilted his brown-gray head at an earnest angle and stared at her with his usually severe face now wreathed with smiles. "Don't take it so hard," he said. "The world isn't falling apart or anything."

("Ours might be," she said. There was a catch in her voice. She looked the other way.)

SESSION 189
SEPTEMBER 20, 1965 9 PM MONDAY AS SCHEDULED

(*Last week we received Dr. Instream's letter of September 13, in which he wrote that he would like to try straight clairvoyant communication with Seth on Monday and Wednesday nights at 10 PM. Dr. Instream also noted that on the evening of August 23, 1965 he and his wife stopped overnight at York Beach, ME, while traveling. It will be remembered that Jane's second envelope test was held on the night of August 23, in the 180th session, and that the test photo featured Jane on the waterfront at York Beach. I took the picture in the summer of 1964.*

(*Dr. Instream would like us to ask Seth why he stopped at York Beach, since he had never been there before. For our part we want to know whether Dr. Instream understands that he was in York Beach on the same night a photo of York Beach was used in a session, or whether he remembers reading about York Beach in previous sessions.*

(*In preparation for her next book, which will deal with the Seth material itself, Jane made an exploratory trip to several county records offices in Elmira; she is beginning an effort to track down Frank Watts. She accomplished a little, and met some helpful people; she enjoyed the quest.*

(*The double test envelope for the 8th test contained a page from an old novel of Jane's entitled* The Adult Time. *She wrote this seven or eight years ago, and it was never published. The page is not numbered. I rummaged through her files and pulled out a page at random. I folded it in quarters and sealed it up.*

(*It was a very hot and humid night but we held the session in our small back room. We opened the windows however. Jane said she felt a little nervous, embarking on the clairvoyant tests with Dr. Instream. She also felt anticipatory. She began speaking while sitting down and with her eyes closed. Her voice was quiet. She used many pauses.*)

Good evening.

("*Good evening, Seth.*")

We will go more deeply into a discussion of the ways and means by which both dream images and other materializations are constructed. For there are various balances, or rather various delicate imbalances, which must be maintained; and there are differences also in the makeup of dream images, which are usually seen only by the dreamer, and some other more physical materializations which may be created by the semi-waking self, and under certain circumstances seen by others.

Nerve patterns are indeed very important here, and mechanisms of metabolism. An understanding of the methods used by the dreamer to construct dream images will, however, allow you to understand more clearly those other constructions. The chemical percentages are important here; that is, the chemical percentages *vary* from those found in the body during what you call normal states of consciousness.

Dream images are composed in part as a result of chemical excesses that are built up normally by the organism in the waking state. Physical materializations are built up by bringing about this condition of excessive chemical action.

It is true that a state can be produced in which such materializations can occur, by artificially producing the chemical imbalance necessary. However, success by this method may or may not occur.

I am keeping your York Beach material until later in the session, close to the ten o'clock hour.

The material of which we are speaking—

(There came a knock on a window from the front of the house. The loud, brittle sound was clearly audible through the closed door. Jane came out of her trance without effort. Our first impulse was not to acknowledge the sound, but since it was unusual we did so. It proved that a TV antenna had been loosened over our porch roof, and a repairman asked us for the loan of a flashlight. We told him we were at work in the back of the apartment, and left the light with him.

(I was somewhat irritated by the interruption, since we use the cramped back room to avoid such incidents. But Jane told me not to worry, that the session was going to be a good one, that she felt Seth coming through well.

(The interruption occurred at 9:11. Jane resumed at 9:15.)

This material will be most helpful in our own sessions, since when we are finished with it you will understand to some degree those conditions which may be advantageous and those which are not.

The electrical composition of the air is important, as you have read, and the periods of even temperature and fair weather are excellent for our purposes.

(Jane's eyes now opened. This was quite early in the session for such a step. They did not open fully; Jane looked casually at me, and about the room, from beneath half-lowered lids. Her eyes closed at the end of the following paragraph.)

The evening hours are best, and it was for this reason that I chose them. By this hour there is apt to be a stability of electromagnetic properties, though of course this is not always the case. Since all things have an electrical and chemical reality, the food that you eat is also important, and it is for this reason that I made certain suggestions concerning your diet.

(See the 185th session.)

These suggestions, as you know, were far from extreme. The exercises that I suggested Ruburt take also aid him in utilizing negative ions. Each individual has various ways in which he or she characteristically handles the protoplastic elements of which the physical being is composed.

The protoplasm is not entirely physical, however, but in a basic manner is a meeting ground between physical matter and inner vitality. Therefore the characteristic ways used by any given personality, in connection with his or her physical image, will also be used in the construction of dream images.

The dream images are indeed extensions, not only of the psychic or inner self, but a definite extension of the electromagnetic and chemical properties that operate through the physical self. It is indeed as if extensions of nerve endings reached out in self-expansion, making new connections, and this is indeed what occurs in the creation of dream images.

I will now suggest your break.

(*Break at 9:27. Jane was very well dissociated for a first delivery, she said. Where in the last session everything had bothered her, even the sound of my writing, tonight nothing bothered her, not even the interruption. Her eyes were closed most of the time.*

(*Jane now told me she thought the "two people" referred to by Seth in the 2nd envelope test in the 180th session, were Dr. Instream and his wife Judy. See page 209. At the time, I had assumed that the two people referred to were Jane and me, since she was in the picture I took. We now know, of course, that Dr. Instream and his wife were in York Beach on the night of the 180th session.*

(*Jane resumed while sitting down and with her eyes closed. Her voice was a little stronger, her pace quite a bit faster. Resume at 9:35.*)

I have a few side notes here.

One. Interruptions in themselves will not bother us once a session is under way. You may follow whatever course you personally prefer, as circumstances warrant.

As far as Ruburt is concerned, <u>uncertainty</u> as to whether or not a session will be held, <u>is</u> disturbing. There will be some circumstances when conditions are not of the best, however, when interruptions <u>may</u> bother. But generally we are beyond such disturbances.

You have noticed, I am sure, that at times visitors to a session are of definite value, for the psychic energy is pooled, and can be of value. The emotional impetus, when it is present, is also of benefit. Now in the same manner you can use and collect such energy when you are in a group, as in your Saturday evening excursions.

There is actually a quite natural and most effective manner of psychic refreshment, and most particularly when the conscious mind is somewhat diverted, as by music and so forth. The intuitions act well under such circumstances, and these intuitions are stored subconsciously, and will show themselves in your work.

There is indeed a knack required here. Primitive peoples use it all unknowing. Unfortunately, in civilized conditions it sometimes needs relearning. All methods of gaining and renewing energy are important, in ordinary living and in our sessions.

Ruburt picked up energy in this way this afternoon, quite spontaneously, and without conscious consideration.

(Here Seth refers to Jane's trip downtown to the records offices, in search of data on Frank Watts. She was somewhat uneasy setting out on her journey, but wound up enjoying the afternoon a great deal.)

There will be more said concerning this matter, since the same sort of mechanism is involved in the construction of materializations, in sessions such as this one, and in the construction of dream images.

A discrimination, preferably a spontaneous and subconscious discrimination, is necessary, but it may be consciously diverted if undue conscious direction is not allowed to rule with a heavy hand. You may consciously give the suggestion to yourself, that you will constructively use such energy, for example, but then the matter should be forgotten and left alone.

The suggestion itself, psychologically, also prevents you from simply being swept away, willy-nilly, by the collective energy. You must understand that use of such energy does in no way suggest monopolizing it. You do not deprive others. Your own actions continue to produce additional energy. This method of utilizing energy is also used in the creation of dream images. The form of the images is not an illusion. You simply have form without mass, to all practical purposes, and there is no contradiction in that statement.

Mass and form may seem synonymous, but they are not. Mass is not dependent upon weight. We may say however that dream images have a <u>density</u> which is formed of electrical intensities, that are partially the result of chemical actions.

You may take a brief break, and we shall consider other matters, and then perhaps return to this material.

(Break at 9:55. Jane was well dissociated; she didn't think much time at all had passed. Her eyes remained closed. Her delivery had been good.

(Jane's eyes closed again when she resumed, in a quieter voice, and with more frequent pauses, at 10:00 PM.)

We will of course cooperate in the experiments with Doctor Instream.

Ruburt may be nervous initially but this will pass. He is actually learning rather quickly, more quickly than I had anticipated. Again, we work with fine distinctions.

The man and woman referred to in the test experiment of August two-three, were the Instreams. We had some difficulty here; and yet also, considering the fact that these tests were new, some success.

For if I did not get the names through, Ruburt did not distort the material in that instance, so that the record shows that I mentioned a man and a woman, and J. B.

(Here Jane pointed at herself rather vehemently. Again, see the 180th session, page 209.)

Ruburt, or Jane Butts, in this case was the emotional connection. The test itself involved however a particular photograph that was of Jane Butts at York Beach, and in which the Instreams did not appear. I was not able to make the distinction clear to Ruburt, for it was definitely not a photograph of the Instreams.

However, on the date the test was given the Instreams were at York Beach. Therefore, the two people came through clearly; and specifically I did not say that you and Ruburt, or Jane Butts, were the two people involved. Hardly an exceptional performance, however evocative enough for a start.

The Instreams did not consider going to York Beach. Neither was their visit a complete coincidence, although it might seem so. All experiences have an electrical reality. Your experiences at York Beach had such a reality, and having met you, not Dr. Instream but his wife unconsciously picked up this connection, and responded to it.

(It will be interesting to learn from Dr. Instream, who was driving the car when he and his wife arrived at York Beach on August 23 for their overnight stay.)

Now, please give me a moment.

(It was 10:11 PM. Jane sat quietly, her eyes closed. Actually her pause was quite brief. Her head was down, a hand to her face. Jane used many pauses delivering the following material, and I will indicate a few of them. I had the impression that she was being careful in what she said, but not that she was particularly nervous.)

These are impressions.

Dr. Instream has within the hour spoken with several people outside of his family, or is with them now.

Specifically two men. *(Pause.)* A chair with a blue seat, or seat cover. *(Pause.)* The men, I believe, were with him earlier rather than at this moment. I believe that he is now standing on the small terrace of his apartment, and is wearing slippers or a slipperlike shoe.

(Pause, at 10:14.) It is possible that these men are inside, however. One of the men rather formally dressed. There is something in the water in the distance, which catches his eye, and upon which he may be concentrating. *(Pause.)*

A stacked-up affair, as of irregular blocks, rather haphazardly arranged. A person, I believe a man, crosses below the terrace. *(Pause.)* Dr. Instream has also been thinking of a book, and perhaps of a specific page.

(At 10:19 Jane took a long pause.)

A passage which has been in his mind. I have an impression of the number 218. I do not know to what it refers. A page number, an address, or simply the digits.

Do you have a test for me?

("Yes."

(I gave Jane the test envelope at 10:21. Again she paused briefly, her eyes still closed. She held the test envelope in her left hand.)

Again, give us a moment.

The impression of several items, of various shape and diverted mass, with separations. Some strong verticals, having to do with two people, and a fall or fall.

("A fall, or fall?")

A fall, or fall.

(I was still somewhat puzzled by the answer, but did not press for elaboration for fear of distracting Jane. I had barely looked at the page of test script when I prepared the double envelopes this afternoon.)

I also have the impression of rubber, but do not know to what this refers. An item of value, and necessary precautions.

Five items. *(Pause.)* Shapes as of hills in the distance; having to do with two people and many designs. One strongly circular, and a space between darks.

I suggest a break.

(Break at 10:25. Jane was dissociated as usual. She said she did not feel particularly nervous while delivering the material on Dr. Instream. Her eyes had remained closed, her voice quiet. She had a vague memory of what she had said.

(See the copy of the test item on page 266. It is an excerpt from one of Jane's early unpublished novels. It can be seen that once again Seth, or Jane, delivered a variety of impressions that can apply easily enough. The script deals with two people. The word "fall" appears once, and is implied in the simile "totter."

(There could be strong verticals, depending on how Jane held the envelope; I do not remember. There are of course separations and many designs. Jane said the station wagon mentioned could be an item of value. Necessary precautions refers to steps the couple take upon learning the imminent arrival of the girl's father, although these are not outlined on the page of test script, but on both preceding and succeeding pages.

(Five items could be the station wagon, a cup of coffee, a pile of bricks,

paint-stained khakis, and the world itself; but this is open to other interpretations, we would say. A strongly circular design I interpret as the world. I interpret the impression of rubber as referring to the rubber band that held the manuscript together in the file drawer. I do not know what to make of the reference to hills, unless it is a rather far-out connection with the "pile of bricks" simile in the script.

(During break I asked Jane to discuss why I picked the particular photograph of York Beach to use in the test for August 23. At the time I made up the envelope the Instreams were already on their way to York Beach; I wondered what lines of communication had been open.

(Jane resumed in a quiet voice, and with her eyes again closed, at 10:42.)

We will end our session shortly.

In answer to your question, Joseph: both you and Ruburt were subconsciously aware of the Instreams' location, and it was for this reason that you chose the photograph of York Beach, though you did not consciously realize the connection.

Ruburt is indeed being very cautious. But he is learning to open up more in these tests, to let more information through. The opening up of the channels is the important thing. Oftentimes information will come through in a rather indiscriminate fashion, and a spontaneous (underline spontaneous) choice of available information is important. A variety of impressions may be received, many valid, but not closely connected enough for your purposes. So it is in the area of distinctions that we must work.

My heartiest regards to all, and I will close our session.

The material on our own test this evening came through as a literal translation of concepts in the script.

("Good night, Seth." A reminder: Seth alone calls for all underlined words.

(End at 10:49. Jane was dissociated as usual. Her eyes remained closed, her voice quiet. Seth's comment on this evening's test came through because Jane and I had been speculating about such a translation of the script at last break.)

SESSION 190
SEPTEMBER 21, 1965 APPROXIMATELY 9:30 PM
TUESDAY UNSCHEDULED

(I made no notes during this session or immediately after. What follows is Jane's own reconstruction of the session, made two days later; for this reason I think it interesting, aside from its intrinsic content, in that it reveals that Jane was able to recall quite an amount of what she said while in the trance state.

(This is the first time she has tried to reconstruct a session from her own viewpoint. As I go along, where necessary I will add my own notes, and these will be in parentheses.)

Our friend John Bradley visited us this evening. We played part of the 170th session, which was recorded and directed by Seth to Dr. Instream. In the middle of a passage Seth suddenly came through, saying: "Why settle for a recording when you can have the real thing?" His voice was quite strong. He seemed in excellent spirits. John had never heard the loud Seth; the previous sessions he witnessed had all been quiet ones. Now Seth began to speak loudly and jovially. Rob made no notes, as Seth told him they were not necessary. These notes are written from memory.

(We had been hunting through the taped session for particularly strong voice effects so that John could get an idea of the power of the Seth personality. Jane was on her knees before the recorder; we had found a strong passage. Her eyes closed and she switched the recorder off as she began speaking as Seth. The transition was so smooth that it was a moment before John and I realized we were no longer listening to the tape. Jane's voice was strong from the beginning.)

John is considering leaving his job and buying a restaurant bar in his home town, Williamsport, PA. He asked Seth's opinion concerning this plan. Seth doubted John would make the move, because of his desire for security for his family, and because of his need for cosmopolitan outlets. These were met in his sales work, but would not be so easily satisfied if he were a proprietor of a settled establishment.

Seth said that no changes would occur in the organization with which John is now connected, Searle Drug, until next February at the earliest. John is planning his job change for next January. Seth said the new project would be a success if John actually bought the business.

(Seth also told John that the data given on Searle Drug, its financial and personal entanglements, plus John's own promising prospects if he remained with the firm through its present crises, still applied. Some of this information goes back well over a year. It is scattered through the following sessions that John has witnessed: 37, 54, 63, 70, 95, 135, 166, in Volumes 1 through 3.)

John also asked Seth if he knew what the trouble had been when John had had a pain in his throat on June 17, 1964; on this date John witnessed the 63rd session. While trying psychological time on June 18, 1964, I had a very startling experience in which I was told by a thunderous voice that John's trouble lay really in a "bad tongue." See Vol. 2, pages 167-68. Seth now explained that this mysterious voice had been his. He said John had cut his tongue on a bone sliver while eating, but because of the human nerve structure in that part of the anatomy the pain had been felt down in his neck.

John made a remark to the effect that he would like some sort of proof of Seth's existence. Seth lit into him, saying that the voice effects were impossible for a woman of my makeup. Seth said he could just as legitimately insist that John prove his existence to him.

(*During this part of the impromptu session Jane's voice became very loud and strong at times; it did not match the effects of the recorded 170th session, but came close once or twice. It was far too loud for the house, in my opinion, with others living so close. Jane's eyes were open for the most part by now, and she, or Seth, often looked deliberately at me, knowing my embarrassment. But this did not prevent another strong blast. At times Jane got to her feet and tipped her head back, as she had done in the 170th session. At these points Seth would remark about using such a position to attain more power, and would talk about how impossible such an effect was for Jane to attain normally.*)

John asked Seth if he knew who he, John, could get to type extra copies of the material. Seth told us that later Dr. Instream would help us out in this respect, although he didn't know it yet. Seth said there was a woman at the college in Oswego who would do the work. Seth also told John to keep looking for someone himself: "The effort will do you good."

Seth said the practice involved in such unscheduled sessions was good for me. In the new experiments with Dr. Instream, involving clairvoyance, Seth said enough valid information would come through to keep up Dr. Instream's interest, even though we would do better later on.

The voice became very loud at times. I worried about the neighbors during our frequent breaks. It was a hot and humid night and our living room windows were of course open. Seth was obviously enjoying himself, and I was very active physically as I spoke for him. My eyes were open a good deal of the time.

A few times the voice reached startling volume. I was afraid that the neighbors would wonder what was going on, and as it turned out my fears were justified. As Seth was speaking a knock came at our door. Almost instantly, it seemed, I snapped out of my trance.

For a moment we just sat there. Then I answered the door. Two neighbors from the house next door stood grinning at us. They had their cat with them. They had heard the voice from this apartment; their place is actually two lots away; a space of perhaps seventy feet separates the two houses.

Our friends were mystified. They had recognized elements of my voice, but because of the volume did not really think it was mine. The girl, Donna Taylor, said she thought we might be in trouble of some sort. Her husband Ed finally decided to come over to see what was going on. Not knowing what to say, I tried to joke that it was the television set, but Donna said it wasn't; their set had been on, and they had checked all the eight stations to see if they could find such a voice.

Rob then said it was an experiment in self-hypnosis for my next book. This certainly was no lie, and the Taylors seemed to accept the explanation. John was having trouble keeping a straight face. The Taylor's cat began playing with our cat, Willy, and we had no trouble steering the conversation into safer channels. The Taylors stayed for half an hour, then left. John Bradley left shortly after. By then it was past midnight.

(I would estimate the session ended at 11:20 PM, with the knock on the door. The Taylors are a nice young couple, newly arrived in Elmira, and do not know of the sessions. When I saw who was at the door I had visions of long complicated explanations, but the self-hypnosis explanation appeared to satisfy them. If they were still curious they did not reveal it. Very few people in town know about the sessions, although this state will be drastically altered next spring with the publication of Jane's ESP book.

(As often happens when witnesses are present, Seth was in a fine and frisky mood; there is no doubt that a witness or two will produce what appears to be abundant extra energy on Seth/Jane's part. More often than not strong voice effects are manifested. Jane appears to be swept up, fully involved in the role, and thoroughly enjoying it. Nor does this involvement produce any apparent fatigue of any kind. On top of this, Seth promised an excellent session at our regularly scheduled time tomorrow night.)

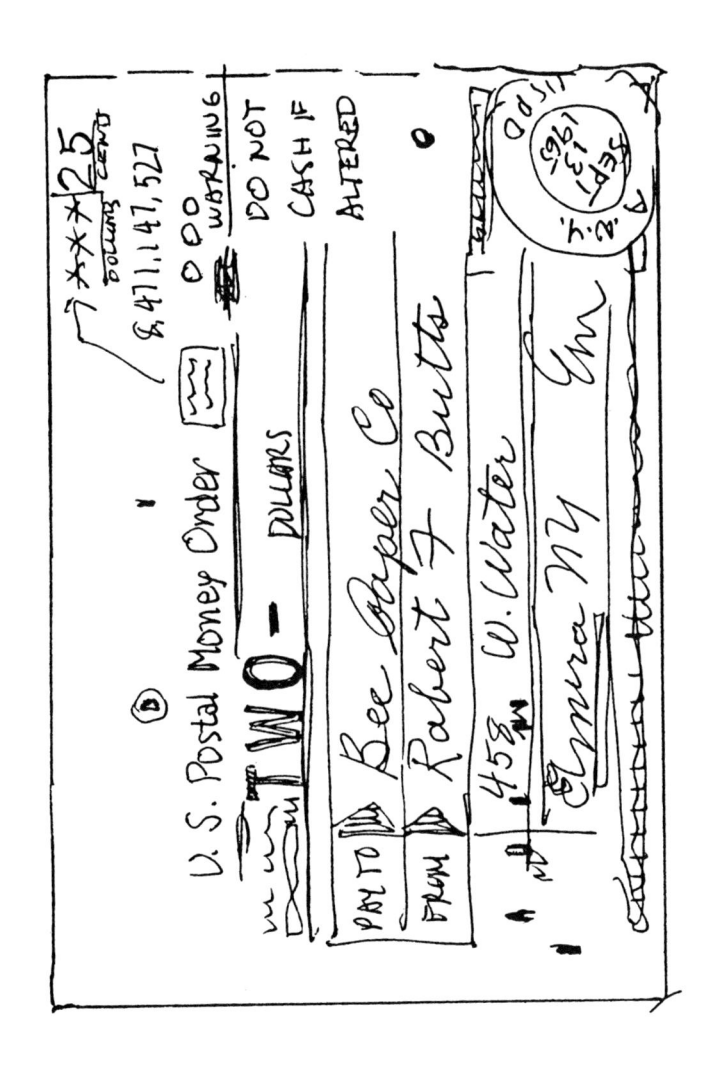

(Tracing of the money order used in the 9th envelope test, in Session 191, September 22, 1965.)

SESSION 191
SEPTEMBER 22, 1965 9 PM WEDNESDAY AS SCHEDULED

(*It will be remembered that in the unscheduled 184th session Seth said that Cosmopolitan Magazine would be interested in an excerpt from Jane's ESP book, but that nothing would happen right away. Jane sent them a chapter on dreams, with suggestions for reworking it into an article. The material was returned today with a plain rejection slip. Seth had stated that Cosmo would return the material, but with a letter expressing interest.*

(*Since we wonder if clairvoyant data involving Dr. Instream will be a regular feature of the sessions from now on, we mentioned this before the session. We also wondered what Seth would have to say about the Cosmopolitan affair, and last night's unscheduled session, witnessed by John Bradley.*

(*See page 277 for a tracing of the money order used in tonight's 9th envelope test. This was returned to me a few days ago; I had written a paper company requesting samples. They sent the samples but returned the 25¢ money order. On the spur of the moment today I decided to use it for the test, and enclosed it in the usual double envelopes. I also enclosed the money order itself between two pieces of thin Bristol, to make it difficult for Jane to unwittingly pick up anything by feeling the shape of the object within the envelopes.*

(*The session was held in our back room. Just before it began Jane admitted, again, to a slight nervousness at the projected clairvoyant experiments involving Dr. Instream. She began speaking while sitting down and with her eyes closed. Her voice was quiet, in contrast to last night's noisy unscheduled session. Her pace was slow, with many pauses. It was another hot and humid night.*)

Good evening.

("*Good evening, Seth.*")

I will be very quiet this evening. Our energy will go into other matters.

Dream images are in a most vital manner extensions of the self. They are projected from the self, extending outward indeed like branches from a tree. Yet they are individual, and have an amount of freedom as even leaves do. And as branches are composed of all those elements that make up the whole tree, so indeed dream images are composed of those elements that make up the personality.

It is obvious that the dream images are not responsible to the ego, however. While they contain within them compositions that are also seen in the physical self, these properties appear in different percentages. As leaves bring vital nutrients to the tree trunk, so also do dream images bring nourishment to the personality.

As leaves drop from the tree, so finally do dream images depart from close connection with the personality. Yet a psychic connection is always maintained to some degree. Dream images are often images which cannot be created for various reasons within physical reality at any particular time. Dream images may appear later however as physical images.

There are seasonal variations, temperature variations, electromagnetic and chemical reactions that all influence the production and efficiency of dream images, and that also influence the effect of dream images upon the individual. There is also, as I mentioned, a close relationship existing between dream images and other materializations, that are not ordinarily regular physical occurrences.

Since the individual creates his own physical image to begin with, then there is nothing so strange about his creation of a pseudophysical body which is not so closely dependent upon the physical system. Again however, such a pseudobody has electromagnetic and chemical connections that originate in the more usual physical image. In your field of activity this sort of connection must always exist.

The field that connects the personality to this kind of pseudoimage is actually formed by extensions of psychic energy. Imagine it, the field, if you will, as a thin but sturdy thread that connects the pseudoimage with the original image. There are some limitations here then as to range. These are not basic limitations, but have to do with the individual's ability to so extend himself. Many dreams involve such roamings on the part of the personality while it is within this sort of pseudoimage.

Much training and practice would be necessary before it would be possible for the personality to be aware of such journeys on a conscious, egotistical level. For like a man walking a tightrope in his sleep, sudden awareness of such a feat could be disastrous, for the delicate balance necessary is not dependent upon egotistical awareness; and such awareness, without warning, could be highly detrimental.

I suggest your first break.

(*Break at 9:22. Jane was dissociated as usual for a first delivery. Her eyes remained closed, her voice quiet. Her pace had picked up considerably. The heat hadn't bothered her, but as soon as break arrived she became aware of it.*

(*Jane resumed with her eyes again closed, and at a slower pace, at 9:33.*)

I feel that I should explain myself to some degree, concerning the infrequent unscheduled sessions that occur, and some of the reasons behind the voice effects, which indeed we do keep under control most of the time.

The unscheduled session is beneficial in that it gives Ruburt practice. The voice effects carry him along so that he gives no attention, or very little attention, to what I am saying, and therefore we <u>usually</u> get a good reception in terms of clear communication.

The Jane ego stands further aside. There is an emotional rapport that also carries Ruburt along when <u>my</u> spirits or moods then also sweep him along; and again the Jane ego is content to stand aside. My emotional makeup comes to the foreground at times, of course. Energy is used for such demonstrations, so that it may seem that the material takes second place. But the practice is to the overall advantage of the material.

There is on occasion an extension of self, whereby the Jane ego can also participate, though in a temporarily subordinate manner. The experience is valuable to Ruburt in that he sees that no invasion is involved; and that when his emotions are stilled there is still an emotional reality, as <u>my</u> emotions come to the foreground.

It is sometimes difficult to maintain the fine distinction that is necessary to <u>you</u>, for example, so that the voice is not too loud. I must use of course a buildup of energy, which is then expended. The rate at which it is expended controls the volume of the voice. There are delicate balances here, you see, so that while I sometimes fool with you in a joking manner, oftentimes the energy simply is not as finely controlled as I would like.

This simply involves practice again, as <u>I</u> learn how much energy is necessary to get certain effects. Since I am using Ruburt's voice mechanisms, certain adjustments must be made as I discover how best to manipulate the necessary mechanisms.

The emotional energy I use as when I show good spirits, are the same energies that <u>propel</u> themselves outward through the voice. This is somewhat more complicated than it may appear. There is a similarity here between the extension of <u>my</u> self outward through Ruburt, and the extension necessary for example in an individual's projection of a pseudoimage.

When others are present there is simply more energy available. Yet again, such use of energy does not imply a depletion. I am not <u>stealing</u> energy from others. In actuality Ruburt uses the energy, for it is in a form which is more accessible to him than to <u>me</u>. There is a pooling of energy in such cases, and in such a pooling of energy telepathic communications are facilitated; for the many selves present, in pooling their energy, extend themselves.

In good circumstances Ruburt then dips into this energy pool, which obviously must contain certain elements of personal experience on the part of the participators. I have meant to give you this information in the past, and shortly you will see why telepathy and clairvoyance occur more readily in the dream state.

Now I suggest a brief break.

(*Break at 9:55. Jane was dissociated as usual. Her eyes had remained closed, her voice quiet. Her pace had picked up speed. She had some idea of what she had been saying, but didn't think she had been speaking for any length of time.*

(*Since it was close to 10 PM, the hour suggested by Dr. Instream for clairvoyant contact with Seth, Jane told me she felt some nervousness, as she had the first time this experiment had been tried in the 189th session.*

(*As during the first experiment, Jane used many pauses. I will indicate just some of them. She began speaking in a very quiet voice. Her eyes were closed, her head down somewhat. Resume at 10:06.*)

Now. We will see what we can get. (*Pause.*) As these experiments with Dr. Instream continue Ruburt will rapidly be more at ease.

It is unfortunate that the <u>idea</u> of tests often disturbs the <u>flexibility</u> that is necessary in order to achieve results. That is, Ruburt, wanting correct information, (*pause*) has some tendency to want it so badly that the ego stiffens, forming barriers.

However Ruburt learns quickly, and in the long run this will not hamper us overmuch; (*pause*) and enough will come through in the meantime, I believe.

Now. These are my impressions. (*Pause, at 10:11.*)

Dr. Instream is now, or has been immediately preceding this hour, or will be immediately following this hour, in a meeting with many people. (*Pause.*) In a fairly large room, with one speaker, and then others for briefer periods of time. A brick building, the meeting not on the ground floor. (*Pause.*) His seat three to five seats from an aisle, nearly but not quite in the center of a row of seats.

(*Jane took a long pause at 10:14, sitting quite still and with her eyes closed.*)

This could be however a theater or theater building, but if so it is not (*pause*) on exact street level.

Someone seems to be wearing an eyeshade, a male.

(*Another long pause at 10:16.*)

Slides or pictures may be shown. I believe he had two visitors today at his office, in particular. One not a student. (*Pause at 10:19.*)

Do you have a test for me?

("*Yes.*")

(*I handed Jane the test envelope at 10:20. She sat quietly, holding it in her right hand, her eyes still closed.*)

Give me a moment and we will see what we can do.

Something two times, in duplicate, or as twins.

I will not give obvious information that Ruburt could pick up through touch.

These are impressions. A gushing forth, such as something explosive, as the rushing of a waterfall. Ruburt thinks of a photograph of a waterfall at your old camping place.

Again, something to do with two people, perhaps several, both males and females. The idea of rock and water and many colors, and a connection with a note. *(Pause.)* A place which you have both visited. Numbers. Too many people for comfort. A border.

Again a multiplicity of design. Initials, I believe R. B. In connection with you, Joseph. Your handwriting on the back. *(Pause.)* Having to do with a familiar place, a tent, and a landscape of a landscape.

I suggest your break.

(Break at 10:26. Jane was dissociated as usual. Her eyes had remained closed, her voice quiet with many pauses. She opened the test envelope.

(The reference to a waterfall puzzled us. Jane then noted that we live on Water St. This may be the connection with this impression, along with Jane's memory of our old camping place. The money order has no connection with camping that I know of. It lay in my drawer, and was not next to or near any other photographs, for instance.

(The large numeral TWO is stamped in red on the money order, as the upper limit of its worth. Since it is for 25¢, there is ample room there for "something two times, in duplicate, or as twins." Two people involved could be Jane and me; she purchased it, filled it out and mailed it for me, along with a note to the paper company that I wrote. "It's a <u>duplicate</u> [mentioned in test] of a money order," Jane wrote later. The paper company is located in New York City. Both of us have been to New York City, and felt that it contained too many people for comfort. The money order has no border. Multiplicity of design, a very general appellation, could refer to the many numbers on the money order I suppose. Jane wrote my name on the order, but it does not bear my handwriting on either side.

(Jane interprets "a familiar place" as Elmira. Since the paper samples I requested were for watercolor paper, I can see where many colors and "a landscape of a landscape" can enter in, since I wanted to test the paper by doing some small landscapes at our landlord's farm. In 1963 we borrowed from our landlord, Jimmy Spaziani, the Ouija board that led to the sessions. See my Introduction, plus various sessions, in Volume 1.

(I regard the test as quite good at this stage, especially the reference to me via initials, and the note, something two times, and a landscape of a landscape. Jane as usual was disappointed.

(Jane resumed in the same quiet voice, and with her eyes closed, at 10:42.)

Since we had an impromptu meeting last evening, we will close our session. However, we will even out so that each session includes the material with which we are concerned, as well as our other data.

The exercise involved here will also help Ruburt in giving the material, and it will help in understanding the operation of the self under such conditions. As such these tests may be considered quite practical portions of the material itself, and we shall use them on various occasions to make certain points.

(Now Jane opened her eyes and looked at me. But they did not stay open for more than a sentence or two.)

I could indeed speak longer, but I will not keep you. I regret causing you any embarrassment, Joseph, despite my humorous remarks to the contrary, and I bid you a fond good evening.

The material which Ruburt sent to Cosmopolitan will be remembered, upon a later occasion, to his benefit there.

My fondest regards to you both.

Ruburt's book will work out very well. And I believe it likely that you will get your kitchen extension.

There is some difficulty, I believe, possible for Ruburt's friend, Blanche Price, in the nature of health.

("Good night, Seth."

(End at 10:48. Jane was dissociated as usual.

(The loud voice during the unscheduled session last night did embarrass me at times.

(I believe the book of Jane's that Seth refers to here is her new project, dealing with the Seth material itself. Jane has been casting about for a good way to present the material, and has about decided upon her approach. She is not quite sure of it however as yet.

(The reference to a kitchen extension concerns our efforts to get our landlord to enlarge our very small kitchen. The house is having a new roof put on now, and the man doing the job is going to speak to our landlord about the kitchen project when the roof is finished. We had about given up on the kitchen idea for this year, but now our hopes rise again. Jane has been focusing on our landlord, whom we like very much incidentally, each day, concerning the kitchen. It will be interesting to see the results.

(Blanche Price is an old friend of Jane's, living in Baltimore. The two women have not met often in recent years; Blanche was Jane's instructor in French at Skidmore College, in Saratoga Springs, NY. Last year while visiting in France Blanche suffered a rather severe stroke, but seems to have emerged without permanent paralysis. We would say she is in her mid-or-late fifties. A few days ago Jane received a copy of a book of poetry of Blanche's that has just been published. Blanche knows about Seth, but little about the material itself.

(Jane plans to copy the excerpts dealing with Dr. Instream weekly, or perhaps

bimonthly, to send to him. If Seth's prediction, made in the last session, to the effect that Dr. Instream will help us out in the matter of copying the material, works out, then perhaps other arrangements will be made.)

SESSION 192
SEPTEMBER 25, 1965 11:45 PM SATURDAY UNSCHEDULED

(This session was entirely unplanned. It was also not consciously expected on my part, although checking over my predictions for Friday and today, I discovered that I had unwittingly made several correct notes concerning it. These correct predictions were quite specific, and included such words as "cave" and "long swim."

(Jane and I went dancing as usual this evening. At one of our favorite spots we met the Gallaghers, Bill and Peggy. It ended up that the four of us returned to our apartment by about 11:15 PM. Jane said she felt Seth "buzzing around", but since I had just caught up on my notes for the three other sessions this week, I begged off. Jane agreed. The Gallaghers were tired and planned to leave soon also.

(Seth announced his presence as the four of us sat quietly talking, at approximately 11:45 PM. Bill and Peggy share the cost of a cottage on Seneca Lake with other members of Peggy's family, and had been taking steps to sell the cottage this fall. Bill dislikes seeing it go, since he uses it as a base for his skin-diving expeditions in the lake, which is one of New York State's famous Finger Lakes.

(Seth promised to keep his voice quiet, which he did throughout the session. Jane sat with her eyes closed for the most part. Specifically Seth asked that none of us take notes, and I was happy to agree. Thus the first half of this session is summarized from memory, with no particular effort made to remember every point covered. I will try to recall just enough to lead into the second half of the session, which I recorded verbatim in my homemade shorthand.

(The first point I would like to make is that Seth told us enough of the clairvoyant material involving Dr. Instream is valid; this will keep up the doctor's interest. The second point concerns the main subject matter of the session, which evolved from a question I asked Seth about the Gallagher's cottage on Seneca Lake. Bill was inspired to ask Seth whether it would be possible to locate Indian artifacts on the lake bottom; he had long been curious about this.

(By this, Bill meant American Indian artifacts, and had in mind stone tools, etc. Seth surprised us by telling us this was quite possible. Then he added that in a certain location could be found bronze artifacts in the lake. There was much here, including some generalized locations and descriptions, that is not recorded. Suffice it to say that Seth made no error in using the word bronze. He also said these artifacts *would date from either the 7th century, or the 17th century.*

(A break came at about 12:45. During it, Bill said he thought the information from Seth was sure to be pretty fragmented. Either that, or such artifacts were not Indian at all. Bill knows something of local history. He told us the 7th century reference would be correct if the Vikings were to be involved, since, he said, this date in history finds Viking evidence in the Great Lakes to the west. As far as he knew, there is no record of Viking activity in this part of the northeast, in New York State.

(Bill also said the 17th century date could be correct if bronze artifacts were shown to be related to the Jesuit missionaries, who were known to be in this section of the country then. Bill has done extensive skin diving in Seneca Lake. Jane and I had heard him mention this rather casually, but knew nothing of the extent of his explorations or deep interest. We had not discussed the subject. Nor has either of us ever done any skin diving.

(Bill was by now so interested that both he and I began to take verbatim notes when Seth resumed, since Bill planned to go diving Sunday. The hour was already late. Jane spoke while sitting down. Her eyes opened occasionally, her voice remained quiet. She smoked. She resumed at 12:55.)

A cove in water, at right angles to a gasoline station. I believe approximately 55 feet, and some boulders beneath here. There is a <u>small</u> object in this cave, but 15 feet approximately beneath to the left are many plants, with strange shaped blossoms; and in the roots, intertwined with the roots of these plants, are some objects of interest to you.

They can only be seen however between I believe three o'clock and dusk.

([Bill:] "At what time of the year?")

October and March, for if the light is not right you will not see them. October 12 to 15 is the best time. They are sunken however, and only portions, very small portions, protrude. One is bronze, one is iron. One is a dagger.

(As she talked, Jane used many gestures. She seemed to try to supplement her verbal descriptions by outlining objects with her hands, as though she was seeing things somewhat difficult to put into words specifically enough. This applied particularly when she was trying to voice descriptions of the geography of the lake bottom. Her pace was comfortably fast.)

They will not be seen looking forward, but looking from the corner of the eye. One has something to do with rubber, though I do not now see the connection. One has something to do with a female, and has a symbol; and the date may be ascertained from it.

The symbol has to do with the moon rather than the sun. I can only see two numbers as far as the date is concerned, and both numbers are 1—one, one. The foliage is waving, and there is a current. The current is a strong and cold one, and becomes colder by the cove.

([Bill:] *"Yes, yes. That's just the way they are."*)

There is some air in the cove.

([Bill:] *"Do you mean cove, or cave?"*)

I use cove.

(*Note the confusion here with the words cove and cave. As nearly as I can recall, I recorded them accurately. As the session continued we felt that Seth was saying cave, but that Jane's lack of marine knowledge could lead her to say cove, for cave. At times of course she distinctly said cave.*)

([Myself: *"Can you give us the location of the gasoline station?"*])

I believe there is an "M" in connection with the station, and perhaps an "A" and a "C". Perhaps something to do with Mack.

Either the man is called Mack—I do not know, or there are Mack trucks. I do not know. But there is a Mack somehow connected with a station, and a child, a female child.

(*Jane's eyes now opened. She looked at Bill and me, scribbling away, and smiled. Her voice remained quiet.*)

I remember saying most clearly nothing about notes.

([Bill, laughing:] *"Well, I can always tear these up. We want to make use of the information if we can, though."*)

I'm simply trying to save Joseph work. The month of May is a good one, but not in connection with these objects. There is a silt that covers much, but because of the currents in May, and sometimes in October, the silt—

(*Jane, her eyes closed, made gestures with her hands, as if to indicate a current or wave that swept clean.*)

([Bill:] *"That's right."*)

—and then you can discover more. The silt is a mineral deposit that gathers because of a collection of nitrogen. The composition of the air has much to do with this, and when the seasons change there is a change in the disposition of the silt.

([Bill:] *"Yes, that's right. I've seen those deposits change many times."*)

Objects hidden then are easier to see. I am on to something else, but I suggest that you take a break.

(*Break at 1:15. Jane was well dissociated, she said. Her voice had remained quiet, her pace had been good. Bill Gallagher was quite excited. Both he and Peggy verified Seth's information about the changes in silting on the lake bottom; Jane was highly gratified to learn that Seth was correct. As far as I know neither Jane or I have come across such specific information; certainly we have never discussed it with the Gallaghers.*)

(Bill now told us that he waits until certain times of the year, when the silt clears up, to go diving. He knows that the formation of nitrogen is somehow related to the dying of algae in the lake, but could not explain it exactly to us.

(Jane resumed while sitting down and with her eyes closed. But she was smoking as she spoke, and her eyes opened occasionally. Her voice remained quiet. Resume at 1:25.)

There is also a spot, and a very important one, that I cannot locate except for the moon position. The rays of the moon in May and/or October, 13 to 15, fall directly above a position in which important artifacts can be found, for there are many artifacts buried within the lake.

This one to which I refer has definitely to do with the 17th century. It is to be found directly beneath the moon's rays at a time when Venus is in the ascendancy, and forms on the surface of the lake an acute angle.

It is however very far down, and to the right of a plane.

(Here, Jane gestured to show that she meant a long flat level of land under water.)

This surface is the home of a rather unusual variety of, I presume you say, fish. But they are different than the fish near the surface, and there is algae here that <u>exudes</u> nitrogen, which is not usual.

This has to do with a chest, and it is of gold. It was a religious rather than a romantic pirate's chest. It had to do with a king, and the <u>death</u> of a queen, and belonged to a royal family, though they never missed it.

("Can you tell us the country of the royal family?")

I have the impression of France.

This was however religious, and intimate to some extent. <u>Personal</u>, I believe you say.

The royal family had many offspring, and there is a connection with a pope, and a bible with gold covers, and a crest. It is however sunken in silt, behind a <u>warm</u> current, and very concealed.

There is a <u>spring</u> here which may serve as a guiding post, if you could find the spring, which is warm.

("Has Bill ever been near any of these locations on his swims?")

One only, and not close.

("Which one?")

There are dangers connected with the last one mentioned, and treacherous currents near the chest. But ways of getting through them which involve two turns to the left, a going-along with the current, a right turn of 23 degrees. But a left turn could cause serious trouble.

([Bill:] "I can smell the trouble already.")

You have a good nose indeed.

([Bill:] "I'd better get myself a good set of fins.")

These artifacts are there. I am not predicting necessarily that they will be found, and I advise caution in any case. The silt can rise—

([Bill:] "Yes, it can.")

—like a sandstorm.

([Bill:] "Oh yes it can. It certainly can.")

If you are beneath it you are safe. If you are amid it, in the middle of it or above it, you are in danger. Its flow is often significant—

([Bill:] "Yes, I'll say.")

—its ways are wise, and if followed can lead to discoveries.

I suggest a break.

(End at 2:35 AM. This proved to be the end of the session even though Seth called it a break. The Gallaghers wanted to have energy for diving later in the day, so called it quits. Before leaving, Bill told us how right Seth was about silt storms; he related a terrifying incident in which he had become involved in a silt storm, and lost his sense of orientation.

(Jane said she had been really dissociated. All of this material about the strange underwater world was new to both of us, and Jane felt particularly good about having it verified so enthusiastically by Bill. It appeared to be at least an excellent example of telepathy, surpassing even the unscheduled 182nd session. It will be remembered that in that one, which the Gallaghers also witnessed, Seth delivered facts about Bill's deceased mother that neither Jane or I were familiar with.

(After the Gallaghers had left, Jane told me that whatever ability she possesses certainly operates at its best when there are witnesses. She also said that a few drinks before a session seem to help a great deal. Counting back, we decided she had had three beers in the course of the evening before the session, although they had been spaced out. Jane feels that alcohol somehow promotes a very beneficial relaxation on her part, for sessions.

(Bill told us that later today, Sunday, while at the lake, he would try to check upon some locations as defined rather poorly by Seth. Both Jane and I urged caution. The turn the material took this evening surprised us. We didn't know what to make of gold chests, Venus in the ascendancy, etc.

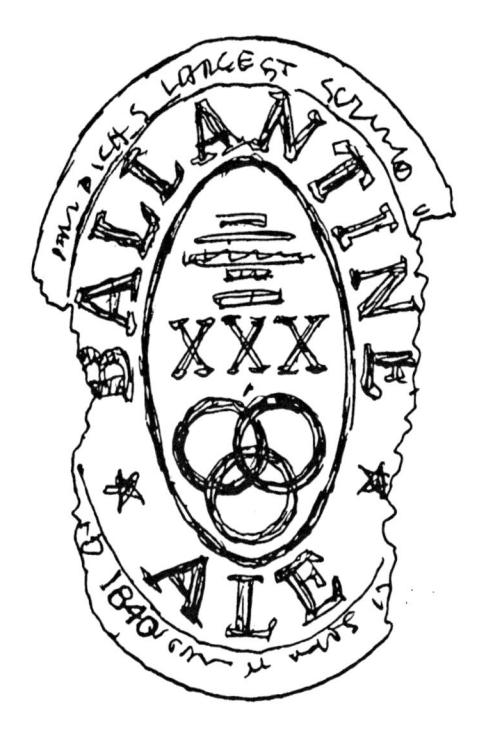

(Tracing of the Ballantine Ale label used in the 10th envelope test, in the 193rd session, September 27, 1965.)

SESSION 193
SEPTEMBER 27, 1965 9 PM MONDAY AS SCHEDULED

(Lorraine Shafer witnessed tonight's session. We hadn't seen her for several weeks. Lorraine now told us that she too had been in York Beach, ME, during the same week that Dr. Instream had been there. Dr. Instream had stayed overnight in York Beach on Monday, August 23; Lorraine had visited the town on Saturday afternoon, August 28.

(It will be remembered that our 2nd envelope test, held during the 180th session, was held on August 23, and that it featured a photograph of Jane at York Beach. Now checking our records, we saw that an unscheduled session was held on August 28. Can this be coincidence?

(The Gallaghers witnessed the unscheduled session, the 182nd. Lorraine knows them superficially, having witnessed a few sessions with them. We find no reference to either Lorraine or York Beach in the 182nd session. It happens that this session was reconstructed from memory; since it was unscheduled I had not been prepared

to take formal notes. Jane and I did our best, recalling it.

(For the 10th envelope test I used a label from a bottle of Ballantine Ale. See the tracing on page 289. Jane and I met the Gallaghers accidentally at a dancing establishment last Saturday evening. I absent-mindedly peeled the label from a bottle as we sat talking in the darkened room, then decided on the spur of the moment to use it for a test. I wondered if friendly impressions might attach themselves to the label. I took care to slip the wet label in a coat pocket when neither Jane or the Gallaghers were looking, and as it developed Jane had no idea of the test object for the session.

(Our encountering the Gallaghers last Saturday evening led to the strange unscheduled 192nd session, incidentally. In that session Bill Gallagher asked Seth about the possibility of locating artifacts in the waters of Seneca Lake. Describing the location of a certain cove, and underwater cave, Seth used as a starting point a gasoline station and the letters M, A, and C. Seth told us these could be part of the name Mack, or were involved with a Mack truck; he was not sure.

(To our surprise Lorraine told us this evening that she is quite familiar with Seneca Lake. She said that in spite of its size there are relatively few gasoline stations on the lake. She also told us that she knows of a Mack's boat livery on Seneca Lake. This livery of course has a gasoline station with it. She gave the location of this station as about 5 miles north of Himrod, on Route 14, on the west side of the lake. Jane and I will relay this information to the Gallaghers.

(The session was held in our large front room. Jane spoke while sitting down and with her eyes closed. Her voice was a bit stronger than usual, her pace faster. Much of the time she sat leaning forward with her head down somewhat. Her glasses were on when she began speaking, actually at 8:58, but she soon removed them.)

Good evening.

("Good evening, Seth.")

May I welcome Marleno to our circle.

It seems that our friends are congregating about York Beach, does it not?

("Yes.")

I will discuss our dream material for a short while, for it is important that you understand it. For in the same way that dream images are projected outward from the personality, so also are thoughts projected, and all influences that extend from one personality to another.

All such projections have an electromagnetic and chemical reality that has its origin within the field of the given personality. This projection of energy is one of the main characteristics of your kind. Dreams and dream images are then projected by the individual in sleep, and also in the waking state, although on a subconscious basis.

So are thoughts constantly sent outward, and other projections which we have not yet discussed. Therefore as the individual sends out these projections, so does he receive the projections of others. As you know, telepathy operates constantly beneath the dictates of the ego, and so is your intellectual climate formed.

It is well known that emotions have a chemical reality, but it is not generally realized that dreams also have the same sort of property. Telepathy is indeed affected by chemical reactions, as dreams are.

(Jane now took a long pause.)

If physical laws were the only basis for actuality, then telepathy would be impossible. But then, dreams would be equally impossible. For in the dream state the personality is molded and changed through actions that do not exist within the physical universe. The personality reacts to dream experiences as it reacts to any other experience. It does not discriminate, as the ego does, between one kind of experience and another.

It is formed equally by those experiences which are purely subjective, and which exist only within the psychological time framework. The subjective experiences therefore result in definite changes within the physical body framework. These changes are not caused because of a physical event, but because of an event occurring within a dream condition which has no reality in your physical universe.

Such subjective events therefore manipulate physical matter through the personality who experiences them. The field of reality for any given personality must and does include all these areas of activity, for they give form and dimension to his existence. I have said earlier that the individual could not exist in a physical universe if he did not also exist in the dream universe. Again, there are chemical and electromagnetic connections that cannot be severed between all these states of consciousness.

If they are severed you would not have a sane unit, but a disjointed pattern not capable of maintaining balance.

I suggest your break.

(Break at 9:16. Jane was dissociated as usual for a first break. Her eyes remained closed. Her pace was good, her voice a little stronger than usual, and with a trace of her brogue. Lorraine was also taking shorthand notes.

(Jane resumed in the same manner at 9:27.)

Now. Any form, even an imaginary form, exists in some dimension as a <u>form</u>.

It may not exist in space but it exists in some dimension as a form, and all forms have structure; and so dream images have structure and form, although they do not exist in your space. And so I have a structure and a form, although I do not exist in your space.

My form may be changed, but so do you change the form of your own thoughts. When you dream of a particular location, that location does then exist in fact. It has a definite reality, although it may not have a physical reality. Because you experience it, and you are partially physical, it does have some basis of reality in physical terms, even though it may not exist full-blown in physical terms.

The connections between dream images and the physical body are always maintained. There is a difference in mass, and a difference in thickness of molecules. Nevertheless the dream location does exist in its own legitimate reality, and its reality is to some extent dependent upon physical reality.

There is a chemical necessity, as I have said, that makes dreaming inevitable. But then these dreams in turn affect the personality in general, and affect the actions of that personality in a physical universe. It goes without saying that telepathy operates within the dreaming state quite as effectively as it operates while the individual is awake. In the waking state it operates subconsciously. But in all times there is no boundary, generally speaking, that exists to separate one psychological unit from another. There are differences between psychological units, and you concentrate upon these differences. Nevertheless one man's dreams affect another's, and that man is in turn affected by the dreams of his neighbor.

I am not speaking, now, of some nebulous indirect fashion. A man is affected by the dreams of his fellows in quite definite, realistic and practical ways. He is affected by them both chemically and electromagnetically, and he in turn also affects others in the same manner.

It goes without saying, again, that these communications follow in the lines of emotional attraction. For one thing, there are also individual differences which operate, so that any given personality will be more open to particular influences, and will tend to ignore others. For while there are no boundaries as such about the self, for practical purposes the self is a core of characteristic actions and reactions with which all environment is manipulated and handled.

These characteristic responses have been built up through past existences, and because the self is not limited the core can at any time expand and project.

I am going to give you a break, so that we shall be in an advantageous position for our Dr. Instream material.

(Break at 9:44. Jane was dissociated as usual. Her eyes remained closed. Her voice continued to display its peculiar brogue occasionally. Her pace had been good.

(Up until now, although the session was being held in our front room, none of us had given a thought to traffic noise. It is interesting to note that when Jane

resumed with the Dr. Instream material, we immediately became conscious of the traffic noise. I was of course aware of my own irritation; Jane concurred at the end of the session.

(*When Jane resumed, still seated and with her eyes closed, her pace was somewhat faster than it had been in previous tests. She used some pauses however, and I will indicate a few of them along with a couple of strategic times. She sat quietly, with her head tipped back as she spoke. Resume at 10:05.*)

We will now see what we can do. Give us a moment.

There is an impression of an incident that occurred, of interest to Dr. Instream, in the middle of this week, possibly around Wednesday, that was unpleasant. *(Pause.)* Involving someone else, but with some connection to Dr. Instream.

As to now, I see him in connection with a railing, of steel or wood. A letter of interest to him that arrived yesterday or today, from a place with high grasses. *(Pause.)*

A variety of shapes such as packages. String of a twine type. I believe he received some bad news this week, and suffered some indisposition. A telephone may be ringing at this moment *(pause, at 10:10)* in his immediate environment.

There is a conversation concerning a schedule, and an automobile ride. He is I believe also thinking of an incident in his past. *(Pause.)*

Do you have a test for me this evening, Joseph ?

(*"Yes, just a minute."*

(*It was 10:12. I had to leave my desk to hand Jane the test envelope. She took it without opening her eyes.*)

Again, give us a moment.

(*As before, Jane's "moment" was actually very brief, much shorter than many of her routine pauses. It was now that I was quite conscious of traffic noise. Jane's voice remained quiet.*)

These are impressions.

A variety of shapes and designs. A connection with a fabric, and something to do with wood, and a house. An impression of several people.

A design repeated, as of blocks. An impression of a journey by automobile. *(Pause.)* A date, perhaps 1965. *(Pause.)* R. B. And another, and the impression of a road or a path, or of lines <u>suggesting</u> a road or a path.

Black and white *(pause)* having to do with a particular circumstance, and initials and many designs. A fuzzy sort of paper, and a smooth one.

I seem to pick up a connection with Christmas or Christmas tree, though I believe this is indirectly connected rather than directly; and something dark of rectangular shape, and also again of a border *(pause)* and something shady, and a sky symbol.

You may as always after our tests take a break.

(*Break at 10:20. Jane was dissociated as usual, she said. She now said the traffic bothered her also. She was not nervous in giving the data on Dr. Instream, or on our own test object. Suffice it to note here that this was Jane's third test before witnesses. An analysis of the test follows the end of the session.*

(*Jane resumed, again with her eyes closed and in a quiet voice, at 10:33.*)

We will now end our session, since we have indeed kept you busy of late.

I am using fine manners this evening, Marleno, and I have not raised my voice—

(*Except now. Seth/Jane's voice suddenly climbed a great deal in volume, very briefly, before subsiding.*)

—since we have had difficulties in that direction. I will indeed therefore close our session out of due regard, although I could indeed continue it indefinitely; and am sometimes tempted to do so. My heartiest wishes to you both.

("*Good night, Seth.*"

(*End at 10:35. Jane was dissociated as usual. Her eyes remained closed. Marleno is of course Lorraine Shafer's entity name.*

(*The label contains a variety of shapes and designs. See the tracing on page 289. The connection with a fabric can be the coat pocket in which I carried the label home. Our table at the dancing establishment Saturday night had a top of simulated wood grain. The house can be our own, the several people of course Jane and me and Bill and Peggy Gallagher; the Gallaghers were with us Saturday night when I picked the label as a test object.*

(*Designs are repeated in the label, but no blocks appear. The journey by automobile can refer to our driving home Saturday evening. There is an 1840 date on the label, but not 1965. I was of course involved with the test object, and my initials are R.B., but this can apply to any test object. We don't know which "another" Seth refers to. The label bears parallel oval lines which can suggest a road or a path.*

(*Neither Jane or I understand the reference to black and white. Having to do with a particular circumstance, initials and many designs, can apply to many things, including the test object. The label is fuzzy on the edges that were torn as I peeled it from the bottle, yet it is printed on a peculiarly smooth paper.*

(*The Christmas reference is an interesting one, and can be seen when one notes that the label is printed in red and green, on yellow stock. Jane said also that to her the XXX symbol on the label means Christmas. We do not know to what "something dark of rectangular shape" refers to, unless it's the shape of the table we sat at in the dancing establishment.*

(*The label has a dark green border. Jane suggested that the "something shady" reference can be the dimly-lit room in which we sat Saturday evening. Jane also said the sky symbol, to her, is quite definitely the circles used in the Ballantine trademark, the three-ring sign. She relates these circles to symbols for the sun, moon, the planets, etc.*

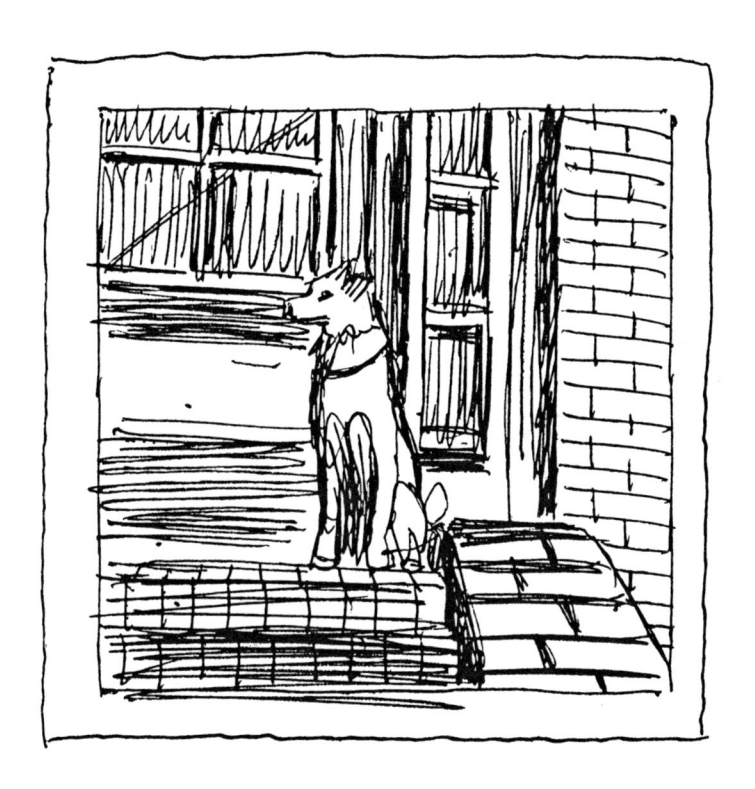

(Tracing of the black and white photograph used in the 11th envelope test, September 29, 1965, in the 194th session.)

SESSION 194
SEPTEMBER 29, 1965 9 PM WEDNESDAY AS SCHEDULED

(We have been reading the article on sleep in the September 18th issue of the New Yorker. Called "A Third Stage of Existence", it deals with REM sleep, or the rapid eye movements that have been shown to occur during dreaming. Since Seth has dealt with dreams to some extent Jane and I have a somewhat different slant on sleep and dreaming, and what is involved.

(For the test object I picked a black and white photograph of a dog Jane had owned when I married her. The dog, Mischa, is now dead. Jane took the picture before I met her, some 11 years ago. See the tracing on page 295. I slipped the photo between two pieces of Bristol, then into the usual double envelopes; the Bristol board prevented identification of the photo's serrated edges by touch.

(The session was held in our back room, and was a quiet one. Jane began speaking while sitting down and with her eyes closed. Her voice was average. Her pace was slow at the beginning but soon picked up speed. She began speaking at 9:01.)

Good evening.

("Good evening, Seth.")

With yourself and Ruburt, I was amused to think that a scientist was conducting experiments on a serious level in order to discover whether or not dreams actually exist.

This is indeed an example of an endeavor of the sort that is too often carried on, with energy expended in a search for a reality that is known by any nincompoop to exist.

The reality of dreams themselves can only be investigated through direct contact. Their reality cannot be probed by scientific devices, for dreams in this respect are as nebulous as the spirit, or soul, or inner self. Dreams are directly experienced. They have no meaning outside of their relationship with the personality.

As far as your system is concerned, they cannot be suddenly made flesh, to dwell among you. REM sleep or no REM sleep, your dreams exist constantly, beneath consciousness, even in the waking state. The personality is constantly affected by them. Their existence has its own dimension which is connected to the physical organism. It is impossible to deprive a human being of dreams, for even though you deprive him of sleep, this necessary mental function will be carried on subconsciously.

Dreams are an example of mental activity that has its origin within the physical organism, but exists in a dimension which is not mainly physical. Dreams are an example of the inner self's basically independent nature.

The eye movements noted in the beginning of REM sleep are only indications of dream activity that is closely connected to the physical layers of the self. These periods mark not the <u>onset</u> of dreams, but the return of the personality from deeper layers of dream awareness to more surface areas.

The self is actually returning to more surface levels of consciousness, to check upon its environment. There is a transference of main energy in deeper dream states, from physical concentration to a mental concentration, actually quite separated from physical connections.

Quite simply, the self travels to levels of awareness, and to layers of the self that are far divorced from the physical areas of mobility. The muscles are lax because activity of a physical nature is not required for the physical organism. Actions are indeed being carried on, and actions which would be considered physical *if* the body was moving, and if the individual were awake. These actions, walking, talking, working, any conceivable dream action, these require energy. The energy that is not being expended within the physical system is used to sustain these mental actions.

The chemical excesses built up in the waking state are automatically changed as they are drained off, into electrical energy, which also helps to form and sustain dream images. Your scientists would learn more about the nature of dreams if they would but train themselves to recall their own dreams, and then study them in relation to their own normal activities and physical events.

I suggest a brief break.

(*Break at 9:28. Jane had been dissociated as usual for a first delivery. Her eyes had remained closed, her pace had been good, her voice average. She resumed in the same manner at 9:29.*)

The scientist of whom you have read, in his experiments attempts to deprive the individual of sleep.

He has worked with human beings and cats. The very <u>attempt</u> to deprive an individual of sleep, however, will automatically set into mechanism subconscious dream activity. The tampering will then change the conditions. The direct experience of the developing dream is what they should be concerned with.

This could be studied to some degree if proper suggestions were given to the individual that he would awaken at the exact point when a dream ends. The dream state and dream conditions could <u>also</u> be studied quite legitimately, and to more purpose, using hypnosis. Here you are working with the mind itself as your material, and merely suggesting that it operate in a certain fashion. You are not tampering with the mechanics of its operation, and therefore automatically altering the conditions.

Dr. Instream might find such a study would bring him much satisfaction. Through hypnosis you can get complete dream recall, with a good operator. You can suggest ordinary sleep, and then suggest that the subject, in his sleep and without waking, give a verbal description of his dream or dreams.

This however would involve many a nightly vigil. A better procedure would be to hypnotize a subject, and you would need a good one, and suggest that under hypnosis he repeat the dreams of the night before. There are many opportunities for an investigation of dreams along these lines, and the results would yield more legitimate information.

The dreams of the mentally ill, using these methods, could also be studied if the affliction, of course, was not too severe. The dreams of children could be investigated in this manner without too much difficulty, and these could be compared, generally speaking, with the dreams of adults. Many differences between the two would be noted.

Children dream more vividly and more often. They return more frequently however to periods of near wakefulness, in order to check their physical environment, since they are not as sure of it as adults are. In deep periods of sleep children range further <u>away</u>, as far as their dream activities are concerned.

The ego, not yet fully formed, allows them more freedom. For this reason also they have more telepathic and clairvoyant dreams than do adults. They also have more psychic energy, practically speaking. That is, they are able to draw upon energy more easily. Because of the intenseness of their waking existence, the chemical excesses build up at a faster rate. Therefore children actually have more of this chemical propellant to use in the formation of dreams.

They are actually more conscious of their dreams, for the ego does not prevent awareness at this stage to the same degree that it will do later.

I will suggest another brief break, as I am keeping the 10 o'clock hour in mind, and would like to start again shortly before the hour.

(*Break at 9:50. Jane was dissociated as usual. Her eyes remained closed, her voice average, her pace quite fast. She also remembered some of the material in a general way.*

(*She resumed in the same manner at 9:58.*)

I have said often that any action changes that which acts, and that which is acted upon; and so in the sort of experiments that are now being carried on to study dreams. The acts of the investigators are changing the conditions in such a way it is easy to find that which you are looking for.

For the investigator himself, through his actions, inadvertently brings about, in specific instances, those results for which he looks. The particular experiment may then seem to suggest conditions which are by no means general ones, but which may appear so. In hypnosis the subject is not as much on guard as a subject of an experiment when the subject knows in advance that he will be awakened by the experimenter, when electrodes are attached to the physical organism, when the conditions of the sleep laboratory are substituted for his ordinary nightly environment. It is impossible to study dreams when an attempt is made to isolate the dreamer from his own personality, to <u>treat</u> dreams as if they were physical or mechanical. The only laboratory for a study of dreams is the laboratory of the personality.

This is not as difficult as it might sound, and I have indeed suggested experiments that would be most effective.

Now, give us a moment and we will see if we can find our Dr. Instream.
(It was 10:06. Jane settled herself in her rocker. Her eyes were closed, her head down, a hand to her face. Her voice was quiet and remained so. She used pauses but they were usually brief.)

These are impressions. *(Pause briefly.)*

I believe that he has left some people, and is alone in what would appear to be some sort of alleyway, perhaps between high buildings, fairly dark with lights nearby.

(Pause at 10:09.) Impressions again, perhaps a round object in his hand. He thinks of papers on a desk, or in a briefcase, that seem to have to do with a particular plan.

Something with checks, perhaps a jacket. And a package which he has received today, or will receive shortly, tomorrow. *(Pause.)*

I believe he has been irritated by a particular person, a male. I do not know… There is a connection, something to do with lights. Perhaps in connection with the man. Does he perhaps live on Light Street? Or his name *(Jane gestured, her eyes still closed)* Light Man—Lightman, or something of that sort. *(Pause.)*

Also something to do with a federal matter. Dr. Instream is thinking philosophically now. Perhaps the round object in his hands has something to do with lights, as a bulb. *(Gesture, and pause at 10:15.)*

Do you have a test for me, Joseph?

("Yes.")

(I handed Jane the envelope. She took it without opening her eyes, then sat quietly, holding it in both hands. Her pause was brief.)

Again, please give us a moment.

Dr. Instream should if possible read the data on your private tests, for on occasion it is possible that some of the Instream material may bleed through, so to speak. This is merely a possibility at times.

These are impressions.

The color purple. *(Pause.)* Something rather neutral, rather than of intimate personal nature. Something partially blank, dots, an assemblage of something, it seems of shadowy form. But vertical and perhaps cone shaped.

Not a photograph. Some kind of lettering *(pause)* and design. Joseph's initials have to do with it, but it is not an object with which he has great personal concern; though there may be a wallet connection, I doubt it.

Perhaps something to do with neighbors indirectly. Mostly design, but with bare portions, and originals rather than exact duplicates. *(Pause.)* A fencelike shape.

I suggest your break.

(*Break at 10:24. Jane was dissociated as usual. Her eyes remained closed, her voice quiet. She said that right after she had delivered the material on Dr. Instream she felt quite tired. She realized she was tired as she heard herself asking me if I had a test for her. When I asked if it was possible for her to change her mind and postpone a test under such circumstances, she said she did not know. Jane regarded tonight's envelope test as pretty much of a failure.*

(*See the tracing of the test photo on page 295. Jane felt the test data contained but few correct impressions. She said the color purple could apply to the brick facing depicted in the photograph. Jane remembered this quite well even though the photo was taken some years ago. Our dog sits before the Bronx, NY, house of Jane's aunt; Jane said she well remembers the peculiar blue and red cast of the bricks. I saw the house once some years ago but have no conscious memory of the brick color.*

(*The photo does have verticals in it, and the dog's form can be seen as cone shaped. Our dog was certainly of personal concern to us, the test object is a photograph, my initials are not directly connected with it as far as being visible, and as far as we know there is no wallet connection with the photo, etc. Thus most of the rest of the data appear as opposite or reverse impressions.*

(*Jane resumed with her eyes again closed, her voice quiet, at 10:29.*)

We will shortly end our session.

Now in regard to <u>our</u> own test this evening: Ruburt, at this stage, should <u>not</u> work on our own test results as he has been doing. He has been concentrating too much on grading our tests.

He has worked at this several hours daily. This is not his job, and it will work against our results. His job is to remain as spontaneous as possible. His work in attempting to tabulize the test results thus far, will only hamper our results. He should be in no way connected with that endeavor.

I cannot repeat this too strongly. He should dismiss the tests entirely from his mind. The tests in the sessions have not bothered him at all to any important degree, except for a natural initial nervousness, and all in all we have been coming along well enough. But at this stage he simply should leave the grading and so forth to you. Of course he may make suggestions as he reads the sessions, but that is all.

I will have more to say concerning this sort of thing briefly at our next session.

(*For the last two days Jane had been trying to work out a system whereby the test results, both hits and misses, could be read more or less at a glance, as opposed to my rather rambling subjective treatment. I think Jane meant tabulate, above.*

(*She had worked out a two-column system that seemed rather good to us, but* neither of us had realized the very intense effort involved would be detrimental. Since Jane's idea would involve listing the material in such a fashion twice a week, and thus keep her involved, we decided to drop the idea, at least for the moment.

(I had planned to ask Seth a few questions at the end of the session. I now realized that Jane was tired, but decided to see what developed. For material connected with the first question, see my notes on Lorraine Shafer, York Beach, and Dr. Instream on pages 289-90, preceding the 193rd session.

("Do you want to say a few words about Lorraine Shafer being in York Beach the same week in August that Dr. Instream was there? Is there any connection at all between the two visits?")

A tenuous one. Marleno knew about your experience at York Beach, and because of circumstances in her own life she visited the general territory. An emotional connection with the sessions did have quite a bit to do with her particular visit to York Beach, however, and there was on her part a subconscious knowledge that Dr. Instream had been there also. I have told you that telepathy operates continually, and has strong emotional connections, so this should be no surprise.

(See the 9th, 15th, 17th, 69th and 80th sessions for material on our York Beach experiences. I believe that above Seth refers to the first three named sessions. These deal with events involving Jane and me at York Beach in August of 1963, preceding the beginning of these sessions by several months.

(Marleno is Lorraine Shafer's entity name.

("Why has our cat Willy been sick so often lately?")

I suggest that you hold this question until our next session, as Ruburt is tired this evening because of his concentration upon the work which I have mentioned. There is nothing serious here, or I would discuss it this evening in any case, <u>since</u> you asked. I will answer specifically at our next session.

My heartiest regards to you both.

("Good night, Seth."

(End at 10:40. Jane was dissociated as usual. Her eyes remained closed, her voice quiet. Her pace had been good for the most part during the session.

(I had intended asking one more question, concerning the source of the material Jane gave on the envelope test. So much of it appeared to be of opposite or reverse nature to the test object that it seemed to fit a pattern.

(We were relieved to learn our cat's trouble was not serious. Willy had been sick rather often during the past weeks. We were puzzled by this, since according to Seth the owners of a pet contribute much to the pet's health through use of their own psychic energy. Since we were so fond of Willy, we had thought we were contributing adequately before the sick spell.)

SESSION 195
OCTOBER 4, 1965 9 PM MONDAY AS SCHEDULED

(This afternoon Jane called her publisher, Frederick Fell, and was pleased to learn that he liked her ESP book very much. The decks are now cleared for publication next April. Jane was also curious to hear Mr. Fell's voice, to see what impressions she might pick up.

(I planned no envelope test for this session. Not because of the poor results of the last test in the 194th session, but to vary the steady test diet. I thought Jane might come to feel under pressure without a break occasionally. I expected the data on Dr. Instream to come through as usual, however.

(Lorraine Shafer was a witness for the session. She had witnessed the 193rd session also. The session was held in our front room, and was not interrupted. Jane spoke while sitting down and with her eyes closed. Her voice was quiet for the most part. She began rather slowly, then picked up some speed.)

Good evening.

("Good evening, Seth.")

I am pleased that Ruburt's mood has somewhat improved. I told him that the affair would work out to his advantage, but again patience is not one of his virtues.

(The last sessions in which Seth dealt with Jane's ESP book were the 178th and the 180th. In both of these sessions, as well as many others, he stated the book would be a success, financially and otherwise. All of his statements concerning Jane's writing sales have proved out so far. Seth first mentioned the sale of the ESP book by name in the 92nd session. See Volume 3.)

Now. First of all, my greeting to Marleno. She is always welcome. There is on her part a block, that operates in much the same manner as Ruburt's ego on occasion, as far as our sessions are concerned. This is caused by an inner willingness to believe, though this is a bad word, in the legitimate nature of my existence; a willingness however that is sometimes so desperate, if you will forgive the term, and so wholehearted, that it sets up automatic barriers on the part of other portions of the personality.

If she were to accept the real validity of the sessions, then she would feel obligated to enter into the affair. She feels too deeply, and so sometimes she backs away, and sometimes she does not. This makes it difficult for me to speak to her specifically, for it is not easy for me then to look into her circumstances. I say this because I would indeed, Marleno, be more helpful, as I have tried to be with the Jesuit and the cat lover. But so far, while you are interested, you have not quite allowed me to probe into your circumstances <u>easily</u>.

(Jane smiled as she spoke. By the Jesuit and the cat lover Seth meant of course Bill and Peggy Gallagher, who have witnessed quite a few sessions. Jane and I soon noticed that Seth did not refer to Lorraine very often, even when she was a witness, and have speculated about the reasons for this. By contrast we have obtained a good deal more information about the Gallaghers, and Jane has been aware of better "contacts" somehow in relation to them. Our thought has been that if Lorraine kept coming to sessions, sooner or later Seth would speak to her.)

I am speaking of these matters since I have intended to do so personally to you, and also because they tie in very well, as you will see, with some of our own discussions. For emotional contacts are what we are working with, and when you block off the contact from your end, then I would not presume, you see, to attempt to break it. My own code of ethics would not allow it.

I do think that these sessions have helped you, generally speaking. The very fact of their existence has been an advantage to you, though you may not know it, and I have hinted at this before. You are wishing for many answers from me, and I have always felt the pull of your inquiries. However at the same time you do set up these blocks; for you are not afraid of the answers, but you are afraid basically that they could be given in this manner.

You may consciously think differently. You want so badly, you see, that the very power of your own desire in these circumstances frightens you off.

(Jane had been speaking rather quietly if rapidly, with her eyes closed. Lorraine, who was also taking shorthand notes, sat close by. Now Jane, her eyes still closed, leaned rather quickly toward Lorraine and her voice boomed out briefly. I confess that I jumped. I didn't have time to observe Lorraine's reaction.)

<u>I am not frightening now, am I</u>? I am indeed as peaceful as a tired old dove with battered wings, and a beak smoothed down. This does not mean that in time you cannot yourself knock down this particular barrier.

Strangely enough, it can be knocked down most easily, if you can think of me in terms in no way occult or mysterious, but simply as a personality engaged in an endeavor which science will soon come to accept, as simply one of the many facts of existence of which they have previously known but little.

Now generally speaking, such emotional responses set up electromagnetic forces. These forces in a large measure form boundaries inside which is a general, or generalized, field or system to which the individual will respond. The emotional blockage sets up barriers however whose main purpose is to protect the individual from anything that he considers at all unsafe or threatening, or simply unpleasant.

It is not a simple question that may be summed up in a statement, such as "attitudes regulate behavior." What is not understood is that emotional attitudes, conscious and subconscious, have an electromagnetic reality that operates very efficiently, either as an open system which attracts new stimuli, or as a closed electric force that is supercharged.

You may now take your first break, and we shall consider these emotional systems in the relation to the personality in the dream state.

(*Break at 9:22. Jane was dissociated as usual for a first delivery. Her voice had been mostly even, her pace rather fast toward the end. A trace of her peculiar brogue had been apparent also, and usually when the brogue revealed itself the voice grew a bit in strength.*

(*Sessions 120-127 deal extensively with the electromagnetic field and related phenomena. See Volume 3.*

(*One of the questions Lorraine had at break, in relation to Seth's statement about helping her, was whether Seth would help through Jane, or through Lorraine herself directly.*

(*Jane's voice was a bit deeper and stronger when she began speaking again. Again her eyes were closed, her pace fast, her brogue more often apparent. Resume at 9:35.*)

First of all, I spoke in terms of helping you through Ruburt. For many reasons too numerous to discuss this evening, I will be working through him only, for I have been working with him for longer than he knows.

There is much preparation necessary for such work. Various kinds of conditions must be exactly met, between those such as myself, and those through whom we speak. Not only general conditions but personal conditions. I meant, very simply, that since you have not been able to be emotionally open, you have often closed up tightly in the sessions. It is not that I could not reach you through Ruburt, and answer some of your questions. In any case it is simply that the answers would do you no good under such circumstances.

Now these same sort of emotional systems operate under all conditions, and they regulate the kinds of experience to which an individual is susceptible or open, and they close out from his awareness those experiences which he has already decided he will not accept. Again, the emotional attitudes have their own electromagnetic reality. This field or system will therefore attract certain experiences, close out others, allow others to come so close and no closer, as is the case with Marleno and our sessions.

Now, this same sort of emotional system operates in the sleeping state as well as in the waking state, though there are differences in that the personality will allow greater leeway in the dream state. But even in the sleeping condition, as should be obvious, the individual accepts and attracts certain experiences and blocks out others. You know that telepathy and clairvoyance operate rather freely in the dream state. However the nature of such experiences is strongly dependent upon the particular emotional system that is characteristic of any given personality.

Dreamer "A" for example may pick up telepathically a small but particular portion of a dream by dreamer "B". Dreamer "A" need not necessarily have an emotional connection with dreamer "B". However there will be at the very least an emotional connection between the event within dreamer "B's" dream, that has strong meaning for dreamer "A". A man may dream of a childhood experience in which he was bitten by a dog. Another man who was also bitten by a dog, may then for example telepathically pick up the original dream. Not because he is necessarily connected with the dreamer, but because the experience will strike at him emotionally, and he will then attract the dream.

Definite electromagnetic actions will therefore occur between the two dreamers, and there may be a spilling over of data, or dream information, before the circuit is closed. You must realize that I am not speaking symbolically. I am speaking in very practical terms. The electromagnetic systems do indeed exist, and when they are open telepathic communications can travel through.

The same also applies to clairvoyance, or to be more precise, precognition, although here we are involved with something more. I have explained how dream images are constructed. You realize that they also have an electromagnetic reality, so there is no difficulty in their transmission from one dreamer to another.

All of these reality systems of which we have been speaking are closely connected. Every thought has this same electric potential. Thoughts are often translated into dream images by a simple transformation. There is little difference indeed, basically, between physical images and dream images, and apparitions, and very little difference between these and thoughts and emotions.

I am keeping our 10 o'clock date in mind, so I will suggest a very brief break. Incidentally, I depend upon you, Joseph , now, to watch the volume of the voice. Do not wait until it becomes too loud. Watch for tendencies, and then we can control it better.

("All right.")

(*Break at 9:55. Jane had been dissociated as usual. Her eyes had remained closed, her pace had been good. I had indeed been watching the volume of her voice, for several times during this delivery I thought I noticed a tendency to escalate in volume. A couple of times I was on the verge of asking Seth to be careful, but the voice quieted each time by itself.*

(*Jane's voice had been pitched quite a bit lower than usual, even when quiet, and this was a bit unusual in that the deeper voice usually grows stronger also. See the 191st session for Seth's explanation of why the voice grows so much stronger at times.*

(*I might also add that we recently learned of other people hearing Seth's strong voice during the unscheduled 190th session. This was the session witnessed by John Bradley. It will be remembered that a young couple from next door heard Seth, and came over to see if anything was wrong. A couple of days ago Jane and I learned that other people in our apartment house heard the voice, and were quite curious.*

(Jane's pace was somewhat slower when she began speaking again. Her eyes were closed, her voice quieter, and she used pauses. She sat with her head down, a hand to her brow. Resume at 10:05.)

Please give us a moment. *(Pause.)*

A bedroom. These are impressions for Dr. Instream. The bedroom is neater than his office.

He is sitting down with his eyes closed. His head is reflected in something oval. *(Pause.)* There is a piece of carpet or rug, and a small black book. He may be using self-hypnosis.

There are voices from another room. Whether they are mechanically produced or not I do not know.

(Jane now took a long pause at 10:09.)

There is a litter of papers, however, that are not in sight in a drawer. He has forgotten about us until very late. He lies down. *(Pause at 10:10.)* He seems to be in a dissociated state, but whether or not it was produced <u>purposely</u> I do not know.

He thinks of a ring, and a peel. He had a phone call at 3 PM today, from a colleague, having to do with something discussed in a letter; though I am not sure that the letter was written to, or by, the individual on the other end of the phone.

The conversation may have had to do with a letter written to another individual. My only other impressions are of a framework and experiment.

(Pause at 10:14.)

Now. Ruburt was upset because of the failure of our last test. Nevertheless, if you have a test for us this evening then we shall do what we can, since it is not good <u>particularly</u> for him to refrain through fear. The tests in the overall will take care of themselves in any case. We shall have too many successes to worry. Therefore, if you have a test for us we shall see what we can do.

("I don't have any.")

Then we will thank you for your consideration of Ruburt. The fact that he was willing enough to allow me to request a test is however a point in our favor.

("I thought it was a good idea to vary the routine.")

This is perfectly legitimate. We will try something else. A situation occurred when Marleno was 15 or thereabouts, that had much to do with her later choices and actions. Her mother was partially involved, although as a consequence. She did not initiate the circumstance.

(*Seth's statement above, about trying something else, surprised me somewhat. What I say here is purely subjective, since I did not write it down at the time it occurred. This afternoon while working I had the rather clear thought that Lorraine would witness the session this evening.*

(*This in itself would be quite unusual, since she had also witnessed the 193rd, last week; never before had Lorraine witnessed sessions so close together by far. I then had the accompanying thought that when I told Seth I had no envelope test, he would suggest that he try something else.*)

We are simply seeing what we can accomplish with these barriers set up as they are, and without attempting to manipulate them ourselves.

The word maple comes to mind. I do not know to what this refers... An address, I do not know. I believe another person was connected with the event, and that it occurred in afternoon, late, or evening. Perhaps in winter or autumn.

Now I pick up the word whiskey, as applying to a later period, and another circumstance involving a man and a late hour, and a dwelling place with a front door precisely in the middle of a front room, and a porch that is shadowed, and back bedrooms with children. But they are not all asleep, and one overhears an argument.

I get the <u>impression</u> of the number 46. Whether this is an age or a date I am not sure, or the number. I merely receive the number.

I will now suggest a break. I will under no circumstances however attempt to probe if I meet with a sincere resistance.

Another child may have been connected with the 15-year-old circumstance.

(*Break at 10:24. Jane said that Seth had her "really out" during the delivery. Her eyes had remained closed, her voice stronger at times, her pace good.*

(*A conversation followed concerning the above data, which was too fast and involved for me to note down fully. Being surprised, Lorraine needed some time to think, for memory to work. At first thought she recalled nothing involving herself as a 15-year-old. Lorraine then began to recall bits and pieces of events which, she thought, might fall within the pattern Seth had been producing in the rest of the data.*

(*Jane said that although Seth did not say so, she felt the data on Lorraine was set in the South. Lorraine agreed, saying that if it concerned an incident she was beginning to recall, it would have taken place in Asheville, NC. Jane also picked up leaf images in connection with a porch on the first floor.*

(*Lorraine had three children then, and they did sleep in back bedrooms of the* apartment house in Asheville, NC, she said. As to a front door precisely in the center of a front room, Lorraine was not sure. She said this could be deceptive. If one looked at the front of the house from the outside, he would see a single door in front, in the center of the house; but this was a door opening into a hallway, with apartments opening off on either side, and thus would not be in the middle of a front room.

(*The number 46 did not mean anything to Lorraine at the moment, and I asked her if it could be interpreted as perhaps the first week in April. Lorraine said the incident she is thinking of in Asheville took place in the spring.*)

(*Jane had but a vague memory of what she had said. She said Seth had not been pushing to obtain the information, and Lorraine agreed. Jane resumed, again with her eyes closed, at a rather fast pace and in an average voice, at 10:35.*)

We will shortly end our session.

The situation to which I referred did occur in the South.

With all due respects to Ruburt, he was right in one respect and wrong in another. The porch to the front was shadowed. He correctly picked up the leaf images; however it was not the first floor. The door was in the center. However, my viewpoint is not precise enough perhaps, but I have the picture of a door precisely centered, leading outward. And I am working here despite the unwitting blocks that are erected. I see something yellow and something rose; and voices <u>rising</u>, and something broken. This is on my part an emotional breakage.

I give my impressions as I receive them, sometimes with connections, and sometimes the impressions are solitary. A mailbox. Black. A rear entry. Something to do with a party, and one child listens, a boy.

Now I have the <u>feeling</u> of a funeral, though this may be symbolic. But there is a connection with a car, perhaps a black one. This could explain the funeral impression. A disturbed afternoon, and an argument, and the strong impression, again, of a breakage.

I believe the breakage was emotional, and yet I somehow connect it with the sound of glasses, whether the man had been drinking strongly or not; this could explain the glasses, which are strongly connected to me here.

You may all take a break or we will end the session.

("*I guess we'll end it then.*")

We will then wish you all a fond and hearty good evening. My best regards to all of you, and all in all we have done well, and I am pleased.

("*Good night, Seth.*")

(*End at 10:43. Jane was again well dissociated, as she had been during the previous delivery. Her eyes had remained closed, her pace had been good, her voice average.*)

(Lorraine thought the date of the incident she had in mind could be interpreted as early in April, probably in 1944, in Asheville, NC. It would, she said, be in the springtime however, rather than in winter or autumn. She said her family had lived on the second floor rather than the first, and agreed with Seth's description, now, of the placement of the front, or porch, door. Seth mentioned "something yellow and something rose." Lorraine told us the walls of the apartment were painted yellow, and that the furniture was of the old-fashioned kind with large rose decorations.

(Lorraine is separated from her husband. Seth's whiskey connection arises from the fact that he was drinking heavily at that time in Asheville; the only time he did so. There were arguments, Lorraine said. If her youngest child, a boy, had listened, he did so at the age of one. Lorraine remembers a black mailbox; the apartment of course had a rear entry also. Lorraine described a party to us.

(There was no black car connected with her during the stay in Asheville, Lorraine said. But she owned a black car in 1960, while living in Elmira, several years before we met her. This is the only black car she has had, or been closely associated with. She did not own it when we met her a few months ago.

(These notes are my interpretation of what was said about Seth's data. I asked Lorraine to make up her own notes for later insertion in the record. She took shorthand notes of tonight's session.

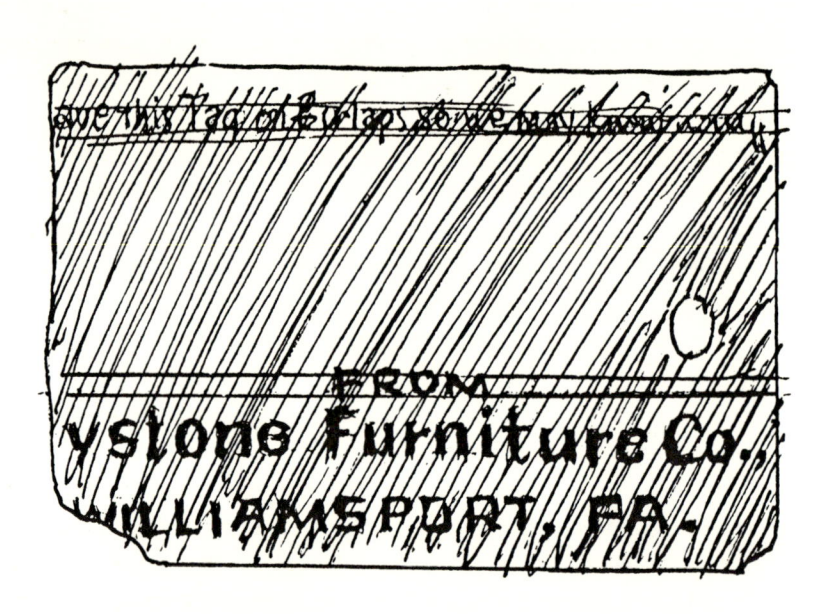

(Tracing of the fragment of the old furniture label used in the 12th envelope test, in Session 196, October 6, 1965.)

SESSION 196
OCTOBER 6, 1965 9 PM WEDNESDAY AS SCHEDULED

(For the envelope test this evening I chose a piece of an old furniture label that Jane and I had peeled from the back of a bureau a couple of weeks ago. See the tracing above. I found the label, or rather part of it, in my studio this afternoon and decided to use it for the test. Since it was lying unobtrusively among my things on a shelf I thought Jane had not been aware of it. She later confirmed this, saying she thought I had thrown it out at the time we removed it.

(The label was brittle and quite brown with age, and broke apart when removed. There was nothing on its reverse side. I thought such an old object might have some interesting impressions attached to it. The bureau it came from is an old-fashioned one that had sat in the garage of "our" apartment house for some years. Our landlord gave it to us, and we fixed it up and repainted it.

(It will be remembered that in the 194th session Seth promised to discuss in the 195th session our cat's rather frequent if brief bouts of illness. Since this was not done however, I mentioned it to Jane before this evening's session. Jane said she had

also thought of it. To avoid interruptions we used the back room, although Jane prefers the larger front room. She began speaking while sitting down and with her eyes closed. Her voice was average in strength, her pace rather fast although interspersed with pauses.)

Good evening.

("Good evening, Seth.")

It is rather important that the reality of these electromagnetic systems be understood, as they are so important in the construction of physical images and dream images, and since they are responsible for the inner communication which takes place beneath consciousness.

These systems are affected by the weather, and they also affect the weather. There is a constant inflow and outflow. The dream, any dream, fits neatly within certain and definite electromagnetic boundaries, and at the same time helps to form the electromagnetic field itself.

No physical matter is without this electromagnetic reality, and no thought exists which does not exist within this reality. Again, I am not speaking symbolically, but quite practically. Emotions, having their own reality within this system, do not affect physical matter indirectly, but cause specific electromagnetic changes within the physical organism.

This, and all such effects, represent one of the most basic ways in which one action causes another action to change. These definite fields operate as channels for inner communications. They may be formed instantly, sweeping out into other directions. They open through attraction. This attraction may originate as an emotional one, but the emotional feeling has its own electromagnetism, and the attraction is in direct proportion to the force of the emotion itself, or to the charge that the emotion may carry.

Briefly, I explained the way in which a dreamer may be telepathically in communication with another man's dream. Not necessarily because he is aware of the <u>man</u>, for in many cases he is not. The telepathic communication arises as a result of an attraction, a personal emotional charge on the part of the second dreamer that allows him to open these channels of communication.

Any experience at all, whether mental or physical, also carries an electric and magnetic reality, so that the experience of any given individual is held in a sort of electric code within the cells. On a subconscious basis the individual is drawn to others who have had similar experiences to his own. He will be more attracted to the various field boundaries to which he himself has been accustomed.

His <u>un</u>conscious communications will also follow this same pattern. This of course includes his dreams. It may be well to remember here that dreams exist even for an individual in the waking state, though he is not aware of them. His mind continues this activity even while the conscious self goes about its daily chores.

These dreams go unrecognized by the conscious ego; but they do _not_ go unrecorded by the inner self, and they therefore exist, and they form electromagnetic channels of their own to which—make that by which—the physical body itself is affected. The physical organism is constantly changed by all stimuli, whether or not the ego is aware of the stimuli. And it is affected by stimuli, whether or not science realizes that the particular stimuli even exists. Therefore, the physical organism reacts to this continuous unconscious mental activity in the form of continuing dream experiences, whether or not the individual is awake or asleep. All of these realities go into the formation of the personality, and unless they are all understood the personality itself will remain a mystery.

You may take your first break, and I have not forgotten the question that you asked me concerning the health of your cat.

(*Break at 9:21. Jane was dissociated as usual for a first break. Her eyes remained closed, her voice even and rather fast, even with some pauses. For much of the delivery she sat leaning forward in her rocker, her head tipped down somewhat, and with her hands clasped as her elbows rested upon her knees. This has come to be something of a characteristic pose for her lately during the sessions; I do not recall seeing Jane ever use it outside of a session.*

(*Jane again sat leaning forward when she resumed speaking, in the same even voice, and with her eyes closed, at 9:30.*)

Now. We shall speak briefly concerning the health of your cat, and Dr. Instream may skip this paragraph if he prefers.

There is a particular type of food that does not set well with him [Willy], although he likes it, strangely enough. Ruburt knows which food it is, for he has suspected it for quite a while.

The pet also sensed Ruburt's own upset when he was, when Ruburt was, worried, and this also contributed. The cat is generally in good health. You are also both in good health at this time. And you, Joseph , should escape your December doldrums this year, and I thoroughly expect that you shall.

(*Jane, as Seth, smiled as she referred to Dr. Instream. Jane does know the suspected cat food, which is a combination of liver and fish. The worry referred to above concerns Jane's interest in her ESP book; it took her publisher some time to let her know he was reading it, and as seen in the 195th session Jane finally telephoned the publisher to get the final okay on the book. Many sessions ago, as many as a hundred or more, Seth told us that animal pets would reflect the psychic health and concerns of their owners.*

(*Many sessions ago also, Seth told me that my Christmas doldrums stemmed from something that happened to me many years ago. I have forgotten the incident, he said. Seth promised to go into it but we became sidetracked on other matters last year. This fall I will make an effort to clear up the matter up before December.)*

Ruburt will find that his own work will now improve. Indeed the improvement has begun. He simply needed a rest, creatively speaking, and the change of seasons will exhilarate him.

Returning to a previous discussion, I would like to make it plain once more that dream images are not pseudorealities. They exist as fact, though in a different dimension from physical reality. Again, no one would deny the reality of psychological experience when it is felt by the waking personality. Yet such experience also does not have a physical reality, to the same degree that a definite physical object has.

It should be emphasized however that dream experiences <u>can</u> have a more lasting and vital effect upon the personality than many so-called physical experiences, for the dream experiences are not blocked nearly as much as waking experience is blocked. The suggestion that also occurs within the dream state works even more effectively upon the whole personality than any suggestion works under ordinary circumstances. And dreams certainly do contain suggestions, and they are reacted to by the personality, not only on a subconscious basis and a psychological basis, but they affect the whole system.

Dream experiences often, very often, change the course of human events. Again, all this takes place through the operation of electromagnetic systems. There is a definite connection between this constant dream activity undertaken by the unconscious self, and what you call inspiration or creative activity.

These apparent inspirations from nowhere definitely come from somewhere, and this somewhere is that inner dreaming condition, which is a necessity on the part of every consciousness, human or otherwise. Here I am using the word consciousness to cover all organisms with awareness. This dream activity seems divorced from the conscious state itself, and came <u>before</u> the conscious state within your physical system. It cannot be turned off, and it will not cease. It will only be noticed, as a rule, when the aware portions of the personality are disconnected from their physical stimulations to some considerable degree.

These dream activities have a pulsing quality that could be compared with the pulsing of heartbeat, and that are quite as vital to the human system. So much telepathic communication is received at this level that the lines of individuality are not as brilliant. Yet individuality does exist here, but it takes a strong organizing system, with amazing powers of discrimination, to handle such data; and it takes the human personality to stand firm upon its own identity while it is, on this other dreaming level, open to so many communications that are not its own.

It is the ego, practically speaking, who attempts to do the distinguishing here; but the inner core of the self, the inner ego of which we have spoken, manages the basic chore. The setting up of the ego represented at once the necessity of boundaries, represented a cutting apart from, a divorcing, and a rigid limiting function. Initially this was necessary while this new sort of creature learned to maintain itself as a separate unit.

But the ego also grows and learns and evolves, and it can assimilate more and more, and accept more, as a portion of its own identity. It is only because your scientists overestimate the physical that it seems to them that man has not evolved to any great degree in the last million years.

I will continue with this later in the session. Now I suggest your break, so that we can keep our appointment with Dr. Instream.

(*Break at 9:55. Jane was dissociated as usual. Her eyes had remained closed. Her pace had been quite fast and sure, with the result that my writing hand was quite tired. Her voice had been average.*

As usual when giving the Dr. Instream material, Jane spoke at a slower pace. By now however the pace was not as slow as it had been during the first few such tests. I will indicate a few pauses and some strategic times. Jane resumed while sitting down and with her eyes closed, and in an average voice, at 10:05.)

Please give us a moment.

These are impressions. He is, or has been, or is thinking of, a gathering of people. Perhaps a faculty affair. A woman close to him in a yellow dress. A clock on a mantel, 4 PM. (*Pause at 10:06.*)

A disturbance of sorts occurred today. He received a letter from a person whose name begins with M. There was a phone call at dinnertime—that is, the night meal. I believe that his office is going to be changed or redecorated or perhaps repainted; some change of this sort in the near future, if it has not already been done. But this is a <u>rearrangement</u> of some sort, that could involve furniture arrangement.

But the office is not the same now, or very shortly will not be as it was when we were there. The change may also involve another person. Dr. Instream may grumble about being routed out, though this might be only temporarily while the rearrangement is being done. (*Pause at 10:11.*)

He stands at this moment against a piece of wooden furniture, and he is drinking from a glass. I believe he is drinking liquor, and he is smiling. This is tonight at this hour, I <u>believe</u>. There are people about. (*Pause.*)

This is in his living room, or one very much like it, with the same view from the windows. The people are dressed formally, comparatively speaking.

Men mainly. He is smiling and chatting. (*Pause at 10:14.*) He has been talking about politics, though this may be university politics. I do not know. He says: "There are large areas of improvement. There are large areas in which improvement can be made."

Someone says, a male: "I'll go along with you on that, George." And I hear someone laugh, this time I think a woman. *(Pause at 10:15.)*

Do you have a test for me?

("Yes."

(I handed Jane the usual double envelope. She took it without opening her eyes, then sat quietly for a moment while holding it in her right hand.)

These are impressions.

A foundation of sorts. A path or road shape not directly centered, with an upward incline. An initial, an area of color, window shapes having to do with two people, but connected with several circumstances, and with a package, perhaps sent from this address.

A diamond shape and crisscross lines, and a voice connected with the item. It seems as if someone stood and spoke outside of what is depicted here. I pick up a connection with a pair of shoes, though I do not know to what this refers, and a fence or border; an enclosure of that kind. Also a departure having to do with an automobile, and perhaps a place with much water.

Ruburt thinks of a photograph taken in Marathon.

I suggest your break.

(Break at 10:22. Jane was dissociated as usual. Her eyes had remained closed, her voice average. Her pace had been a little slow. She was not, she said, nervous while giving the Dr. Instream data. She said: "I did seem to see him standing with his mouth open in a characteristic pose, with a drink in his hand." Jane said the impression was not too clear, and that she also had some impression of the living room and terrace of the Instream apartment, which we had seen in July 1965.

(Jane told me she was nervous, however, when it came to our own envelope test. She did not think I had a test for her. She said it was hard to say exactly when she became nervous, but that it was probably as I handed her the test envelope.

(Marathon is in the Florida Keys, perhaps 40 miles north of Key West. It is a beautiful place and Jane and I spent a winter there several years ago. We do have photographs of the place.

(Seth's impressions do appear to be far-ranging, in connection with the old bureau and its label. Jane and I can make some connection with some of the material, but in the light of what follows we decided to wait. We will also try to verify some of the impressions through our landlord, Jimmy Spaziani. We do not know how much he can help, since he has owned our apartment house but a few years.

(Jane resumed with her eyes closed and in a quiet voice at 10:31.)

We will speak but briefly. <u>Originally</u> the bureau belonged to a woman to whom it was delivered at this address. She left your town and went to Florida, and left the chest.

Ruburt picked up the Florida connection, and this led him to think of his photograph. I always distinguish between our lines of thought when this happens. We will perhaps discuss this sort of test at our next session.

Now however I will end tonight's session. My heartiest regards to you both.

I believe that the woman lived in your apartment, and that the chest was used by others after the woman left, and before you obtained it.

("Good night, Seth."

(End at 10:34. Jane was dissociated as usual. Her eyes remained closed, her voice quiet.)

OCTOBER 8, 1965 FRIDAY   REPORT BY JANE BUTTS

(Tonight Bill and Peggy Gallagher came to visit us. Bill told us that he would have to leave for a few minutes to pick up an advertisement at the bus terminal and take it to the newspaper office, the Star-Gazette, where he works. On the spur of the moment Peggy suggested that we all try to pick up impressions concerning the ad, while Bill was gone. Bill himself would not know the contents of the ad, which was in an envelope, until he opened it at the paper.

(Bill said that he would try to think strongly of the ad. He left here at approximately 10 PM and returned about 10:35. Rob, Peg, and I had all written down our impressions, and none of us knew what the others had written. None of Peg's were correct. Many of mine, about 11 impressions, were correct, and some of Rob's.

(My score would seem to be above chance. I did not seem to pick up impressions about the ad itself, however. I seemed to pick up impressions of Bill at the newspaper office, and follow him as he went about his chores. I had no idea at the time that any of my impressions were correct. Indeed I suspected that they were all wrong. I seem to work with words rather than images, that is, I pick up word impressions, I guess, rather than pictures.

(The following is an exact copy of the impressions as I wrote them on my slip of paper. The impressions themselves are in caps, and directly beneath the correctness or incorrectness is noted.

1. A SUDDEN TURN

(Correct. On entering the newspaper building Bill went into one particular office and left, making a sudden and sharp turn to go upstairs.

2. FEELING HE STARTS TO GO UPSTAIRS

3. OR STOPS TO TALK TO SOMEONE THERE
(Correct on both points. Bill went upstairs to talk to the men in the Ad department. Though I have been in the newspaper building, I did not know that these offices were upstairs. Bill's own office is downstairs, as I knew, and if I thought about it at all I assumed that all his business took place there. I had no idea that Bill had any connection with the upstairs offices at all, since the editorial work is done there, and he has nothing to do with that at all. Peg, who works up there, has told me often that she never sees him upstairs.

4. THREE PEOPLE IN PARTICULAR IN HIS OFFICE
(Correct, though this was the upstairs office. The three people were a Mr. Connor, who Bill definitely did not expect to see, and his two children.

5. THE THREE PEOPLE IN THIS POSITION:

(Correct. They stood speaking in the given position.

6. SOMETHING TO DO WITH THE SEASONS
(Correct. Bill spoke about the "sunny climes" in particular in contrast to our autumn weather, as he intends to go to Puerto Rico for his vacation and the discussion had to do with the differences in weather this time of year.

7. THE AD BLOCKED, FIRST LINE FOUR WORDS, THE WAY IT WILL BE ARRANGED ACTUALLY IN THE PAPER
(? The ad hasn't appeared in the paper yet.

8. CIG
(Correct. Bill insists this is a direct hit. He said that the term sig is always used in the ads, and is part of the language of the ad department. They discussed which "sig" to use, and the word "sig" was inserted, though no signature was then written in. Though sig means signature, the word signature itself is never used, Bill said. Phonetically the words are the same, cig and sig, though mine begins with a C.

9. CIDER
(Wrong.

10. BOTTLE
(Wrong.

11. A PAIR OF SHOES OR SHOE SHAPES
(Wrong.

12. MINE - O - GRAPH
(Wrong. The ad had to do with a stere-o-phonic. There is some word similarity.

13. SPECTACULAR
(Wrong.

14. MAN WITH A BEARD CONNECTED WITH IT (THE AD)
(Wrong as far as Bill knows.

15. EARNEST TALK WITH A MAN ABOUT LINEUP
(Correct, and not anticipated by Bill.

16. 15 SOMETHING
(Wrong.

17. A TOUR
(Correct. Bill and another man discussed a specific tour taken by the other man a few years ago to Puerto Rico.

18. SUDDENLY UNDER TENSION
(Correct. Bill had an unpleasant encounter with Mr. Connor earlier in the day, and he was thinking of quitting his job because of it. When he found Mr. Connor in the office after regular hours, and unexpectedly, Bill was upset and instantly tense.

19. USES WORD PADRE
(Near-correct. Before Mr. Connor's entrance, Bill was joking with another man. On purpose he pronounced the word Ponce as P O N K A Y, which sounds very much like padre.

20. BRAZIER
(Wrong.

(Note: I am completely unfamiliar with any ad terms, and did not even know that lineup was such a term, much less sig.)

OCTOBER 8, 1965 FRIDAY   REPORT BY RFB

(While Bill Gallagher was putting on his hat and coat at 10 PM tonight, preparatory to leaving our apartment for the bus terminal, I wrote down two impressions of headlines. I was not in a trance state. Bill did not see these until he returned at 10:35 PM; he told me both of them were incorrect.

(After Bill left Jane and Peggy sat talking while I read. As she talked Jane jotted down her impressions. I interrupted my reading to put myself into a light trance state, and then wrote down four more impressions. Three of these proved to be correct. I used the trance state rather casually, and later wished I had written down more impressions; but I was interested in getting back to my reading.

(My impressions follow just as I wrote them down. They are in caps, followed by interpretations.)

1. COME TO OUR BIG TIRE SALE

2. NOW IS THE TIME, DON'T DELAY

(Both incorrect. I made these before Bill left the apartment. The ad was printed on Tuesday, October 12, 1965. The actual headline consisted of the single word NOW!

3. HANDLED BY A LARGE FAT MAN

(Correct. The above impression and the following three were made in the light trance state. Bill said the description fits the stereotyper at the newspaper, and that the two of them discussed the ad this evening. Murphy, the stereotyper, whom I have never met, is according to Bill a large, rotund fat man. I have not been inside the newspaper building since Jane and I moved here five years ago.

4. HEAVY TWINE AND GREEN PAPER

(Incorrect. Here I referred to the wrapping of the ad when Bill picked it up at the bus terminal. Bill said the ad was wrapped in brown paper and sealed with brown paper tape.

5. BETWEEN TWO LAYERS OF CARDBOARD

(Correct. Bill said the material for the ad, [the plates], was protected by two layers of heavy cardboard.

6. 4 COLUMNS

(Correct. Bill said the layout suggested for the ad was for four columns. When he got to the office and tried to make a layout for four columns however, he found it to be too crowded and switched to a five-column layout. The sigs he arranged at the bottom of the ad.

(With this impression, as I sat with closed eyes, I seemed to receive a picture. I saw fairly clearly a four-column layout set in type; at the top was a plate for printing a photograph, with headline lettering on either side of the photo. I could not distinguish the subject matter of the photo. When Bill returned he asked me to diagram what I had seen. To the viewer's left on page 321 is a copy of the drawing I made for him, to the right is a sketch of the actual ad as printed. On Friday night Bill told me my sketch was pretty close to the layout he finally decided upon at the office, and talked over with the stereotyper. My impression was of the metal printing plate, not the final printed ad. The metal appeared to be clean and unused and shining.)

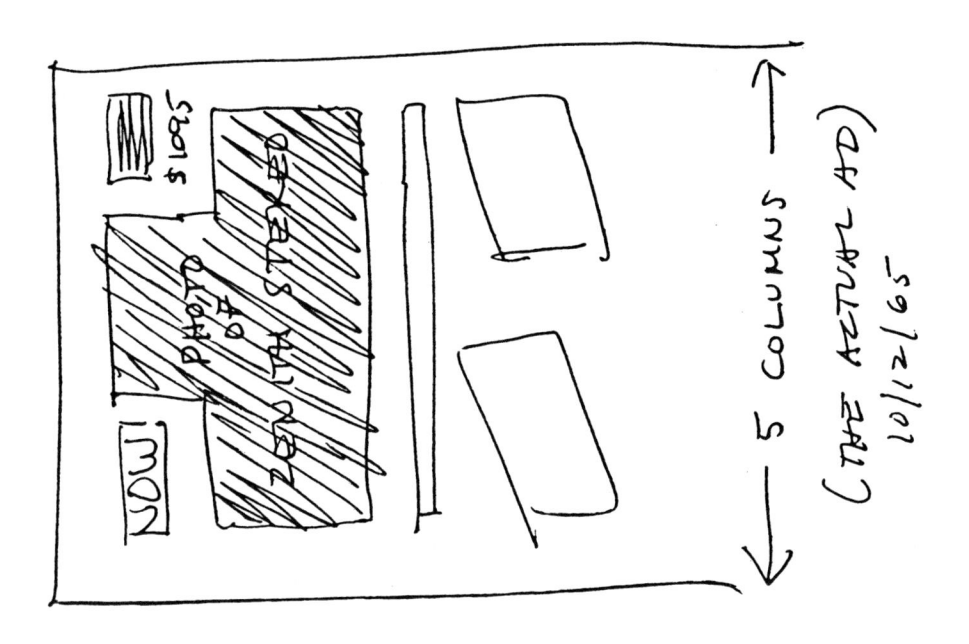

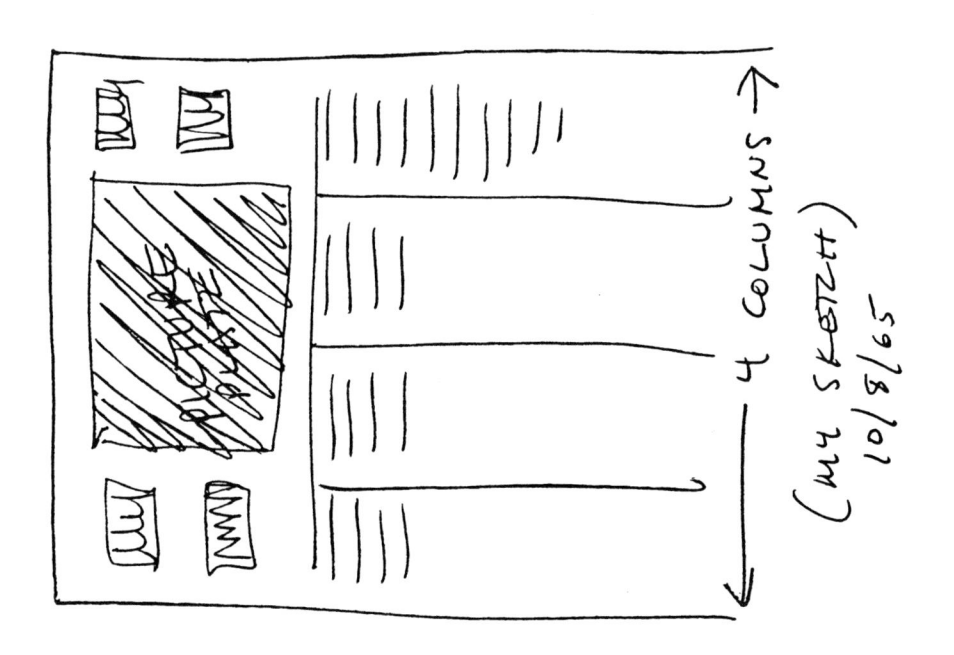

SESSION 196

(Tracing from my note pad of our title suggestions for Jane's book on ESP and the Seth material.)

SESSION 197
OCTOBER 11, 1965 9 PM MONDAY AS SCHEDULED

(Today Jane was quite upset because she still hasn't received a letter from her publisher, Frederick Fell, even though Mr. Fell reassured her about the ESP book when she telephoned him last Monday, October 5, the day of the 195th session. In that session Seth also offered reassurance to Jane.

(For the test this evening I chose a page from my notepad. Jane and I have been trying to think of a good title for her book dealing with Seth and the material, since she has begun work on it. See the tracing on page 322. The page is on white paper, and the writing on the tracing is done with the same pen I used to make the original notes. I sealed the folded page in the usual double envelopes, also inserting two pieces of Bristol board for stiffeners. It's our 13th envelope test.

(The session this evening was held in our back room and was quite peaceful. Jane spoke while sitting down and with her eyes closed. Her voice was average, her pace rather slow in the beginning.)

Good evening.

("Good evening, Seth.")

Now. These electromagnetic changes form their own <u>kind</u> of pattern, which has mass but no weight, or weight so slight as to be indistinguishable.

The mass, generally speaking, is a denseness formed by the varying intensities. There are mathematical precisions and formulas here. There is a ratio between the mass, which is usually considerable, and the weight, which is barely noticeable. These electromagnetic frameworks could be considered as skeleton forms within physical matter.

The electromagnetic reality within the human organism has considerable mass, but the entire physical weight amounts to 3 to 6 ounces at the very most. Again, the mass is composed of electrical intensities. I have told you that all experience is basically psychological, and that it is held in coded form within the cells. One electrical pulsation can represent an emotional experience. The importance of the experience to the individual will be responsible for the intensity with which it is recorded.

(Again, see sessions 120-127, in Volume 3, for material on the electromagnetic field and related subjects.)

All of an individual's experiences, even those of which he is not aware on a conscious basis, therefore are part of the electromagnetic reality that forms this particular individual's electromagnetic identity. It exists within the physical matter of the organism during existence within the physical system. While the experiences which form this framework and compose this individual's identity are obtained through his interaction with the physical system, his electromagnetic identity is not dependent upon the physical field.

During his life within the physical system attractions with it are of course maintained. At physical death this connection is severed. Polarities are changed in reverse fashion. The individual identity, composed of its electrically and magnetically coded experiences, is therefore intact. I say intact, for to all purposes this is so. When the polarities are changed however in reverse fashion, the present ego follows its attraction to the subconscious, and the two are more or less united.

It goes without saying that there are electromagnetic connections between the ego and the subconscious, within the physical system. Again, we speak of the ego and the subconscious as separate merely for the sake of convenience. They merely are interchanges and mass identity centers where highly intricate self-translations take place, and where various transformations occur.

In the past we have spoken briefly concerning a tricky subject, the relationship of intensity and the nature of distance. The electromagnetic identity of any given individual contains the past identity systems, again in coded form. In other words, the previous personalities of past lives.

(See the 125th session in Volume 3, among others.)

They are only available however under certain circumstances, for each of them is coded within a specific intensity range. They exist simultaneously with the present personality, but the present personality <u>as a rule</u> cannot pick them up, so to speak. Sometimes there is a bleedthrough however. Also, the chemical nature of certain emotional experiences may cause a freak electrical storm within the identity system, so that a past life may suddenly be recalled.

I have mentioned that any action has an electromagnetic reality, and so thoughts and dreams as well form this identity system.

I suggest a brief break and we shall continue. You should get a charge out of this material, if you will excuse a poor pun.

(Break at 9:26. Jane was dissociated as usual for a first delivery. She ended the delivery with a smile. Her eyes remained closed, her voice quiet. Her pace was fast after a rather slow start.

(Her voice was a bit stronger when she resumed, again with her eyes closed, at 9:32.)

In telepathic and clairvoyant experiences, the electromagnetic reality <u>pattern</u> is what is transmitted. It must then be transformed into a pattern that will be distinguished by ego awareness, if the individual is to be consciously aware of having received such a message.

Often such messages are picked up and translated by the subconscious. The information is used and acted upon without conscious approval or recognition. In almost all cases however, there must be an emotional attraction, for this is what allows for the transmission. Indeed, this is what makes the transmission possible.

The ego chooses channels of reception with great discrimination; and, again, it censors anything which it feels is a threat to its own dominance. In sleep however many dreams are of a telepathic nature, with strong clairvoyant overtones. It is the ego's persistent discrimination in choosing the stimuli to which it will react that in a large measure determines the nature of physical time as it appears to the personality. The ego, because of its function and basic characteristics, cannot make swift decisions as can the intuitive self. Therefore it perceives events in a peculiar manner, almost in slow motion, so that the whole effect is of a series of separate events, one happening before or after the other.

The intellect is a part of the ego, and its development is important. Therefore the appearance of separate events trains the intellect. Otherwise full use of the intuitions would be relied upon and the intellect would not develop, for the intellect is an important feature in the further specialization of individual consciousness and identity.

You are midway here. In the future the ego and the intellect will expand sufficiently so that they can contain and use and appreciate all the other functions and portions of the self which they now mistrust. Individual identity will then expand to include a greater variety of impulses and stimuli, which do not necessarily come from the self, and yet maintain specialized identity.

The ego will become more of an organizer in general, letting in literally a barrage of experiences, and organizing them into meaningful patterns. Now the ego fears such experiences, and censors them and holds them out because it is not certain of its strength, or its ability to mold them into significant patterns.

As the ego becomes certain of its strength, then it will allow the self to expand. I mentioned in our last session that the scientists did not realize that man has indeed evolved since the development of the human brain. For it has learned to form literally millions of new connections, meanings and concepts, new gestalts that have indeed made man something quite different than he was. All of these are new electromagnetic patterns which are now indelibly a part of the race.

The size of the brain has little to do with any of this beyond a certain point. The number of electrical connections are important however, and even old portions of the brain are affected by them. The old portions of the brain are <u>not</u> the same as they were. Physical examination of them only discloses their condition in the present. The growth of the cortex greatly affected the more primitive portions.

I am keeping our date in mind, and therefore suggest a brief break.

(Break at 9:54. Jane was dissociated as usual. Her eyes remained closed, her pace fast, her voice good. She resumed in the same manner at 10:01.)

I would like to remind Ruburt, again, that I told him that Peggy Gallagher would be of help in our sessions, long before she was a friend.

The affair the other evening worked out well. It was spontaneous, the atmosphere was friendly, and the Gallaghers' attitude is an excellent one. There will be other and better such communications between the four of you.

(See the report by Jane and me at the end of the last session. Bill and Peggy will be leaving next week for a vacation in Puerto Rico, and the four of us have already made plans to try some telepathic/clairvoyant communications. The plans are simple; at session times next week Bill and Peggy will attempt to concentrate on Jane, Seth and me, with a view to seeing what Seth can pick up.

(In the 63rd session of June 17, 1964, Seth said that Peggy Gallagher's subconscious abilities were well developed. Peggy is a feature writer for the local paper. Jane was working at the Arnot Art Gallery then, and the two became casual acquaintances. However the friendship between the four of us did not begin to develop until early this year.

(It might be interesting to note here that Peggy was hypnotized by Dr. Milton Erickson in late March of 1959, during a meeting of the Finger Lakes Clinical Hypnosis Association at the Mark Twain Hotel in Elmira. Peggy attended the meeting in her role of reporter, and volunteered as a subject. Before about twenty people Dr. Erickson put her into a deep trance quite easily, with the result that Peggy had complete amnesia for a ten-minute period. After she learned of the Seth sessions Peggy searched the files of the newspaper for a copy of her article on the experience. It was printed on April 2, 1959.)

When Ruburt learns a few lessons, he will be able to tell when his impressions are correct. Most of the wrong ones are not <u>necessarily</u> errors, but he has not made the proper connections, or gone far enough, but stopped short in processes of association. For the basic valid impressions are not picked up by the ego; and, again, must be properly transformed into data that can be understood. And this often emerges as associative material, that must then be deciphered. He is in training, so to speak.

Now, give us a moment, and we will contact Dr. Instream.

(Jane paused at 10:07. She sat quietly with her eyes closed. Her head was tipped down, her hands to her face.)

These are impressions. Mud, and water, and umbrellas. An inkwell. He may be writing. He has been concerned with a schedule. (Pause.)

Five objects in particular, and one of them is a gift, or was a gift to him. A cluster of events he considers too many. The number 12. He is very cautious this evening.

He thinks of someone whom he considers in the same light as a daughter. His wife may be allergic to dogs or hair. I think of a dog with wet hair, a shaggy one. *(Pause.)*

There was a 4 o'clock appointment today, or he thinks of a 4 o'clock appointment for tomorrow. His hypnosis experiments have a snag that will be overcome.

He has walked outside, and it is rainy and dark. He smokes outside as he walks. Tomorrow is a special day for him in some manner. *(Pause at 10:16.)*

Do you have a test for me?

("Yes."

(As usual I handed Jane the double test envelope. She took it while her eyes remained closed.)

These are impressions.

Five. An afternoon. The color yellow. An unusual circumstance. Something to do with two people who have a dog.

An arch shape. Designs that go in one direction, diagonals. The number 4, or four numbers. *(Long pause at 10:19.)* White. An F and a W, and a table and chairs.

A time several years ago. Something hot, that is a warmth, as of a hot day.

I suggest your break.

(Break at 10:20. Jane was dissociated as usual. Her eyes had remained closed, her voice quiet, her pace rather slow.

(Once again Jane considered the test a failure, and attributed it to her being upset today. As it developed we did not ask Seth for specific information on the impressions, so I do not know whether they were merely too far-ranging for our purposes, or simply errors. I saw possible connections with a few of them, and will note them for the record.

(The room, my studio, in which I wrote the suggestions for Jane's new book title, has yellow painted walls. The notepaper is white.

(The material on a dog reminded me that the Bristol stiffeners I enclosed tonight's test paper in were the same two in which I had enclosed the test photo for the 11th envelope test, in the 194th session. The photo was of our dog, Mischa, now dead. It was taken several years ago or more, on a hot day in the summer; Jane was also with a man whose first initial was W on that day.

(If impressions can attach themselves to the test object itself, they can attach themselves to any other object; so once again it appears that the problem for Jane is one of discrimination. She was disappointed at the results of this evening's test especially when comparing it with the good results of last Friday's spontaneous affair with

the Gallaghers. See pages 316-321.

(Jane resumed in a quiet voice, with her eyes closed, at 10:30.)

I do have a few suggestions, though Ruburt may not particularly approve of them.

I will no longer ask you if you have a test. You will simply at your leisure hand me a test when you have one for me, at any time in the session. You may, in other words, interrupt. Do not tell Ruburt the results of the test immediately.

He may read them when they are written up. I believe this will be of benefit, at least for the present. In fact, this is an excellent suggestion, and will aid in achieving greater spontaneity for us.

He has been upset, but this situation will soon be taken care of. It is this, plus the fact that he worries about his score, that is bothering us now. It has not bothered us to any great degree in the Instream material. Though all the connections have not been hits, enough has come through to show validity; though with training Ruburt will improve in allowing me to come through more specifically.

We will now end our session. My heartiest regards to you both. I believe a rather bizarre event will occur, regarding the Gallaghers, at approximately five o'clock during their vacation.

("Good night, Seth.")

(End at 10:37. Jane was dissociated as usual. Her eyes had remained closed, her voice quiet. Her pace had been average.

(It will be recalled that Seth himself [or Jane?] initiated the idea of asking me if I had an envelope test at each session. The first such test was held in the 179th session, and Jane knew about it before the session began. In that session however Seth also said it would be better if Jane did not know whether I planned a test before any particular session.

(In the 180th session however, Seth's comments led into the second envelope test, and in the 183rd session Seth queried me outright as to whether I had a third test for him. This process set up a pattern which we have followed ever since.

(As stated before, the Gallaghers leave for a vacation in Puerto Rico next week; the four of us have planned some clairvoyant tests. Perhaps Seth will be able to tune in on the bizarre event involving the Gallaghers before they return home.

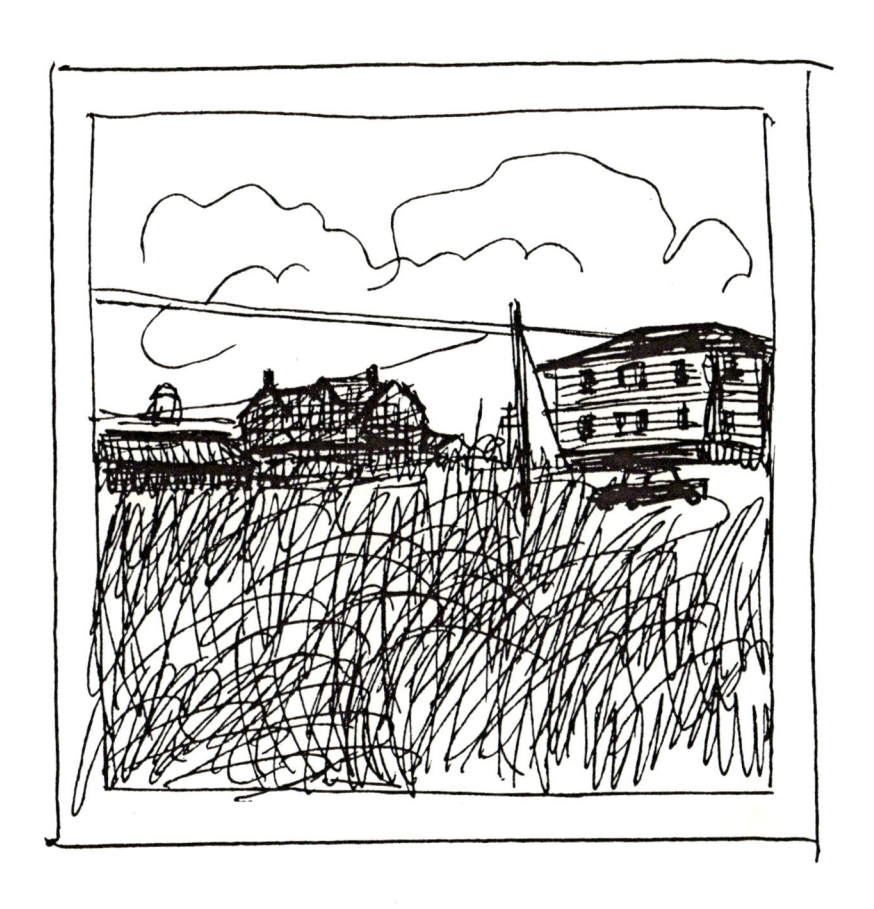

(Tracing of the photograph used in the 14th envelope test, in Session 198, October 13, 1965.)

SESSION 198
OCTOBER 13, 1965 9 PM WEDNESDAY AS SCHEDULED

(Yesterday we received Dr. Instream's letter of October 11, in which he asked that Seth try giving data on one location and one object in the clairvoyant tests.

(Not having heard from her publisher yet, as he had promised she would by now, Jane wrote and mailed to him a pretty stiff letter. However, she did not appear

to be in the upset mood she had been in prior to the last session.

(This afternoon I made up the usual double test envelope, including a pair of Bristol stiffeners. The envelopes contained a black and white photo of York Beach, ME, taken there last summer, that is the summer of 1964. It is of a view I scouted from our motel window. I took it for reference for a future painting, and consists mainly of a mass of tangled marsh grass in the foreground; in the background rise a couple of average-looking houses, a telephone pole and some wires. I obtained excellent detail in the rhythmic pattern of the waist-high grasses, which was what I wanted.

(I wasn't decided whether to ask Jane to hold an envelope test. On the one hand I didn't want her to feel I was pressuring her for a test every session; on the other hand I wondered whether she would think I was taking it easy on her if I skipped the test. So I thought I would see what developed in the session.

(The session was held in our back room and was not interrupted. Jane began speaking while sitting down and with her eyes closed. Her voice was quiet, her pace slow at the beginning, with pauses.)

Good evening.

("Good evening, Seth.")

We have not discussed the inner senses in some time.

You should by now realize that they have an electric, magnetic reality also, and that the mental enzymes act as sparks, setting off these inner reactions.

In the dream state these reactions are more easily triggered. This is the result of a lowering of egotistic guards, for the ego sets up controls that act as resistance to various channels, so that many connections are closed. All of these systems are interconnected. They all operate simultaneously. However, the personality is certainly not aware of their existence on a conscious level a good deal of the time.

The inner senses are connected then to the physical mechanism. Sometimes inner perceptions may be touched off as a result of stimuli received through the outer senses. In many cases however the stimulus comes from the deeper levels of the self, where however it may be translated into terms that the personal subconscious can use.

In such circumstances these perceptions may find their way to the ego, appearing as inspirations or intuitive thought. It is obvious that many such intuitions appear when the personality is in a dreaming state or in states of dissociation. The intuitions themselves, while seemingly mental, are action, and as such they produce changes in the physical organism, both chemical and electromagnetic.

The reality of such intuitive thoughts as electromagnetic actions has not been understood, and is quite vital to any comprehension of the human system.

I have said before that thoughts exist in such a dimension. Constructive thoughts do not simply affect the system for good in some sort of a generalized fashion, nor do destructive thoughts simply happen to affect the system directly.

The effect of any thought is a quite precise and definite one, that is set into motion specifically because of the nature of its own electromagnetic identity. The physical system operates best within certain electromagnetic patterns, and is adversely affected by others. These effects change the actual molecular structure of the physical cells of the organism, for better or for worse, and because of certain laws of attraction a habitual pattern will operate. A destructive type of thought, then, is dangerous not only for the present state of the organism, but dangerous in terms of the future.

Poor health is indeed caused mainly by habitual destructive thought patterns which directly affect the physical system, because of the particular range within the electromagnetic system in which they fall; and despite any objections I will stick by this statement. The bad health, for example, does not occur first, resulting in unhealthy thoughts. It is indeed the other way around.

For such habits operate not only in the waking state but in the sleeping state also, where the personality is even more open to suggestion. A vicious circle is therefore formed. It is often broken however, and in many ways.

I suggest a break and we shall continue.

(Break at 9:20. Jane was dissociated as usual for a first delivery. Her eyes remained closed. Her voice grew somewhat heavier and stronger as the delivery progressed, and her pace speeded up.

(Seth began talking about the inner senses almost as soon as the sessions began, in December of 1963. By the 20th session he had mentioned many of them. By the 60th session he had gone into some detail on 9 inner senses, 11 basic laws of the inner universe, and 3 properties of physical matter, along with the many other subjects included in the sessions. Check Volumes 1 and 2.

(More inner-sense delineations are to come, according to Seth. With a list of the above categories in mind however, it is clear which senses and laws apply to the material in the sessions following, up until now. I have often meant to remind Seth to mention the specific senses along with the material under discussion but have not done so.

(Jane resumed in the same fast manner, with her eyes closed and in a good voice, at 9:30.)

For these thoughts set up charges that oftentimes cannot be used effectively by the physical organism, and when excesses of such charges occur an illness develops. This is not to say however that illness can be treated using electromagnetics though in the future, the distant future, this may be practical.

Illnesses must be treated primarily however by changing the basic mental habits, for unless this is done the trouble will erupt time and time again in different guises. However, the system obviously has the ability to heal itself, and every opportunity should be given so that it is allowed to do so. To my knowledge nothing is known about the healing effect that often occurs in dreams themselves. For a wholly destructive attitude of mind has been changed overnight in the dream state to a constructive condition, and the whole electromagnetic balance has been changed.

("Not too fast."

(Jane's dictation was quite fast along in here, and I finally had to ask for relief. This is the first time such a situation has developed in some time. Usually it takes place when witnesses are present.)

Surely investigation should be done to probe into this matter. In such a case negative ions form an electrical framework in which healing is possible. Such healing dreams come most often when the inner self deeply feels a sense of desperation, and automatically opens up channels from deeper layers of the self, that have been closed for all effective purposes.

We find here an almost instant regeneration, a seemingly instant cure, a point from which the organism almost miraculously begins to improve. The same happens however in less startling cases where, for example, a merely annoying condition of health will suddenly disappear.

Now we come to see one of the main points of this discussion. These therapeutic dreams, with practice, can be brought about through self-suggestion. To some extent this is not unknown. Various old cults have used this method, but it can be quite practical in modern life.

(Jane's voice now hovered on the edge of loudness. Her pace was still good, her eyes closed.)

The suggestion itself, you see, being action, has its own electromagnetic reality, and since the suggestion would be a constructive one, it would already begin to set certain healing processes into motion, and spark the formation of others. This can be used to your advantage in daily life.

Such inner therapeutics also occur however at various levels of consciousness where they may be sparked by exterior stimuli of an esthetic or pleasing nature. Other exterior conditions have also their effect. To involve oneself in large groups, for example, is beneficial often, not simply to take attention away from the self, but because a larger range of electromagnetic realities are easily available.

It is obvious that some individuals seem to have a better effect upon other individuals, and what we have said should explain the reasons for the differences.

The overall health of the individual and the delicate balance of electromagnetic properties are important, for when the organism is set deeply in destructive patterns, then this may be also felt in the dream state, so that destructive dreams <u>add</u> to the overall unfortunate state.

Dreams are indeed symptomatic of the personality's overall condition at any given time, but they also help form that condition. The connections here are extremely complicated, and yet use of suggestion in bringing about constructive changes through dreams can be of great benefit.

We shall have more to say concerning this subject, for practically it is of considerable importance. I will now suggest a break, and we shall have a try with our Dr. Instream.

(*Break at 9:50. Jane was dissociated as usual. Her eyes remained closed. Her voice had been good, her pace quite fast at times. She had been aware of the deeper and stronger quality of her voice.*

(*Jane said she hadn't been in a poor or depressed mood lately so much as a period of transition. Having finished one project, the ESP book, she was beginning a new venture, the book on the Seth material itself. At the same time she was casting about for another endeavor. Whether it would prove to be short stories, a novel or poetry, she did not yet know.*

(*Jane now resumed at a slower rate, in a quiet voice and with her eyes closed, at 10:01.*)

Dr. Instream understands, I am sure, that we are not only involved here with inner perceptions, and with translations that must be made as data is given by me to Ruburt, but we are also working within human limitations, and of course with human potentialities.

This is all fairly new to Ruburt, and he is doing very well. We shall make an effort to be more specific. But one must always read large print as a training before small print can be read with care or precision.

Ruburt is extremely cautious. This will not work to our disadvantage however, for his cautiousness in these matters acts as a strong balancing mechanism, so that he learns to deal with inner perceptions stage by stage. His personality is not overwhelmed therefore. We have taken his ego into consideration at all times, so that he can consciously assimilate what he has learned, as is preferable. At times this may mean that we progress slowly, but the progression is steady and firm.

Now give us a moment.

(*This is the eighth Dr. Instream clairvoyant test.*

(*Jane paused at 10:07. She sat with her eyes closed, her head down and her hands to her eyes. Her voice was quiet and she used pauses, a few of them long.)*

A blue vase *(long pause)* of glass on a stand or table in a smallish room. I will give this as the particular object. *(Pause.)*

Here are some given impressions. A hat on a tall rack, a single rack with offshoots on it. A message having to do with a boy. The message directed to Dr. Instream. Perhaps the initials B. M. *(Pause.)*

The boy either 12 or 22 years old, with a farm somehow connected with his family or the message.

A chip on the blue vase, on the left and toward the bottom. *(A long pause at 10:13.)* An indelible pencil in Dr. Instream's pocket, with black lead. The pencil with a brand name on it, something like Connecticut.

Do you have a test? I will ask you.

("Yes.")

(I handed Jane the double test envelope at 10:15. I had decided to pass up the test for this session, and certainly had no thought that Seth would ask me for one.

(This is the 14th envelope test. Jane took the envelope without opening her eyes, as usual, and sat quietly for a moment while holding it in both hands, without bending it, etc. She used pauses while delivering the test data, yet spoke confidently.

(As she delivered the first phrase below, I had the rather strong impression that it referred to the Dr. Instream test material, but I cannot say why I felt this.)

Also a connection with a message, and the color green.

The impression of a framework of thin lines, with some cube formations. The mass rising vertically mainly. *(Pause.)*

A photograph this time, without a border. *(A long pause.)*

Something to do with a circle, and white and leaves. Dark leaves against white. Afternoon. *(Pause.)* A place which you have both visited, and water nearby.

A mistake of sorts connected here somewhere. Two people, and a look out.

I suggest a break, and Ruburt may open the envelope.

(Break at 10:20. Jane was dissociated as usual. Her eyes had remained closed, her voice quiet. She said that when she heard Seth ask me for the envelope test, she became nervous, for as Jane she had no intention of asking for a test. Then, Jane said, when she realized she did feel nervous, and that she was sitting stiffly, she relaxed and let Seth take over.

(See the tracing of the test photograph on page 329. Most of Jane's impressions can apply to the photo. A "framework of thin lines" is an apt description of the patterns formed by the high marsh grasses in the foreground of the photo, with the houses rising in the background as "cube formations... rising vertically."

(The test object is a photograph, but with the standard white border.

("Something to do with a circle" is interesting, in that our motel at York Beach,

where this photo was taken, is situated on a circular driveway in back of the beach hotel that fronts on the ocean. In the photo the marsh grass comes out as "dark leaves against white," and the photo was taken in the afternoon of a bright day. I recall this easily enough because I had to wait until the sun was in the correct position to give a good contrasting result in the black and white photo that I wanted to use for reference.

("A place which you have both visited" is of course York Beach where the photo was taken, and "water nearby" is the ocean perhaps 75 yards away.

(Jane tells me that "a mistake of sorts connected here somewhere" could refer to a mix-up concerning the room we had rented at the motel, but I do not recall this personally. It was nothing serious, Jane said, but a bookkeeping error on the part of the motel room clerk, to the effect that our room had been reserved for someone else, in advance; we were to be moved to another room, she said, but the transfer never took place. There was no unpleasantness involved.

("Two people" can be Jane and me, just as I recall that in the second envelope test, which also concerned a photograph of York Beach, the two people mentioned could be us. See page 206.

("And a look out" is interesting to us, because I spent some time for a couple of days looking out our back motel room window, studying this particular view before finally taking a picture of it. This involved checking the appearance of the marsh grass at various times of the day to see when the light would be best, then waiting for a sunny day to increase contrast, etc.

(Jane said she felt she had learned several things at once during this test. While Seth was giving his data on the photograph, she said, she was also aware of several images of her own. It was as though she heard what Seth was saying, then conjured up her own separate set of visual images. Jane said she is particularly aware of this because as a rule she does not see images at any other time.

(Jane said the key point here is that although she had these images of her own, she did not give voice to them as part of Seth's data; she was able to appreciate the difference. She said it is difficult for her to learn to use herself to the proper degree in interpreting Seth's material, without interfering with it.

(While she was giving Seth's data, Jane said she had images of a childhood playground in Saratoga Springs, NY, with houses nearby, but recognized this as her own data and did not give it as Seth's. She felt sure the test object had a northern, as versus a southern, background, but did not say so because Seth did not say so.

(All in all, Jane was pleased with the results of the test. Much of the time in the past she had been quite critical about test results. She now resumed in a quiet voice, and with her eyes closed, at 10:30.)

We will shortly close our session.

A note here to Dr. Instream. This material is more illuminating because

Ruburt is in training, so to speak; because the <u>ways</u> in which the personality receives, interprets and translates inner perceptions are more obvious <u>now</u> than they will be at a later date.

The development will make obvious certain stages by which the personality approaches such material, and this should be valuable simply from a psychological viewpoint.

I realized that Ruburt would do fairly well this evening on our own test, which is why I suggested the test, and also suggested that Ruburt open the envelope.

My heartiest regards to all.

Ruburt will be in fine fettle by Saturday in regards to financial matters, and his kitchen. Both affairs will be settled by then.

("Good night, Seth."

(End at 10:34. Jane was dissociated as usual. Her eyes had remained closed, her voice quiet.)

FRIDAY, OCTOBER 15, 1965 TWO DREAMS BY JANE BUTTS

(Since Seth gave us the material on therapeutic dreams last Wednesday, I began suggesting that I would experience one, as I was in a bad mood generally speaking and had been for a week; also I felt poorly with aches and pains etc.; nothing serious but annoying.

(Friday morning after writing for two hours, suddenly I felt very sleepy and could hardly hold my eyes open. Since I never take naps in the morning I tried to continue working but finally gave up, and went to bed. At the time I wondered about the peculiar sleepiness, wondering if it had any connection with a trance state.

(At 10:30 AM, I checked the clock and I awoke at 11 AM, so the following two dreams took place within the half-hour period. The first dream was entirely forgotten until I had completed writing my notes on the second dream, then I recalled the first one.

(The first one was not pleasant. The second one left me with strong feelings of joy and discovery, seemingly out of all proportion to the dream itself.

(This is the first dream. I was in bed, and then I realized that I heard voices in my head; was not at all sure that this was a dream. The voices were very loud, independent, each quite different from the others, and I believe, all male voices. I was frightened because I couldn't turn them off and they seemed to go on as if the people they belonged to had no idea that I could hear so clearly. However, I do not remember what they said. The volume was startling in itself. Finally I shook my head and yelled out. It was as if there was a radio in my head that kept switching from station

to station.

(The voices continued. Then I realized that my small transistor radio was at the head of the bed, that the voices were coming out of two speakers on it. I switched it off, relieved to find such a simple solution. But the voices kept on. Now I got out of bed [in the dream], went into Rob's room and found that another radio sat on the bookcase where the Seth material is kept, and that the voices were coming from this radio also. As I reached out to turn the radio off, I received quite a severe, though harmless shock. As a result I was afraid to touch the radio again, or yank the cord, so I left it and went into my room, the living room. Here the dream becomes unclear. Perhaps there was an electric storm outside, and electricity of some sort in my room. I don't recall that the voices bothered me now or if I heard them, though I had not turned the back radio off. From this scene I went directly into the second dream. The earlier fear was gone.)

SECOND DREAM

(I am in our living room. It seems very dark, with two rather than three windows, and the middle one is blocked partially. I look again and now it is bigger and brighter than it ever was; the third window is back, but now it is moved out further, extending the room several feet. [Actually this must have to do with our hopes of having our kitchen enlarged.]

(Then at this end of the room I discover heavy dark wooden doors. Opening them, I find a lovely table-and-chair set of simulated wood, and I tell Rob that we can use them in our new kitchen.

(A noise catches my attention. Investigating I see that new people are moving into a back apartment in our apartment house. [There is no such apartment.] I remember that I had forgotten the existence of this apartment and am angry with myself. The apartment is very large, about 10 rooms, lovely dark woodwork. I am doubly angry at myself when I discover a lovely kitchen and bath between this apartment and our own, since we could have used these rooms ourselves, paying extra rent for them.

(The new family is large. The members operate an excellent clothing store inside the apartment, in the center. There is a staircase leading down to a side street. Clothing is arranged on shelves, and so forth. A sale is planned. Then I realize that I did know the people who lived in this apartment before also, and had forgotten. I am aware that I knew them in a dream, rather than in normal waking life.

(The men in the family are dark-complected, handsome men, olive skin. We all get along well and like each other very much. We stand laughing by the staircase. I'm curious about some other apartments, also in this building, and owned by our

landlord also. I am happy and anticipatory, looking forward to seeing these apartments. Then on the staircase, in a pile of neatly-stacked clothing I discover a lovely dark green jacket with fur collar and zipper that is mine, and I remember now that I put it away last year for the season and forgot it until now. Another article of clothing catches my eye. I think it is mine for a moment and realize it is not.

(I laugh. These people all like me very much. I leap with more than normal grace down from the banister. One man puts an arm out to assist me. Again, full of joy, great joy, it seems, I look forward to looking at the other apartments. Then I remember that it is nearly lunchtime, and Rob will be home. I decide to go home myself and then return to look at these apartments.

(Outside there is still another apartment house that belongs to our landlord. A door is open. I look inside, see furniture, and know it is not vacant. Now it is raining slightly. I drop my cigarettes, pick them up, then discover that I also have an extra pack I did not know about. One pack is wet, but will dry. The other pack is only slightly wet.

(A paperboy comes across the yard and calls me by name. I do not know who he is, but think that I must have known him sometime in the past. Now I begin to realize that the whole thing is a dream. I think of looking at the other apartments now, before the dream is over, but realize that if I do I run the chance of forgetting this part of the dream, and I want to write it down.

(Someplace in here I dance quite happily, am filled with the joy of discovery, and am quite as happy as I have ever been in my life. In the dream I also know that this dream is like another I had previously and had forgotten.

(I awoke, still full of good spirits, my previous mood completely vanished. Until I wrote this dream down, I did not even remember the first one. The mood of the second prevailed.)

THE SETH AUDIO COLLECTION

RARE RECORDINGS OF SETH SPEAKING through Jane Roberts are now available on audiocassette. These Seth sessions were recorded by Jane's student, Rick Stack, during Jane's classes in Elmira, New York, in the 1970's. The majority of these selections have never been published in any form. Volume I, described below, is a collection of some of the best of Seth's comments gleaned from over 120 Seth Sessions. Additional selections from The Seth Audio Collection are also available. For information ask for our free catalogue.

Volume I of The Seth Audio Collection consists of six (1-hour) cassettes plus a 34-page booklet of Seth transcripts. Topics covered in Volume I include:

- Creating your own reality – How to free yourself from limiting beliefs and create the life you want.
- Dreams and out-of-body experiences.
- Reincarnation and Simultaneous Time.
- Connecting with your inner self.
- Spontaneity–Letting yourself go with the flow of your being.
- Creating abundance in every area of your life.
- Parallel (probable) universes and exploring other dimensions of reality.
- Spiritual healing, how to handle emotions, overcoming depression and much more.

FOR A FREE CATALOGUE of Seth related products including a detailed description of The Seth Audio Collection, please send your request to the address below.

ORDER INFORMATION:
If you would like to order a copy of The Seth Audio Collection Volume I, please send your name and address, with a check or money order payable to New Awareness Network, Inc. in the amount of $59.95 plus shipping charges. United States residents in NY, NJ, PA & CT must add sales tax.

Shipping charges: U.S. - $5.00, Canada - $7, Europe - $15, Australia & Asia - $17
Rates are UPS for U.S. & Airmail for International - Allow 2 weeks for delivery
Alternate Shipping - Surface - $8.00 to anywhere in the world - Allow 5-8 weeks

Mail to: NEW AWARENESS NETWORK INC.
P.O. BOX 192,
Manhasset, New York 11030
(516) 869-9108 between 9:00-5:00 p.m. Monday-Saturday EST

Visit us on the Internet - http://www.sethcenter.com

Books by Jane Roberts from Amber-Allen Publishing

Seth Speaks: The Eternal Validity of the Soul. This essential guide to conscious living clearly and powerfully articulates the furthest reaches of human potential, and the concept that each of us creates our own reality.

The Nature of Personal Reality: Specific, Practical Techniques for Solving Everyday Problems and Enriching the Life You Know.. In this perennial bestseller, Seth challenges our assumptions about the nature of reality and stresses the individual's capacity for conscious action.

The Individual and the Nature of Mass Events. Seth explores the connection between personal beliefs and world events, how our realities merge and combine "to form mass reactions such as the overthrow of governments, the birth of a new religion, wars, epidemics, earthquakes, and new periods of art, architecture, and technology."

The Magical Approach: Seth Speaks About the Art of Creative Living. Seth reveals the true, magical nature of our deepest levels of being, and explains how to live our lives spontaneously, creatively, and according to our own natural rhythms.

The Oversoul Seven Trilogy (The Education of Oversoul Seven, The Further Education of Oversoul Seven, Oversoul Seven and the Museum of Time). Inspired by Jane's own experiences with the Seth Material, the adventures of Oversoul Seven are an intriguing fantasy, a mind-altering exploration of our inner being, and a vibrant celebration of life.

The Nature of the Psyche. Seth reveals a startling new concept of self, answering questions about the inner reality that exists apart from time, the origins and powers of dreams, human sexuality, and how we choose our physical death.

The "Unknown" Reality, Volumes One and Two. Seth reveals the multidimensional nature of the human soul, the dazzling labyrinths of unseen probabilities involved in any decision, and how probable realities combine to create the waking life we know.

Dreams, "Evolution," and Value Fulfillment, Volumes One and Two. Seth discusses the material world as an ongoing self-creation—the product of a conscious, self-aware and thoroughly animate universe, where virtually every possibility not only exists, but is constantly encouraged to achieve its highest potential.

The Way Toward Health. Woven through the poignant story of Jane Roberts' final days are Seth's teachings about self-healing and the mind's effect upon physical health.

Available in bookstores everywhere.